I0867423

When I Open My Eyes

dance health imagination

When I Open My Eyes

dance health imagination

Miranda Tufnell

Triarchy
Press

Published in this edition in 2023 by:
Triarchy Press
Axminster, UK
www.triarchypress.net

A catalogue record for this book is available from the British Library.

ISBN:
Print: 978-1-913743-75-8
Ebook: 978-1-913743-76-5

First published in 2017 by Dance Books

Cover image: Antonia Bruce, Harvest, maize rootball. Cyanotype on treated paper, 2015.

Throughout this text the names of participants have been changed to protect privacy.

Contents

Acknowledgements

In the shaping and direction of this book, I am hugely indebted to the many people who read, commented and edited with me what at times seemed an impossible undertaking. In particular Chris Crickmay generously gave ongoing critical and editorial support. I am immensely grateful to my sister Zoe Tufnell, to Filipa Pereira-Stubbs, Niamh Dowling and Victoria Hamilton for their thoughtful reading and commenting on the emerging text. Keith Doyle kindly took on the laborious copy edit. I owe thanks to Dr Gavin Young and to Dot Main, practice nurse for their engagement and support for the Breath of Fresh Air project. Also thanks to Meg Peacocke and Alice Oswald for their poems, to Chris Drury, David Ward, Kay Syrad and Antonia Bruce for their contributions of images and text. To Michael Reinhart, Tomo Brody, Pari Naderi, Christina Kipp and Edmund Blok for their wonderful photographs. Many thanks also to Kate O Hearn who helped with permissions and to Liz Morrell whose design brought this book to life. I owe much to my collaborators Brenda Mallon and Tim Rubidge, for sharing the journey, invaluable colleagues and allies in conversations and work in developing the Breath of Fresh Air project. And I am deeply grateful to all the artists who have shared their practice in this book – and to those whose work is not represented here but who have been working for many years and with immense dedication to develop this field. Above all I am grateful to all those whose glorious creativity emerged through their illness, who gave their trust and taught me to see the astounding beauty of each and every body, and inspired the writing of this book.

Foreword

I knew Miranda many years before she came to work in our rural practice in Cumbria. I had seen her dance and I knew how much movement mattered – what it meant for her. I did not then realise that she would be able to bring that meaning to the patients in our practice.

I sang and was aware of Alexander Technique (F.M. Alexander having developed his technique to overcome problems with own his voice as an actor). I also knew how powerful the arts could be – for me, particularly, music. In 1993 my 13-year-old son had a very severe head injury which left him badly brain damaged. Some months after this I was having a singing lesson on Schumann's Dichterliebe. At the end of the lesson I was suddenly overcome by a terrible sadness and remembered James had had an accident. The point of this story is not my remembering, but that whilst singing I had been able completely to forget the accident, something which had never happened until that moment.

Art has the power to move us (it is significant that this English verb means to 'take us somewhere else in our emotions' and also 'take us to a different place'). I knew through the work of the British neurologist Oliver Sacks in *Awakenings* that many patients with post encephalitic Parkinson's disease had been unable to walk and yet, if music was played, could dance. I believe it is a common experience that many who stutter can sing flowingly.

Meanwhile as a GP I had come to feel frustrated by the direction that modern medicine was taking – involving itself increasingly in measuring bits of patients – blood pressure, body mass index, cholesterol etc. Decades before Einstein had said 'Not everything that can be counted counts, and not everything that counts can be counted.' Nonetheless we went on counting. Most of the doctors I knew felt the limitations of this mechanistic view of illness. Wise doctors were only too aware that there was not 'a pill for every ill' and that the divide between mind and body was not only false but very misleading.

Miranda talks of us becoming increasingly out of touch with our bodies as we lead lives more and more confined indoors in front of computer screens. At the same time I was seeing patients who had come to see their body as the enemy – they felt they had been betrayed by their bodies whether this was because of cancer or diabetes or arthritis or all the other chronic illnesses many have to live with.

Miranda was able to show me that movement and the Alexander Technique was a method whereby the patient could use their own body to overcome, particularly musculoskeletal pain, but other problems too. I was delighted to find a way of working that enabled patients to care for themselves and not become, as many with chronic illnesses understandably do, dependent on others to put things right.

At that time (the 1990s) we had an unusually enlightened Family Health Services Authority in Cumbria, and they approved the idea of our practice employing Miranda as an Alexander Technique teacher. I believe she was the first ever to be employed within the NHS.

Miranda refers to her project 'A Breath of Fresh Air'. It was very exciting for me to see patients who, I felt, had become stuck – or at least *I was stuck* in my ability to help them – finding ways through movement to overcome the difficulties they had had with mobility and to be lifted out of the dark, sad places they had come to inhabit. Not only was this very heartening but it was very instructive to see how mind and body interacted. Nothing is ever 'all in the mind' – whatever is in there will affect your body, and what is happening to your body is likely to have a profound impact on your mind.

Miranda's work in the practice and particularly her project showed me how patients could use their bodies to help heal themselves. I am not pretending that their arthritis, or whatever illness they had, went away but they learnt to cope with it better and to view it differently so that they no longer saw their body as the enemy.

I hope this book will be read by health professionals and particularly by GPs who have contact with so many people every day and that those doctors may be inspired to use different ways of helping people. This in turn will require many more to be doing work like that described in this book. And I hope it will also inspire many of those working in the arts and particularly dance and movement to involve themselves in healthcare.

Dr Gavin Young
Temple Sowerby, Cumbria
March 2016

Preface
my story of movement

Gorse

Mars must be the god of gorse. Sinewy
enduring, these stems that can wrest sap
from a dry bank and burn furious and clean,

There's not a month when gorse won't muster
a pinch of light, but now it's March, each hard bush
is bunched with gold, a hammered brightness,

yellow blossoms crowding among the forged
steel blue spines of a new season.
Faultless and harsh, their windborne essence.

Nostrils aren't enough for it: gulp the perfume
through your open mouth, the bittersweet
of being alive, of still being alive.

Meg Peacocke

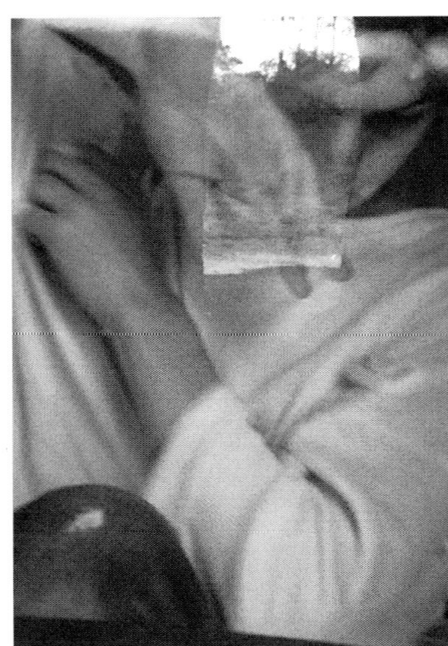

This morning at dawn I take a friend's dog for a walk. Her tail swings joyously as she bounds through the grasses, every part of her body is alert, reading the air for scents, for sounds and for presences I cannot perceive. The morning is exquisitely still. Spider threads travel the grasses – delicate highways that break against my body as I pass through. I go out early every morning from a need to feel the new day. The world at this early hour is undisturbed, the edges of things softened, blurred yet somehow linked. Birds sing, dew or raindrops sparkling on leaf and twig. There is a fragrance in the air – all feels untouched, renewed by the quiet of night. I breathe in the stillness, the freshness that is everywhere.

For over forty years I have been involved in the worlds of dance and performance, health and therapeutic bodywork. It has been a lifelong passion to explore the nature of the body – that complex anatomy of sensitivities, histories and chemistries that we call ourselves. It has been a search to find a more embodied and connected way of being in the world.

Growing up first in the Cambridgeshire Fens and later in an old farm high up in the Yorkshire Dales awoke a passionate love and hunger for wild places, where I felt close to the elements, to the forces of life. Ours was a house of words. My parents were both writers and our homes were full of books in which I immersed myself, relishing language and words for their goblin life, for the voices and worlds they revealed. And I felt strangely aware of wordless undercurrents, invisible movements that seemed to be speaking beneath, whatever I sensed or perceived; forces and energies hidden within the adult world to which my child's body responded yet for which I had no words.

I was one of those children for whom school was a dreary nightmare. The sense of joy and connectedness I experienced outside in nature vanished; no time for wandering or reverie in the noise and clatter of classrooms; no time simply for listening, for seeing without in some way reducing, interpreting, the multi-faceted world of my senses. The natural world seemed to retreat and hide itself away from my confused and timetabled mind. I remember the loneliness of that absence, and a growing sense of not quite being present – of life going on at one remove. Many people are speaking of how our schooling trains a particular aspect of mind, prioritising words, language and linear thought in contrast to the myriad, shape-shifting world of our senses. As Alan Johnson so aptly commented, 'we educate from the neck up and mostly to the left side.'

But I continued to revel in books, and embarked on a degree in English. As time went on I found myself increasingly cocooned inside myself, and strangely isolated from the world about me. One evening, my head over full from a day in the library and my body dulled and myopic, I tripped and fell off the pavement into a busy road. It shocked me that I was becoming so out of touch with my body and with my surroundings. On a wild impulse, I auditioned for a dance school out of a headlong desire to reclaim a sense of connection, to escape from what Tom Myers has termed the dis-ease of our age, 'kinaesthetic dystonia', a loss, or numbing, of the vital ability to be informed by our senses. I began dancing to feel again and to emerge out of a numbness that somehow enveloped me. Dance, I hoped, would open the door back to a vividness known in childhood – a sense of belonging to the wider world.

I threw myself into the rigours of the dance training. Initially I was intrigued, realising my right foot had no idea what my left foot was up to. I loved the challenge of learning this new language, this mapping of so unpredictable a territory as my own body. But soon I felt that I was becoming deaf to other dimensions, and to an inner call for feeling, for freedom. Confronted daily by the glare of studio mirrors I felt myself like Andersen's ugly duckling – awkward, graceless and yet again dispossessed. So I left dance school feeling that was the end of my dance career.[1]

However my interest in dance was rekindled as I became aware of a seismic shift that was beginning to happen in the dance world, from learning through imitation – teaching a style (jazz, ballet, Graham, Limón) – to more exploratory and improvisational approaches that drew on the subtleties of movement that arose from within the experiencing body. I studied T'ai Chi with its delicate nuanced understanding of breath and the flows of energy throughout the body. Contact Improvisation came into my life with its focus on gravity, weight and momentum, a wilder dynamic movement practice. And I began what has been a lifelong passion, a study of experiential anatomy through Release teaching, initially influenced by Simone Forti, Nancy Topf and Mary Fulkerson. These practices began to open a way into perceiving the living architecture of the body and the myriad energies and movements at play within.

Yet I found I still could not raise my arms without pain in my neck and knew I had to find something else. Coming back to England from New York in 1976, I began to teach improvisation, make performances, and to immerse myself intensively in the Alexander Technique.[2] These parallel events were for me the doorway I had been seeking. In the quiet and non-directive touch of my wonderful Alexander teacher, Bill Williams, I began to perceive more clearly the nuanced and subtle complexity of my body, to sense the way everything that happened, each thought and feeling, resonated and reflected within me. I began to experience my body as a living river, the confluence of many streams, where every tissue and cell responded to thought, feeling and event – all we see and feel mirrored in this matter we call 'the body'. Through Bill's quiet touch, my attention began to settle and the tangled storms of feeling and emotion to find coherence.

I see Bill Williams as my first dance teacher. Through him and the listening stillness of his hands, I began to sense the wellsprings of movement arising from inside me. My whole approach to the body and dance underwent a quantum shift. I learnt to listen from the inside to the body as myself, notice the changes of tone and quality, micro movements that subtly but profoundly shaped how I felt in myself and how I perceived the world around me. If I could breathe, widen the field of my attention, and take time to notice how pain or shock resonated in my body, I found a sense of rhythm, rather than

[1] I was not alone in my seeking for other kinds of training for the dancing body. In the USA the Judson movement among others and Butoh dancers in Japan were each exploring body disciplines outside traditional dance and performance.

[2] Alexander was an actor. Losing his voice compelled him to investigate how patterns of tension affected his entire body, and could not be relieved by simply addressing throat or voice box. His technique develops awareness of the unified field of the body and mind.

overwhelm, of internal space and possibility, rather than habitual contraction against difficult circumstances.

Bill taught me to drop below the surface of everyday awareness, and to realise that, as I slowed down my body softened, and I began to notice shifting constellations of sense impressions, memories, dreams, thoughts and images. I began to make dances that I hoped would make visible something of this elusive, metamorphic nature of being alive. Making performances has been a way of excavating this territory, and it brought me into contact with artists in other fields whose interests seemed to parallel my own. For me the beginnings lay in stripping back what seemed at that time the grand gestures of dance to explore the subtleties of everyday movement. Walking – examined, played with in rhythms, patterns, turns, pauses, accelerations – revealed a surprising and delicious complexity. I was fascinated by the small yet momentous and deeply personal shifts of quality in the experiencing body, which I sought to make visible through light and shadow. In particular I was interested in how fractionally close the extraordinary, the astoundingly beautiful, lay to what was conceived of as banal and ordinary. In those heady days of breaking against tradition everything was material for dance. And along with this ran a passion to dissolve the hierarchies of dance, and make it accessible to all and everyone. Every body dancing.

In the late seventies, I met Chris Crickmay (a visual artist and ex-architect) and began a long-term collaboration which continues to this day. Together we made a film for the Open University on dance for 'non-dancers' called *Dance Without Steps*. This seeded a trajectory of work that we came to call 'body and imagination'[3] – a cross-arts exploration of diverse creative strategies, the focus of which was sourced in the sensing body and movement, and extended through drawing, painting, writing, and making.

It has always seemed to me that as imagination and creative energy flow through our sentient bodies, we connect and engage more fully with each other, and with the world about us. I remember the extraordinary beauty of an elderly man standing motionless and alone in a room with arm upraised; I remember a blind man on the stage of Sadlers Wells running, spinning, arms outstretched, face radiant with joy. These precious moments when a person's body becomes illuminated, and everyday movement transforms into what we call dance; moments when soul becomes visible in body, and a person most vividly alive.

I spent many years working in and out of London, teaching and making performances, interspersed with periods in Canada where my then partner Hugh Brody, an anthropologist, was involved in land claims. I was deeply moved by how Native peoples, so profoundly dispossessed from their territories, language and way of life expressed their belonging and entitlement to land in the courtroom through stories, songs and dances. It influenced the way we later initiated health projects in communities in Cumbria and Northumberland.

[3] We subsequently wrote two handbooks for creative practice: *Body Space Image: Notes towards improvisation and performance*, and *A Widening Field: Journeys in body and imagination.*

Coming back to England we moved as a family to an old mill on the edge of the Cumbrian fells. Getting to know a landscape over time, through weather and seasons awakened me to the shifting parallel rhythms and tones in both land and body. I trained and taught at an Alexander school and later studied cranio-sacral therapy, seeking through both these disciplines to deepen and refine my understanding of the body – of the shaping forces of movement, of life and of health. The Chinese say we become ill when we are out of touch with the rhythms of nature. The quixotic vitality of that northern landscape taught me to listen and observe in new ways and nourished my ongoing exploration in body, health and imagination.

In Cumbria I was fortunate to meet Dr Gavin Young, a visionary GP who was prepared to offer me work within his surgery. For fourteen years I worked part-time as an Alexander teacher with people who had a wide range of muscular-skeletal problems. It was a rich and stimulating time, meeting and working with people who would not ordinarily engage with a practice such as the Alexander technique. Increasingly I was aware that developing awareness of the body had a profound effect on how a person managed their lives. Regaining a trust in the body strengthened a person's sense of self, and restored their innate capacity for well being.[4]

Yet in my work in the surgery, I became increasingly aware that for some people more was needed. I remember a young woman I will call Jennifer who had been severely injured in a motorcycle accident. Her partner had been killed and she had undergone extensive surgery to her pelvis and legs. Working to re-establish movement, to help Jennifer walk with less pain, was only one piece of a jigsaw that might enable her grief and despair to ease, and for her to recover pleasure in life again. Her attempted suicide propelled me into more direct action, and Jennifer began to come regularly to the studio at my home and together we moved, drew, made things, moved, wrote poems and laughed. Art making of any kind offers a creative space where imagination is engaged and new (and often surprising) images and stories appear. These open up new perspectives for a person – restore a sense of connection and purpose in living. For Jennifer finding other aspects of her body, voices, characters, energies, brought about a sea change in her life. Through her I felt how deeply the creative spirit, latent in us all, could bring back a sense of joy and trust in life again – a route to health in the full sense of the word.

Working with Jennifer helped me shape a bridge between my own creative work as a dance-maker and artist with the everyday health needs of my community. With the support of practice nurse Dot Main, Dr Gavin Young and Tim Rubidge (a close friend and experienced dancer), we set up movement and creative projects in rural Cumbria and Northumberland. We hoped these would address the wider issues of people's well being – their imaginative world as much as their ailing bodies. Of all the work I have engaged with in my career, this project that we came to call the 'Breath of Fresh Air', inspired

[4] The osteopath James Jealous has suggested that: 'healing is not a resolution of the past but lies in allowing the future to come in to the present'. 'Allow ... to come in ... the present', these qualities of quiet receptivity are so easily overridden in our current pressured climate where the demands of specified targets and outcomes dominate.

and touched me most deeply. Daily I witnessed the creativity, humour, tenderness, and human kindness within the groups, as people came to trust and listen to their bodies, moving together, writing poems, painting dreamscapes and sharing together. (An account of one of these projects forms the first chapter of this book).

I continue to work both with groups and one-to-one, listening to the unique ways our bodies move and express our life experience, and exploring ways to give form to these wordless realms. In recent times, myself and other dance artists have set up a network to share and develop practice – we have called it the Knowing Body Network, knowing from and through the body.[5]

There is a growing body of artists and movement practitioners working in this field of arts and health, and I have had great pleasure in working with some of them. The space of this book can contain only a few of their voices in what is passionate and life enhancing work. Short term funding, the vagaries of arts policy and the isolation in which many of these dedicated practitioners work make this work intensely vunerable. In writing this book and sharing windows into a few contexts, my hope is that it will support and strengthen the cause for others to take up the flag for this precious work within what is becoming an increasingly pressurised and reduced health sector. Socrates chastised doctors of his era for attempting to heal the body without first engaging the soul or essential nature of a person.[6] Dancers and artists working creatively with the body can do much to strengthen a person's capacity for wellness – for feeling alive and whole in ourselves.

> To be great, be whole; don't exaggerate
> Or leave out any part of you.
> Be complete in each thing. Put all you are
> Into the least of your acts.
> So too in each lake, with its lofty life
> The whole moon shines
>
> Fernando Pessoa

[5] The Knowing Body Network.

[6] See Shaun McNiff *Art as Medicine: Creating a therapy of imagination.*

Introduction
a medicine within

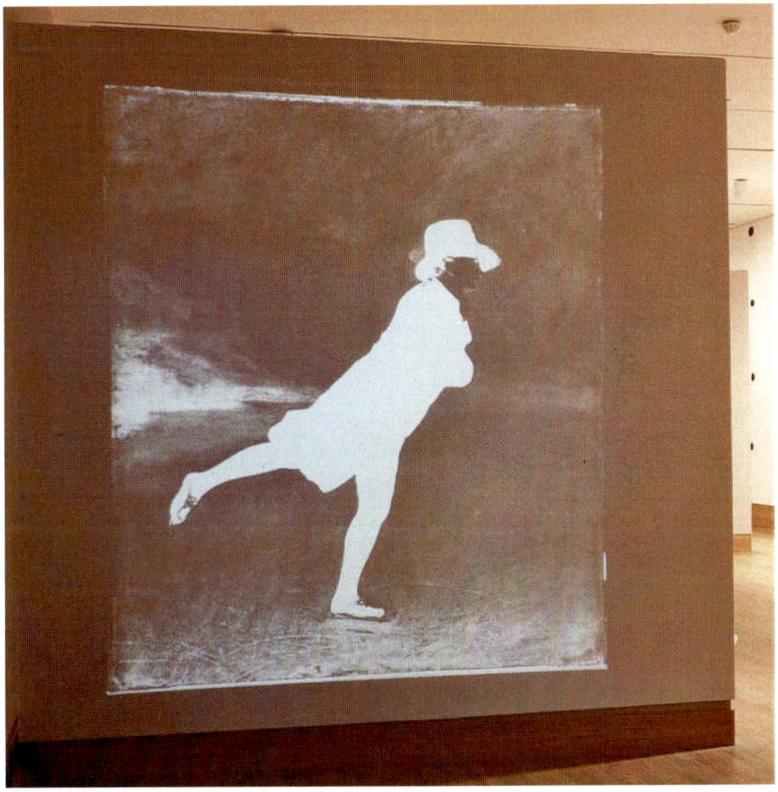

The real voyage of discovery consists not in seeking new landscapes but in having new eyes.
Marcel Proust

This book is a gathering of voices and stories from artists, patients, and health professionals working in the field of arts and health. These stories speak to ways in which arts, and particularly dance practice, can work alongside and in support of our beleaguered and overstretched healthcare system. There is a growing though disparate body of evidence from experienced and skilled movement practitioners who navigate an always complex, sometimes controversial, but often fruitful interface between clinical care and the creative arts.

Around the world there are movement projects for people living with mental health problems from depression, dementia and eating disorders, to dance projects in stroke units, in rehabilitation, in palliative care, with boy soldiers, with refugees, with mothers and babies. There are movement projects for people with trauma and for those who have been tortured where the pain is beyond any words. In a time when the NHS is under increasing pressure there is much the arts, and particularly dance, can do in bringing people together and supporting them to care more effectively for themselves. The stories in this book often began as stories of isolation and illness but grew into stories of strengths discovered, of hope and of well being. It is my own hope that this book will fan the flame of these developments and encourage practitioners on both sides (clinical and artistic) to look further into the value of this work and the contribution it can make.

Looking after ourselves

Many people feel out of touch with their bodies – anaesthetised, as it were, from that which is closest and most vital to them. Many of us treat our bodies as a complex consumer commodity unsuitable for home repair, take little care of it and cart it to the NHS when it doesn't seem to work. Yet our relationship to our bodies underpins every aspect of our lives. When we lack a felt awareness of our bodies, we lose connection with an innate bodily intelligence that underpins how we look after our health and well being.

Dr Malcolm Rigler, a GP who pioneered the use of the creative arts in his surgery, commented that a central concern in general practice is inspiring people to care for their own bodies, something he felt artists and dancers were uniquely able to help with:

> I always wanted to do all I could to help patients fully appreciate and understand the fragility and complexity of their own bodies, but I wanted this to go beyond biological facts and simple health education. I believe we could sow the seed of total enchantment with the human, help us find meaning in life and so value ourselves, our neighbours and the community in which we live.

Illness can be a wake-up call to remember what has been forgotten or ignored in the stresses and strains of life. We all need to keep in touch with whatever makes life worthwhile.

To feel well is not a given – every moment offers us creative choices in how we perceive, breathe, respond and shape our worlds. Developing trust in our bodies, refining physical awareness and cultivating a language for what we feel strengthens our capacity to look after ourselves more imaginatively and effectively.

In the last century Alexander, Feldenkrais, Mabel Todd and many others pioneered somatic approaches to the body that developed body awareness in order to recover function and healing.[1] Their work revealed just how much we can affect our health through more conscious awareness of the body; that the body is infinitely more responsive and mutable than we have believed. An embodied and creative arts practice offers a context for play and exploration of what we feel, thereby refreshing our language, stories, and perceptions.

In every culture and in every medical tradition before ours, healing was accomplished by moving energy.
Albert Szent-Györgyi[2]

Life is movement. All the tissues of our bodies depend on the circulation and movement of energy, information, nutrients and waste within us. All traditional healing practices affirm the need for movement to sustain life processes – movement of breath and lungs, of digestion, of heart, blood and fluid circulation. Every cell in our body exists in fluid communication with the whole – muscles, bones, ligaments, organs and fluids form a streaming continuum in which lack, or loss, of movement in any particular area causes loss of plasticity, loss in renewal of tissues and loss of responsiveness. Paralleling these are the movement of our thoughts, sensations, emotions and feelings. Our relationship with the world is in effect a dance of interchange and response to the constantly shifting conditions of our inner and external worlds. Homeostasis is the ability of any organism to maintain internal equilibrium by adjusting physiological processes. Becoming more aware of our bodies, attuning to the myriad of internal sensations is a first step in calming the mind and helping rebalance these subtle chemistries of our bodies. Candace Pert, a neuroscientist whose book *Molecules of Emotion* has done much to develop understanding of the body-mind continuum, describes the body as 'a flickering flame'. Caring for ourselves involves listening to and getting to know this sensing, moving body that we are.

Movement... the language of the body

To speak of dance for many people conjures idealised images of the body, which conversely evoke a sense of our own body as graceless and failing even as we long for the ecstatic freedom of Nijinsky's leap. Yet there are as many ways of moving and dancing as there are styles of clothing – each belonging to particular peoples, places, moments of history – such as ballet, jazz, Afro, club. But beneath the techniques and traditions of these different styles exists a dance in which we all move: a dance that becomes visible the

[1] It was losing his voice that propelled Alexander to discover his technique for mind-body integration. For Mabel Todd, a riding accident that broke her back led her to her seminal book *The Thinking Body* and the development of Ideokinesis.

[2] Szent-Györgyi was a scientist working at the Institute for Muscle Research which later became the National Foundation for Cancer Research.

moment we are still and listen, a dance that expands within the rhythm and quality of our conversations, in the movement of our bodies each day as we are drawn this way and that – as we turn, bend, rise, walk, dream or fall to stillness. The glamorised images of dance of which we are all familiar blind us to another kind of 'dance' – the subtle riverflow of movements (thoughts, sensations, emotions) that shape each moment of how we perceive, feel and manage our day-to-day lives.

In a session, I watch a woman crippled with hip pain and scarcely able to walk. She lies on the ground, seemingly still, and yet, as her fingers slowly uncurl and her arm extends, I become aware of a small dance unfolding its music through every part of her – gestures of extraordinary delicacy and expressive poignancy. She tells me later it was a dance for her son who drowned several years previously and it was only within the movements of her body that she could begin to express pain that was otherwise overwhelming.

Healing through dance is one of the earliest known expressions of the arts. The inner melodies that dance and movement awaken can restore a sense of pace, rhythm and coherence. Movement offers a language where words fail, bridging the gap between the buried inner territories of our feelings and the landscapes and people who form our world. Above all the creative sensitivity awakened through movement brings a trust in what our bodies' feel, (sensations, intuitions, instincts), rather than avoiding feeling as many of us do, and so wakes up a sense of connectedness.

Finding our way

When we are not well we often question what we can do to 'get better'; many people want to be actively involved in their own recovery and not just passively receive treatment administered by another. But the particular pace and pleasures that nourish and sustain us are unique to each person's life experience. We may not know what will restore connection and pleasure but the free play of creativity offers a context for exploring, imagining and feeling – a context where the absorption in something other than illness invariably opens out the stories of how we conceive our self and our lives. We discover buried and forgotten aspects of ourselves, small things overlooked, small voices calling out for unmet needs, stories and memories that reconnect us to a sense of purpose and meaning. Medicine does not have time to delve into what makes life significant, but sustenance of the soul is vital to health and wholeness.

Illness often follows in the wake of a loss or period of stress when our immune system is compromised. When we feel low it is often difficult to value ourselves enough to look after ourselves and this neglect may precede further and more serious illness. Like Ulysses trying to get home there are times in all our lives when we experience what feels like the drying up of a stream, a 'withering field'[3] when we feel disconnected from the waters of life. An art's practice that listens and engages through senses and body brings us vividly

[3] The osteopath William Garner Sutherland coined this evocative phrase when talking about loss of health.

into the present moment infusing new content into our lives therebye nourishing us emotionally, strengthening self-esteem and lifting our spirits.

The arts cannot solve our problems, but they invite us to question, explore and discover other aspects of who we are – aspects that are not just to do with our immediate difficulties or illness. Dance, movement, has the capacity to bring us into a more personal, imaginative and creative relationship with our body-self, re-connecting us to what is well despite illness, and so bringing about easier conditions in mind and body. The free play of creativity opens a door to buried resources strengthening our capacity to meet and adapt to change.

The need to be heard, to express ourselves, to have a voice, is fundamental to well being and a sense of self. Everyone has the need to tell their story and to have it valued. We need intelligent listening and know how differently we feel in ourselves when we feel heard and recognised for who we are. It might be said that this is the realm of therapy, but the role of the arts in expressing what matters for us predate that of therapy by thousands of years. Our individual and collective experience of illness and dying is harsher and lonelier when this basic human need is unfulfilled.

Away from the familiarity of home and in contexts where there is often little time to communicate, losing a sense of self may be inevitable – we become patients, administered to, looked after, but rarely heard, or heard at the level at which we hear and recognise ourselves. One woman said of herself: 'I wanted to go in a dustbin.' It is this loss of a sense of value in one's life that this work seeks to redress.

Artists working within the field of the arts in healthcare may be perceived as delivering soft outcomes in contrast to the targeted outcomes and predictions demanded of mainstream medicine. Though an arts practice does not seem to engage with these focused outcomes, it invariably goes far in strengthening a person's well being and thus their capacity to self care.

Perhaps the most important aspect of what movement and creative expression can do is to reconnect people with what they love and has mattered to them in their lives. It is difficult to convey the feel of this work, the softening, grounding and energising effect on participants that it can bring about. Something of the process of learning to inhabit one's body and simultaneously to give form to one's personal world through imaginative activity can change the tone of a person's life dramatically. In circumstances of trauma or ill health, this brings to the fore what has been crushed or fragmented by illness – the wider field of a person's life and well being.

> And should the world itself forget your name
>
> Say this to the still earth: I flow
>
> Say this to the quick stream: I am
>
> Don Paterson, *Orpheus* (2006)

A Breath of Fresh Air

Come and find new ways to breathe and relax and discover more ease in mind and body. Find pleasure in relaxation. Find ways to feel better in yourself and gain control over your symptoms. There will be a variety of creative activities to help reduce stress and tension resulting from longterm illness, injury, pain or depression.

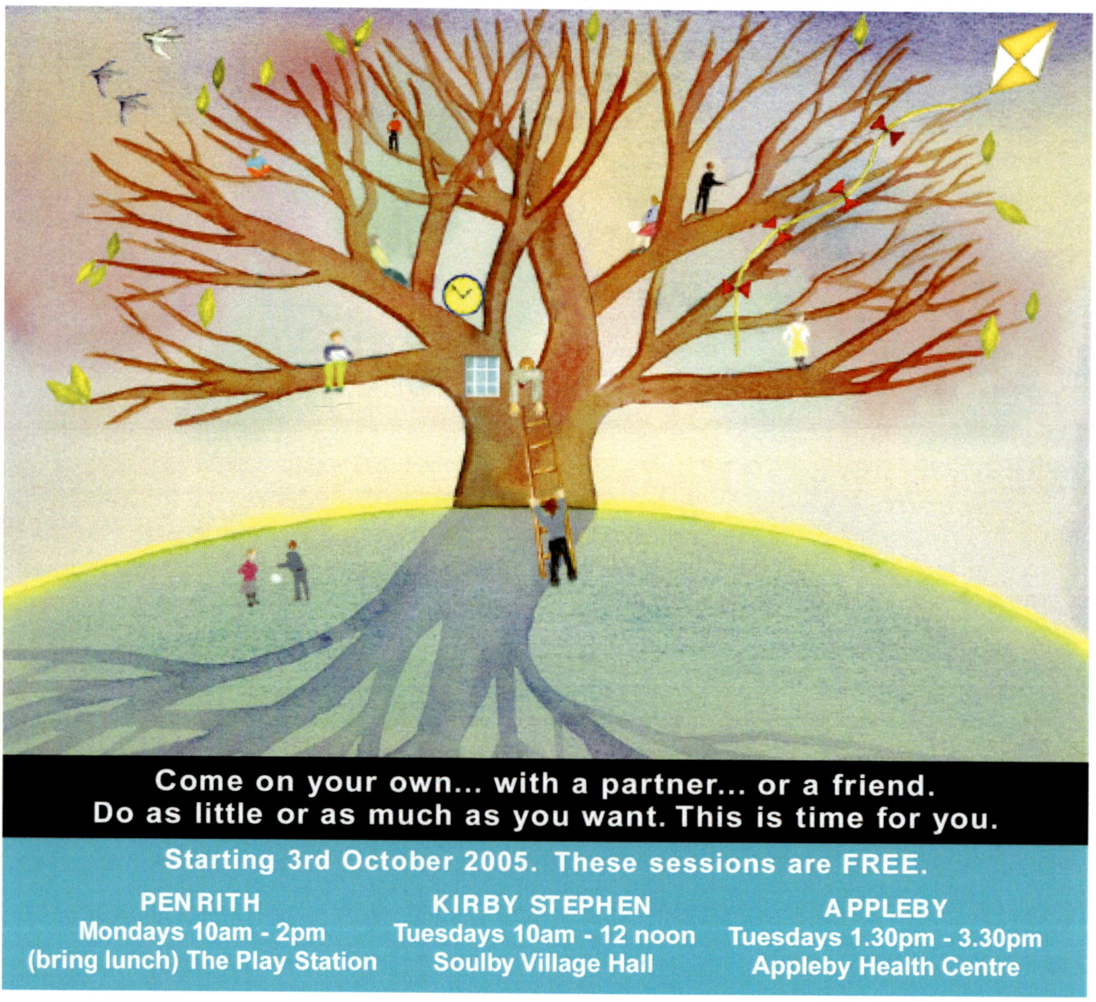

**Come on your own... with a partner... or a friend.
Do as little or as much as you want. This is time for you.**

Starting 3rd October 2005. These sessions are FREE.

PENRITH
Mondays 10am - 2pm
(bring lunch) The Play Station

KIRBY STEPHEN
Tuesdays 10am - 12 noon
Soulby Village Hall

APPLEBY
Tuesdays 1.30pm - 3.30pm
Appleby Health Centre

Miranda Tufnell is an Alexander teacher, cranio-sacral therapist and dancer who worked at Temple Sowerby surgery for 14 years. Brenda Mallon is a writer and psychotherapist who has worked for 20 years exploring dreams, creativity and loss with both individuals and groups.

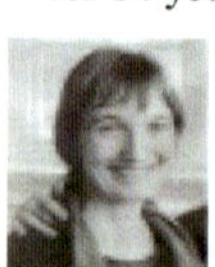

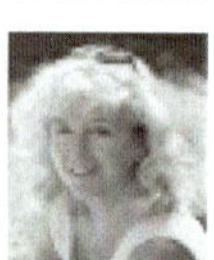

If you would like to join,
please telephone Miranda on: 0777 9153689

'A Breath of Fresh Air' is part of a Body Stories arts & health research project.

A Breath of Fresh Air

an account of a project

Brenda Mallon and Miranda Tufnell

The most authentic thing about us
Is our capacity to create, to overcome
To endure, to transform, to love,
And be greater than our suffering.
We are best defined by the mystery
That we are still here, and can still rise upwards.

Ben Okri, *Mental Fight*

Background

This chapter is a revised account of an arts and health project in rural Cumbria and Northumberland. The project was intended as a pilot study which we hoped would be followed by more sustained work.[1] For three years, we worked in a range of contexts and with diverse groups, each group evolving a particular format and name. In the final stages we called our sessions A Breath of Fresh Air.

The project grew out of my own therapeutic work in Dr Gavin Young's surgery near Penrith. I was joined first by Tim Rubidge, a dancer, and Jilly Jarman, a musician, and finally by Brenda Mallon, a writer and psychotherapist. I am hugely indebted to the generosity of these collaborators who dived, questioned and reflected with me. This text draws on all of their contributions.

Our intention was to complement existing NHS services. In setting up the project Tim and I spent a year talking to a wide range of professionals in both health and social services including schools, libraries, GPs, physiotherapists, community and psychiatric nurses. We wanted particularly to reach those for whom currently there was no other provision and who would not ordinarily engage with an arts activity.

These were categories of patient that a GP felt could be helped by an arts and health project: people suffering with anxiety and depression, with medically unexplained symptoms, people with long term health conditions who were despondent, isolated, and

[1] The project was jointly funded by Northumberland Health Action Zone and the Arts Council of England.

who had 'lost hope', carers in danger of burnout, and people needing support in their recovery from illness or surgery.

At different times we ran projects for people identified as suffering from stress, hypertension and depression, with heart problems and those living with chronic pain. For people living with poor health in isolated rural communities, there was little to help them keep heart with their lives. Our aim was to provide support and resources for people whose health might otherwise spiral further downwards.

In talking to our various steering groups and healthcare professionals, it was difficult to assess who of their patient group particularly might gain from our work. Everyone was keen for us to support particular groups. We felt we could work with almost anyone but this made it difficult to convey to the medical teams what our content might be – and thus the appropriateness of their referral. Our policy became as much as possible to run open groups where people with very different needs and mobility could come together. In the overall project six different venues were used, some with more than one group, with sizes varying from four to twenty.

When Tim and I began our work in Cumbria we rarely used the word 'dance' as it conjured idealised images of the body/self for people who felt physically compromised. None of the people who came to our groups wanted to 'dance'. Indeed, they perceived dance as irrelevant to their health needs; yet all wanted an easier relationship to their bodies. This caused Tim to identify our evolving role as one of 'ambassadors for the body'.

We were acutely aware, throughout this project, of the deep alienation and shame associated with the body, and the delicacy of encouraging participants to listen to their bodies without activating potentially overwhelming memories of trauma. In its final year, we renamed our project A Breath of Fresh Air[2] as we hoped that each of those involved would find ways to breathe and feel strengthened in their lives, and that the sensuous play of creativity would reveal images and stories that would restore feelings of power and purpose in each person's daily life.

Our aim was to establish informal workshop settings where there was time for people suffering from various kinds of mental and physical poor health to come together and discover a more positive and creative relationship to their bodies and to their lives.

What follows is a collage of ingredients that includes accounts of what we did and why, along with the voices of both participants and practitioners (artists and health professionals).

> **Lucy**: 'I liked coming because you could be completely yourself – you didn't have to put a face on – you didn't have to get smart – it was just good – I liked it – it was good to talk to people who understood – and you were yourself and if you did feel you wanted to shed a few tears and have a cry it didn't matter... I went out the other night with some friends and

[2] We discovered that for some, our company name Body Stories evoked images of abuse. Our initial worthy title was Moving Towards Health but we changed this to the more colloquial Breath of Fresh Air.

they were all talking about their work and what they were doing ... and I just felt sad – I felt I couldn't talk properly because they all went out to work, their lives were completely different to mine, and I felt sad and a bit useless. But those sessions[3] were so nice – you could just be yourself and I knew it was OK. Nobody was judging you and I wasn't thinking or trying, and it was nice to have that few hours.'

Dr Gavin Young, GP – extracts from an interview with Miranda Tufnell

I think my role as a GP is to help everyone involved to make sense of what is happening – to try and get them so they understand why 'this illness, this awfulness' has happened to them. Because if they can understand it gives them some ability to manage it themselves, which is what I would like them to do, and they themselves would feel better if they could do that....

I think the other thing that is very important is the idea of a doctor as a teacher – or maybe a sharer of information would be better – to help people be able to make decisions. I think there is an increasing desire not to be the passive recipient of medicine ....

The problem is that the delivery of healthcare becomes terribly target orientated ... hundreds of different things we are supposed to measure – that doesn't sit easily with a patient-focused system of healthcare.... How can I be your personal doctor and attend to what you come to me with if I'm busy thinking I've got to complete all of these score things on a great chart...? You have to be able to manage all those tasks, without losing the humanity, and attend to why the patient has come to see you....

The deeper things within human beings are difficult to measure ... and because they are not measurable doesn't mean they don't matter – indeed they are immeasurably important.

[3] A Breath of Fresh Air.

Dot Main, practice nurse – extracts from an interview with Miranda Tufnell

I was delighted, really delighted, that someone was thinking along these lines of providing something more ... that we as health professionals haven't got the time to provide. I could see the benefits in many ways – particularly for people with chronic disease and their carers – so they had somewhere to go on a regular basis – that was consistent – that eventually felt quite safe – somewhere they could perhaps become themselves more and start to enjoy things, apart from thinking about their illness and how they were coping. Through this project you were giving them other ways of coping with their illness. You were helping them find themselves again ... something which was lost...

There is such a time problem in general practice. Even twelve months ago we had a little more time to give, but now I feel that there is increasingly less time. So much is demanded of people working in primary care. I do feel that if it becomes a case of ticking boxes and making sure we have got all this information to audit in order to get money to be able to care for people, I think it becomes wrong – you are not looking at the person as a whole, you are just making sure you have their blood pressure recorded, making sure they have had their last cholesterol done – making sure their long-term sugars are up-to-date – you are not actually looking beyond that to see always *why* it might not be quite right, *why* this might not be working out, or *why* the blood pressure might be high or the sugars running high ... there is no time to ask questions sometimes – to say for instance 'How are things at home?' 'What is happening with little Johnny?' or 'How is your husband or partner?' – the questions that matter.

Get well card made by workshop participant

'I've written myself a get well card – when I was relaxing – I kept seeing these eyes – and they were looking out and looking bright – and that was really lovely because I think I am just starting to realise that it's good to be alive – which may sound very simple, but it wasn't that long ago that I didn't really care if I was or not – so I wrote myself a get well card.'

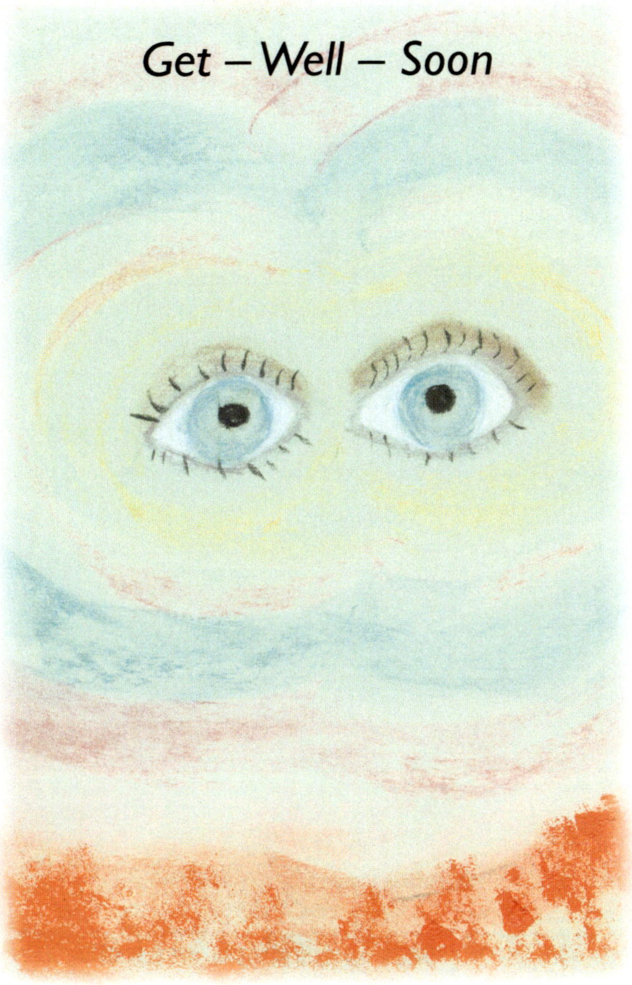

Get – Well – Soon

Three simple little words and eleven letters
A well made gesture that is said so often
– but what does it really mean?
Get on with it
Get your act together
Get up and stop moping around
Get a grip

Well – what is your problem?
Well, if you had a life that is as tough as mine ...
well what will people think?
Soon be better – there, there
Soon forget about your problems
Soon be back to normal.
What does it really mean, 'get well soon'?

Getting in touch with your real self,
Getting into a slower gear,
Getting back to enjoying my basic loves.
Get back into a lifestyle that cares for me
as well as my family and friends.

Well – Well is a feeling I feel every Tuesday
and can last the whole week.
Well, Well, Well, I do have an artistic side.
Well is as deep as I want to go.

Soon ... soon everyone will enjoy a more peaceful Helen.
Soon people will want to be around me again.
Soon I will stop worrying about what my husband thinks of me.
Soon I will accept and enjoy me for just being me.
Get-well-soon
I intend to.

Getting going

> The placebo effect is about enabling patients to rediscover their self-healing powers. [The task of the GP] could involve supporting and nurturing people at a low ebb, while enabling those same patients to develop their own role in self-treatment as they become stronger.
>
> Dixon & Sweeney, *The Human Effect in Medicine: Theory, Research and Practice (2001)*

All who came to the groups were suffering both mental and physical distresses. Many felt the NHS could offer them nothing more. Their stories were of loss, of lifestyle, of work, of friendships, of self-esteem, of fear and helplessness, coupled with a sense of having become profoundly isolated. In these circumstances many had given up and had lost the confidence to get out and try something new. So we were delighted when people responded of their own initiative to our posters and arrived into our sessions.

Conditions people came with:
cancer, ME, chronic pain, auto-immune illnesses, bipolar, eating and obsessive compulsive disorders, back pain, chronic depression and anxiety.

One problem had often led to another causing a downwards spiral into other health problems. Chronic health conditions can be accompanied by shame at 'failing' to get better. Those with poor health often strive to meet the expectations of others and feel judged for their inability to overcome their changed circumstances. With ill health the body often becomes something unpredictable and feared for how it may react: violent shaking, dizziness, sudden spasms of pain, inability to breathe. There is the shame of not being able to cope with everyday tasks, of being easily and often suddenly overwhelmed. For many who came to our groups the stresses of poor health had caused them to retreat and hide away from a world that seemed to exclude them in their difficulties. With illness many of the activities that give pleasure, meaning, and self-worth are no longer possible. We hoped our Breath of Fresh Air initiative might in some way reverse these inward, downward spirals.

Lauren's Story

When Lauren first came to the Breath of Fresh Air project she walked stiffly and looked to be in extreme pain. She was thirty six years old, the mother of a ten year old and a three year old. She had had full time jobs, worked on a farm and in a pub, did her shopping, cleaned her house and enjoyed life, went out with friends.

A series of accidents and illnesses culminated in the auto - immune illness that utterly changed her life. Imagine every day you are in pain. You can't carry your shopping and it's hard to make the journey to the shops anyway. Your friends slip away from you because you can't join in the usual social activities and besides, when your friends look at you they see the pain etched in your exhausted face. It's hard to look after your children but you do, only sometimes Lauren hurts so much she cannot manage to pull a comb through her hair and she has to ask someone else to do that for her. Also, sometimes her body goes into shock because of the pain and she starts shaking and it can last for twenty minutes.

'It can be at bit embarrassing,' Lauren said, in her understated way, 'like when it happened at school. It was not nice for my little boy.' The little boy, with his shaking mother, stood at the school gates until the tremors stopped. Though Lauren was in a crowd of parents she felt isolated and that sense of isolation impacted both on her emotional life and on the lives of her children.

Establishing a group

> No man is an island, entire of itself; every man is a piece of the continent, a part of the main. If a clod be washed away by the sea, Europe is the less
> Any man's death diminishes me, because I am involved in mankind; and therefore never send to know for whom the bell tolls; it tolls for thee...
>
> John Donne, *Devotions upon Emergent Occasions,* 'Meditation 17'. This famous quote was written as a meditation on illness.

The experience of illness, as Lauren's story above, is often one of isolation, of feeling left alone and having nothing to contribute to others. Developing participation with people who are vulnerable is inevitably a delicate process. Everyone arrives as an individual with a particular history, often with apprehensions about joining a group, being among strangers and being able to manage what may be asked for. Taking time to feel out people's interests, concerns and needs was vital in establishing confidence in participating in something as unfamiliar as an arts project. Yet once braved, being part of a group can in itself be an important step in recovering a measure of well being. A group becomes a kind of family, where people feel at ease and comfortable together.

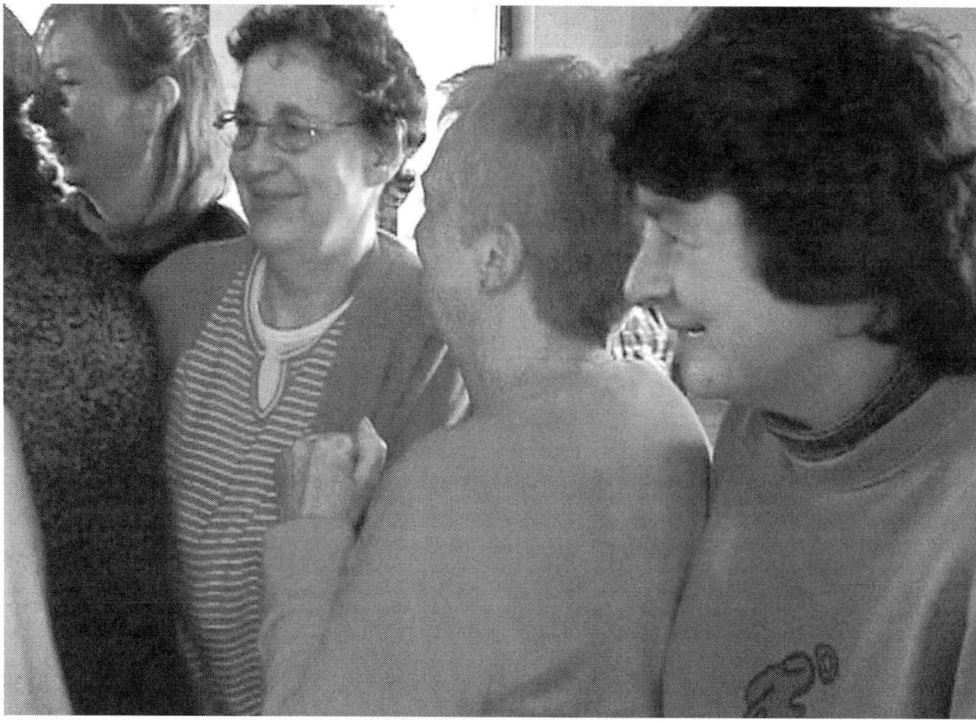

In many circumstances people's health was so poor that continuity of attendance was impossible, yet it was important to hold a space, even if only two were able to turn up. People living with chronic ill health experience repeated disappointments and loss of hope – being reliable and steady is vital among those whose own world can feel very fluctuant and unstable. The sharing of life experiences that arose through creating with others was one of the most potent and moving aspects of the work, a moving out of isolation into a discovery of shared experiences, which created powerful and sustaining bonds between participants.[4]

On our first day, Tim and I brought branches of richly coloured autumn leaves, which we set in a glass vase in the window to catch the sun, alongside a bowl of fruit. This made a rather dowdy village hall feel more hospitable. It was a cold but bright day and people arrived with some apprehension and scepticism about what they might be expected to do with two artists. We began sitting in a circle and introduced ourselves with observations about the weather and inquiries about where people had come from, asking each person what they would most like help with from the sessions. All spoke in different ways of their stiffness, coldness and pain in moving. Even in that first meeting, others responded and offered suggestions, which made a warm and friendly start.

[4] In South Africa there is a concept of *Ubuntu* which roughly translates 'I am because we are'. A person is a person through and by means of all the others they are connected to. There is no concept of a person in isolation. We all actively co-create and sustain each other.

What people said they hoped to gain from the sessions

To breathe and move more easily … to know how to loosen up and ease pain … to walk/ move without pain … to remain active … to manage problems better … to relax … maintain a level of fitness … I'd like to be ordinary again, I want to be me, the old me … to feel better, be able to express myself and find the real me … to stop feeling so agitated.

Some initial responses

> **Helen:** I really didn't know what it was about – I really didn't know what it would do – at that time I was struggling just getting out of the house, so the whole thing was a major feat just to get here and be among people – I certainly didn't want to open up and tell anyone who I was or what had happened to me – I found it very stressful, the first week especially.

> **Keith:** I came to the sessions when they first started. 18 months before that I lost my wife. I suppose I was going through the usual stages of trying to come to terms with it. It was around that time that lots of things went wrong and caused a lot of grief... I had deteriorated after my wife died... I had cancer scares and one thing or another... I kept myself inside my cottage, hiding behind my walking stick and not really wanting to open the door to people or life... I felt pushed away.

For many the loneliness of illness had brought on mental and emotional difficulties. Members of the group commented that one of the benefits of attending the sessions was 'to get to know other people' and 'to revive social skills'. Severe pain cuts people off from their previous abilities, often they lose the person they once were and have to find a way of living which is dramatically different from their previous existence. Many people become painfully isolated.

In Latin the word 'patient' derives from pathos or suffering,
and it refers to a passive state, yet we find the same root in passion,
and the word compatible, to suffer, or endure together

joining

'Happier people are healthier people'

In an early meeting about our project, Dr Gavin Young spoke of how many of his patients viewed their body as the enemy, something feared in its vulnerability and dysfunction. He hoped that we dancers might find creative approaches to help people feel, enjoy and learn from their bodies. We also hoped that bringing people together into groups might ease the depression, isolation and sense of exclusion that poor health can bring about. We wanted to find ways of making the body both accessible and at the same time something of inspiration and of beauty, and to use movement and imagination to support the potential well being of each individual. Pain or poor health profoundly undermines our relationship both to our bodies and to everyone around us – our families and friends. When we lose these essential connections, our sense of identity and of personal worth is profoundly diminished. William Garner Sutherland, the founder of cranial osteopathy, describes this as 'a withering field', when body and mind cannot let in the vital life force or find the resources to heal.

> The magic elixirs of life ... wonder, nutrition, humour, faith, nature, exercise and community ... hope, passion, relaxation, family, curiosity, creativity, wisdom and peace.
>
> Patch Adams, *Gesundeit* (1998) – Patch Adams is an American doctor, clown and social revolutionary.

Health is not simply absence of disease but involves a complex and elusive weave of physical, emotional, mental and spiritual elements. To the Greeks healing implied service to the Gods, a reconnection to forces greater than the individual. In Norse *haelen hal* – 'health' – means wholeness, a call to connect the part to the whole, to expand into a fuller, richer engagement with life. Our health and well being lies in the quality of our relationship to ourselves and to those around us, in the joy, laughter, wonder, curiosity and compassion with which we meet events in our lives. Each of us needs to make sense of our suffering and to find ways to express and share the uniqueness of our experience.

Describing what she liked about the sessions, Laura wrote: 'Going in feeling a bit sad and then coming out happy. It's like a ray of sunshine. Everyone gives each other a bit of sunshine and support.'

We were moved to witness the ways in which each person was gradually able to move beyond their difficulties, expand into the creative space of a session People wanted time to be themselves without the usual constraints of being a mother, a father, or the many roles we have in our lives. As Helen said: 'Tuesdays are the highlight of my week because it's just for me! It allows me four hours of total focus on me. I have no guilt that I should be doing something for others, doing things I wouldn't have time to do usually.'

Creating together

> You could say that creativity is fundamental.. and what we really have to explain are these processes that are not creative. You see, usually we believe that in life the rule is uncreativity, and occasionally a little burst of creativity that comes in that has to be explained. But...creativity is the basis, and it is repetition that has to be explained
>
> David Bohm, Nobel prize-winning physicist

'To create' in Latin means simply to make. In ancient times creativity was seen as the province of the gods, its sense being of the origins of the universe – worlds formed and growing in the awakening and discrimination of elements – light from dark, land from water, earth from air and the wild diversity of species. Creating with others takes us on journeys together into the unknown, like Darwin's voyage on the Beagle, we follow moment by moment wherever senses and imagination are drawn. We explore, discover, take risks, make mistakes, adapt, transform and along the way find new and often surprising characters, images, and narratives.

Creating in any medium awakens our senses and our stories. Creative space offers a context where people are free to explore, share and find form for what really matters to them. Where words fail, creating in any medium offers a means of expression that helps a person reconnect to the wider field of their life experience. Away from the familiarity of home and in contexts where there is little sensory stimulation or time to communicate, it is easy to lose this vital sense of self and of agency.

We always began each session gathering together in a circle and checking in. Each person had the opportunity to talk about how they had been since the last meeting, how they were feeling and to share anything that was important to them. People shared their fears and worries as well as their high points. This part of the work was invaluable. It gave us the opportunity to gauge how people were feeling and to respond to their needs. Whilst everyone had the chance to speak there was no compulsion, if someone didn't feel like talking or wanted to say just a couple of words, that was fine. Even silence gave us a measure of how a person might be feeling. Because of the vulnerabilities of participants we always worked in pairs, one leading, the other observing and able to support anyone with particular difficulties.

In building up the trust and support of the group it was important to recognise individual needs. The sharing and communication between members however brief was vital in establishing a measure of trust in what might emerge through the creative process and prepared the ground for the subsequent sharing with partners. As part of this sharing process we stressed the importance of confidentiality within the group.

'I like the opening circle as it lets everyone centre themselves
and speak of any worries.'

Finding a theme

After everyone had 'checked in' we moved on to the theme of the session. In choosing a theme we sought to establish common ground between people with very different health issues. Each session we created a 'centre piece' on the floor in the middle of the circle which illustrated what we would be working on. We used bones, branches, leaves, mosses, stones, shells, paper butterflies – this offered a visual metaphor where people's thoughts, reflections and questions could settle.

The themes chosen always explored some aspect of health and the body. We might demonstrate how a part of the body worked – with visual aids, illustrations or with a skeleton. We explored the anatomical relationships of spine, head and neck, breath, feet, and encouraged people to develop their own sense of any part, its movement and relationship to the whole. Through this the details of anatomy became felt and personal, stimulating people's stories and personal images. The vertebrae of the spine as stepping stones, or pathway, creating length between the head and pelvis, the head as look-out post... weather vane... tree house, we sent messages through the arms, tap-danced the toes, imagined conversations between body parts – always exploring ways to open up people's felt sense of their own bodies and to free up habits of stress or tension.

We looked at people's dreams and favourite stories, and explored different aspects of relaxation. We aimed to make each session informative, conversational, exploratory and fun. There were lots of opportunities for people's questions and comments, and personal insights or experiences about their own bodies.

In one session we brought acorns, nuts, seeds, and grass heads and talked about winter and the need for darkness and rest; we shared thoughts about a seed and new beginnings, and of conditions needed for growth. Each person chose something from this autumn basket, and then step by step through movement, making and writing, imagined its growth – what it might become – and what gift (quality or energy) it might offer them. These processes gave room for each person to make their own journey into story, association or memory.

From the very beginning, **M**, a retired policeman, shared his love of bees and beekeeping for which he was well known in the Eden Valley. He spoke so often and so lovingly of

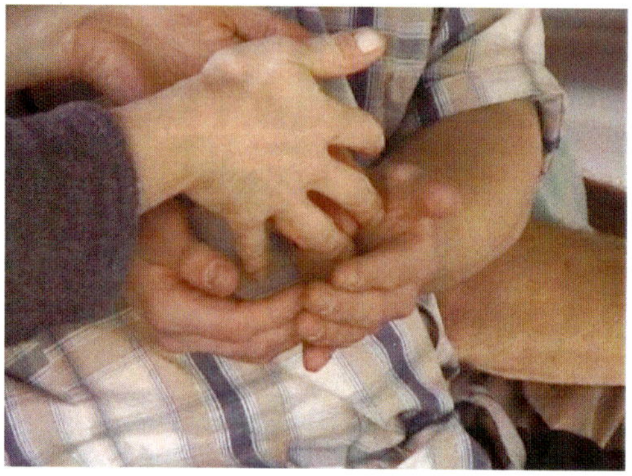

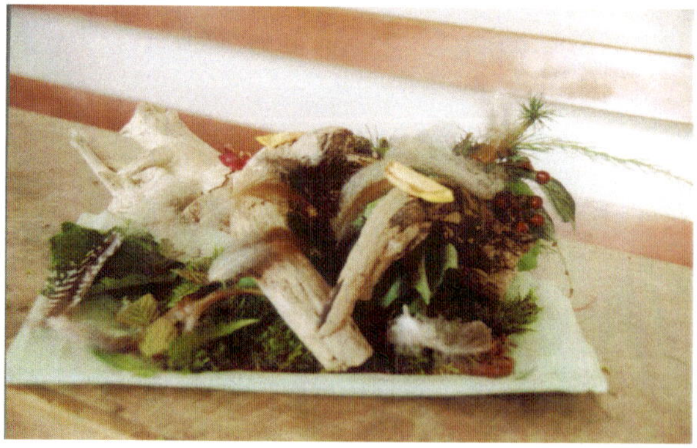

them it was as if the bees came with him to the sessions – perhaps because he was no longer able to be active with them. His hands were swollen and pale from diabetes, yet he 'spoke' in movement, describing the details of how he would trim the wings of the queen before swarming – an action he could no longer perform.[5]

Keith was the oldest in our group; an accident in the Second World War had badly damaged his right arm. His 'good' left arm consequently had to compensate and worked hard. Bone grafts taken from his leg for his arm had caused other problems, his right foot had lost its reflexes and he was frequently in pain. The accident had also caused severe hearing loss which made being in a group both a joy and a struggle. Yet in a session after he had moved this is what Keith wrote:

> ***To my arms***: 'I have reason to be glad for my hands and I realise more and more the way they have served me – if I could draw I would put my two hands together as Thanksgiving – the Indian or Japanese way. I have gradually become more aware of their skills – their functions – and the enchantment they have provided for me – I liken them to branches of trees in touch with each other – passing messages with each other – but able to act alone – blending into the body... marvellous in their activities – the hands and arms through which we express grace and happiness.'

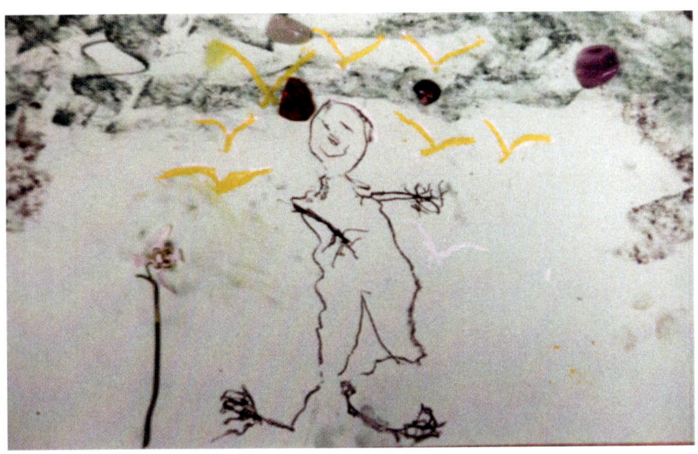

> ***To my feet:*** 'Hey, what about us down here? It's shameful the way you treat my mate and me. We're much more important than your fat belly,

[5] Dot Main, practice nurse: 'As a diabetic patient he had lots of problems with circulation in his legs and his arms and hands – he wasn't able to do what he once could and was becoming quite clumsy. He found that coming to the project helped him so much – just with the gentle movements that you helped him to do – and also I think it helped him think about things in a different way. He just couldn't believe how much better he felt. He said it was wonderful – he actually came to tell me that. So for him it was important to have that place to come once a week as he knew that you would be there to reassure him as well and support him. That's important.'

your genitals or any big idea of your head. You can't even stand, walk, run or dance unless we're up to the mark and we're tired of being ignored except when you occasionally cut our nails because you've nothing better to do. Those nails were once proper claws in better days, you know. But now, you don't even wash us often enough, though we've spent the day kicking about in dirt and dust. And as for getting a decent pair of socks to wear we've no chance, except maybe at Christmas! So we're demanding, in future, better attention and much more respect from you. Otherwise we'll let you down.'

Movement towards health

Our sessions always began with an aspect of the body. Many people were in pain and restricted in their capacity to move. Each day we took time focus on breath, on settling and stillness; this slowly developed people's ability to listen to their bodies without fear. Waking up in the senses – taste, sight, hearing, scent, touch – connects a person to their surroundings, which like mindfulness practices can begin to free the mind from habitual anxieties.

Breathing in… breathing out… letting the outside in… letting the inside out

We found that as people began to trust and notice more of what they felt in their bodies a gentler rhythm emerged, a quality of receptivity, which opened up the possibility of change at many levels. Most importantly the musicality of movement offered a way of experiencing the body as more than its symptoms and illnesses. Each person could move as much or as little as they wanted or felt able. Often we suggested participants close their eyes to delve deeper into sensory awareness. In the initial stages, some members were embarrassed about moving, feeling that they might be 'judged' or be found wanting because they were not 'dancers'. This embarrassment seemed to dissolve swiftly once people felt at ease within the group.

For people living with chronic pain, movement can be feared and posture fixed in an effort to avoid further aggravation. Slowing down, connecting gently to the rhythms of breath and visualising slow movement can be a powerful tool in restoring a sense of ease and capacity to self-manage (research confirms that even imagined movement can increase blood flow).

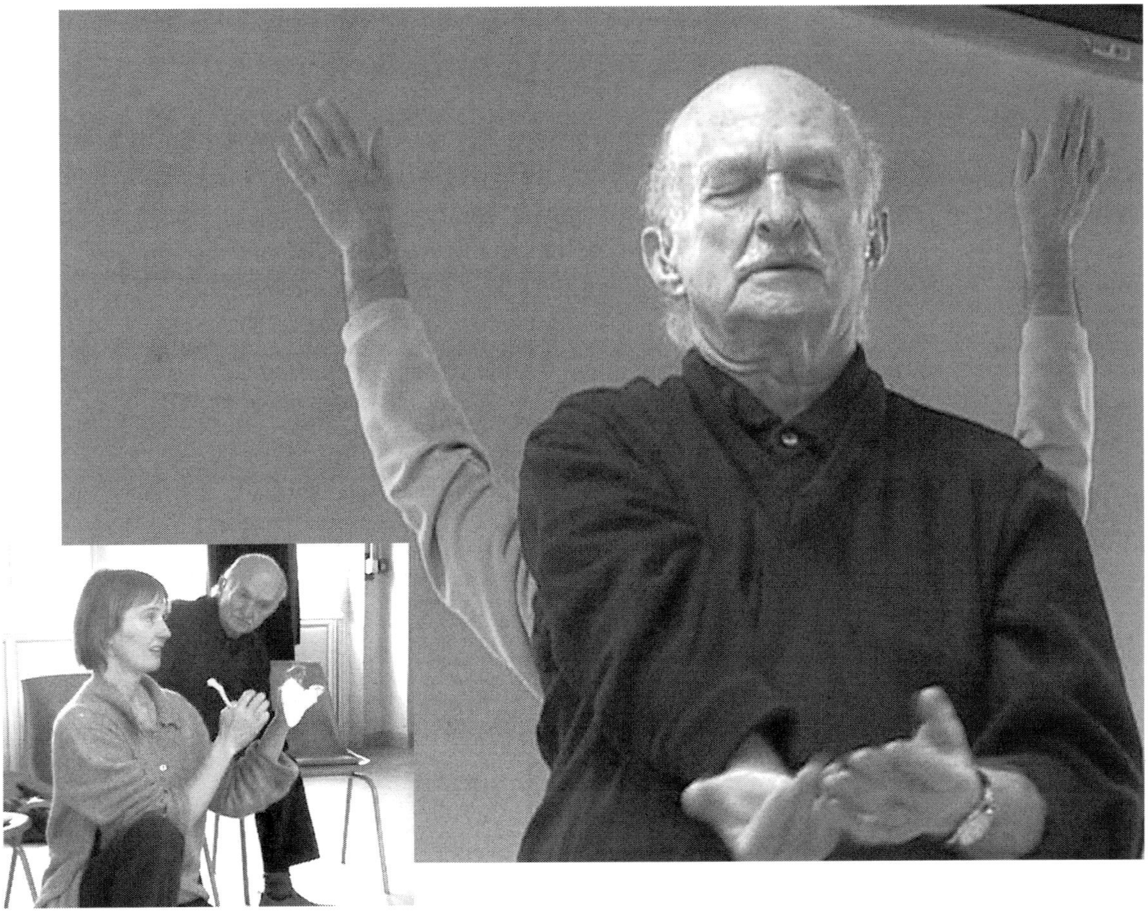

A palette of possibilities: things we did

We explored and invented ways to help people relieve patterns of tension or stress. Movement 'conversations' were popular in our groups; between parts of the body; or with a partner. Sometimes people shared a favourite story, a famous character, or treasured place. Sometimes people spoke of movements they loved to watch: horses rolling in the grass... swallows diving through the air... falling rain... washing on the line... In sharing, each person would speak and add a gesture or short movement phrase to evoke their words that others of the group mirrored, added to and passed on.

One day Tim brought a bag of pebbles from the beach, which people arranged and rearranged in clusters and then placed around the room. We talked together about the moon and tides, and tides and rhythm within the body. From this we invited people to connect with two stones placed separately in the room, and to imagine their different qualities – and then to make a 'dance of two moons' exploring 'what happened between'.

Another day, after a walking warm-up, Tim brought a book of paintings by Howard Hodgkin. This grew into a conversation about how Hodgkin used colour and what might be its equivalent in the body, which led to an improvisation based on 'painting' the room and the spaces between people with movement-colour.

We regularly shared information about structure and function in the body. People enjoyed getting this information – we explored the anatomy of how we breathe, of the spine and head-neck relationship, of shoulders and arms

Our intention was to cultivate a sense of wonder and curiosity about the body and encourage people to connect in a more personal way with how their body felt and moved (rather than simply through exercise or 'rehabilitation'). Many people began to take the initiative and invented new ways to manage their symptoms.

> **C** had long-term back problems and sciatica. She seemed depressed, and was edgy in her behaviour to others. After a slow meditative 'dance' focusing on the moving length of the spine and the connections of limbs into the spine, she chose a stone from a basket of objects as in some way evoking her dance. She said it reminded her of 'going to the beach as a child and gathering treasures from all around her – shells, pebbles, driftwood... all those pieces coming together... a bit like me.' She was smiling and more open when she left the session and for the first time stayed for a cup of tea with the rest of the group.
>
> **D** had heart problems and diabetes; she spoke of her heartache around her daughter, who had died several years earlier from drug abuse. Yet she shared movement renderings of her daily household chores – knitting, cooking, cleaning – which all the group joined. 'What would people think if they looked in the window and saw us now!' she exclaimed with both humour and delight.

Arm dances

Feeling out each part... elbow... wrist... fingers... shoulder Exploring... possible...
impossible... movements... Sensing impulses... letting each arm 'dream'...
have a voice: greeting... holding... flying... restraining Imagine a conversation...
between left and right arm between arms... and the rest of the body
Allow... disagreements... surprises

Take colours *... draw or paint the arm 'stories'...*
Imagine each arm has a voice... what does it say? ***make a short poem*** *from its 'words'*
As a group **gather up words** *as a movement score:*
rouse... relish... raid... risk... rattle... be reasonable... rakish...rinse... roll
Be grizzly... grumpy... galloping... gutted... grotesque... gentle...
These collective words encouraged people to explore a palette of energies; calling out new qualities in the mode of Simon Says.

People's responses We asked people to say something about what happened to them when they moved, relaxed and focused on their bodies:

Lucy: 'I think I felt more about my body since coming to the classes and moving as I don't think I did before – you made me think – how it works... I used to look forward to it – I used to think 'that was my time' I used to completely switch off from everything and I did benefit from it. And you weren't judged for it.'

Susan: 'I loved the movement – both the feeling of it and the feeling of where your arms were and the ease in which they moved – and also with this arm, which is my good arm, I had several interesting and good sensations with it – including the memory of pain in my wrist – it was like pain but it wasn't ... some of the fibres started moving in ways that they never normally moved ... there was new movement in that – and that was interesting – it was a spontaneous dance – it was lovely.'

Fiona: 'The movement was lovely – just doing it and receiving it – I saw it more in terms of sailing – the wind and sails and sea – it was certainly amazing and the music – it was like we were different notes of music almost ... I find it very hard to relax and trust.'

movement

From a session on breath

Marie: 'I was surprised by the dancing, the slow movement gradually rising from the exhausted body – so you should not be surprised to see the colours in my carnival wings – not arranged in any order – not the usual careful planning – colours precisely placed to match the prism of a rainbow – but you can see the whole kaleidoscope of my carnival wings – huge fruit flies still carrying their colours ... the flight for the carnival dance.'

> Remember dancing no need for words
> Dancing is not writing even though words may dance on the page Just
> spots before the eyes – fine contradiction this Remembering terror
> exercised by movement
> Years ago now ... on the living room carpet
> Dancing away the terror – welcoming the dawning of a new birth.

Amy

In and out breath of life

In and out, precious, precious breath

From the core of my being... in and out... sacred breath

Sprit of life

I breathe, I breathe in, I breathe out, tasting the colours of life, finding my balance like a dancer moving with the breath

Like a willow moving in the wind

Twisting and reaching out, bending and swaying

Getting restricted and tied down but infinitely flexible, changeable, bending with the breath, breathing into restrictions – breathing out bursts of colour... changing with an ever-changing landscape.

Keith: 'In the first place I can do far more with my body – even in a grotesque way taking part in the dance sessions with one leg and one arm kaput – it's a bit difficult – I got a lot out of what I did in the end and certainly began to be conscious of various parts – how they depended on each other and how I should be looking after them a damned sight better than I was doing... I hadn't really thought about my own body – if I saw myself walking down the street I probably wouldn't recognise myself. Then you begin to say, "Hello… this is me – this is my arms, my leg" and you begin to become to terms as if it's a stranger.'

Music, as accompaniment, and making music together

Jilly Jarman, a musician who worked with us the first year of the project, would bring percussion instruments into the sessions: rain sticks, flutes and bells. We would use music as a 'light and lively' interlude where the rhythm is bright and energetic and simple enough for everyone to join in. We also sang songs and chants that we made up on the spot and tried out different vocal sounds to make 'soundscapes' that paralleled what was going on in the physical movement.

> Music creates a theatrical space where one is allowed to be extravagant, beautiful, and outrageous and to delight in the similar transformation of others.
>
> Jilly Jarman

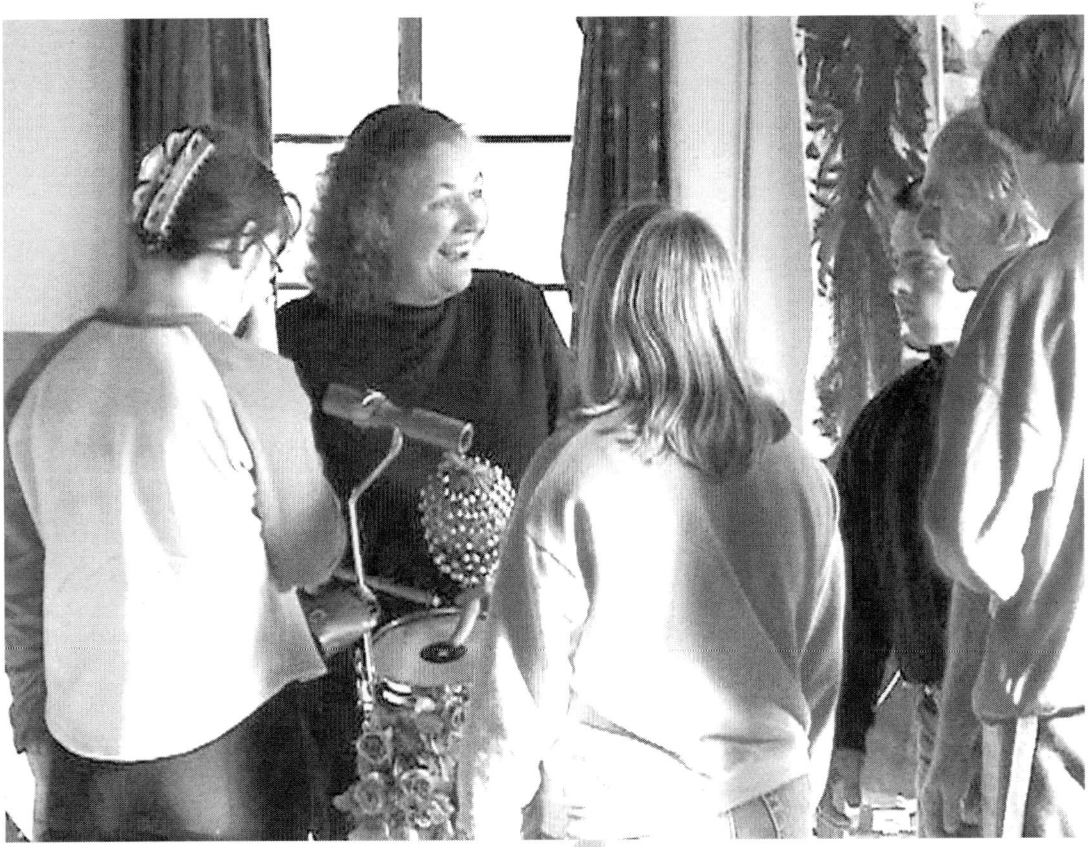

Music can set the tone and mood of a session – it invokes movement and creates a convivial space that brings people together. Harmony and rhythm are restorative in their own right and have a powerful effect on the body. Music helps to transform a simple gesture or movement into a richer, creative expression. It helps an individual connect their own creativity to the group as a whole and reduces any sense of awkwardness or embarrassment.

Music is a great resource in this work. However, it was also important that music did not drive or *impose* a mood or rhythm; each person needed to be free to find their own pace and energy.

> **J**: 'With the music and the movement and the breathing and just the rhythm [itself], you feel like you are relaxing and moving upwards – it is so beautiful and light; I loved it.'

> **H**, paralysed from a stroke and hunched in her wheelchair, suddenly comes to life, hauls herself onto her feet, and waves her walking stick in the air in response to the pulse.

> **Jane**: '[Music] makes you more aware of all the things that are in music that are in the body too, like vibration, rhythm, cadences, harmonics. Mostly I don't notice my body – the music makes you wake up inside and hear details and surprises, things you didn't know were there. It feels like finding a 'musical body' that is dancing inside, not my everyday plodding body that hurts if I move too fast or that gives me headaches.'

> **Patrick**: 'I know that exercise 'lightens' mood, but this is showing me a way that gentle movement and music strengthens and relaxes body and mind.'

> **Bob**: 'What I'm gaining is a feeling of equilibrium with my body as it is now.'

Time for stillness, reverie and relaxation

> Yet it is in our idleness, in our dreams, that the submerged truth sometimes comes to the top.
>
> Virginia Woolf

In our groups, relaxation was popular and formed the basis of much else. Our modern world is addicted to speed – the person who goes slow, dawdles, meanders, daydreams is chivvied to return to a fast pace where will and effort rule. Developing a capacity to relax, rest and be still are vital aspects to restoring balance in the body. Bed rest is the prescription for many illnesses yet all too often we neglect the need for internal silence and stillness. Only when we get ill may we notice a deep undertow of fatigue, and realise how our body (and soul) like a shy child has been seeking our attention for a long time.

All healing and meditation traditions emphasise the role of breath in quietening the thinking mind. For people with acute conditions, the struggle to manage day-to-day can be stressful and exhausting. As plants draw in and rest through the winter darkness we too need to be able to quieten, settle towards silence and stillness to get back in touch with the rhythms of body and being. Being able to rest was vital in helping people reconnect with the wellsprings of their lives; one person commented that spring only came after the long stillness of winter.

> Humans are the only mammals that don't regularly nap.
>
> Bonnie Gintis

A guided relaxation focused people's attention, deepened body awareness and developed a sense of space throughout the body. To relax is not to collapse, become passive, but rather a time for quiet awakening, and listening to whatever drew attention in the body. Participants spoke later of the value of stillness in creating a sense of possibility, of opening, and of feeling their bodies soften easing patterns of stress and pain.

Practice nurse: 'I had a young girl in for an injection but she was so tense I could not do it. I wished she had been able to manage her tension – had been coming to your project.'

Time to settle and get comfortable in the body, time to notice sensation, frees the mind from habitual ways of thinking about events or problems. Connecting to the body brings us into the present moment and into a more instinctual, intuitive way of seeing and being. Softening and relaxing wakes up a greater capacity for noticing what is going on inside and out[6] which helps feelings to loosen, flow and transform.

Taking time to relax body and mind was a crucial part of each session. Each person chose somewhere in the room to lie down. In winter when the room was cold they had to cover themselves with blankets! We guided a journey through the body which developed the theme of the session. This gave people a time for reverie, to digest whatever had happened and prepared the ground for further making and writing.

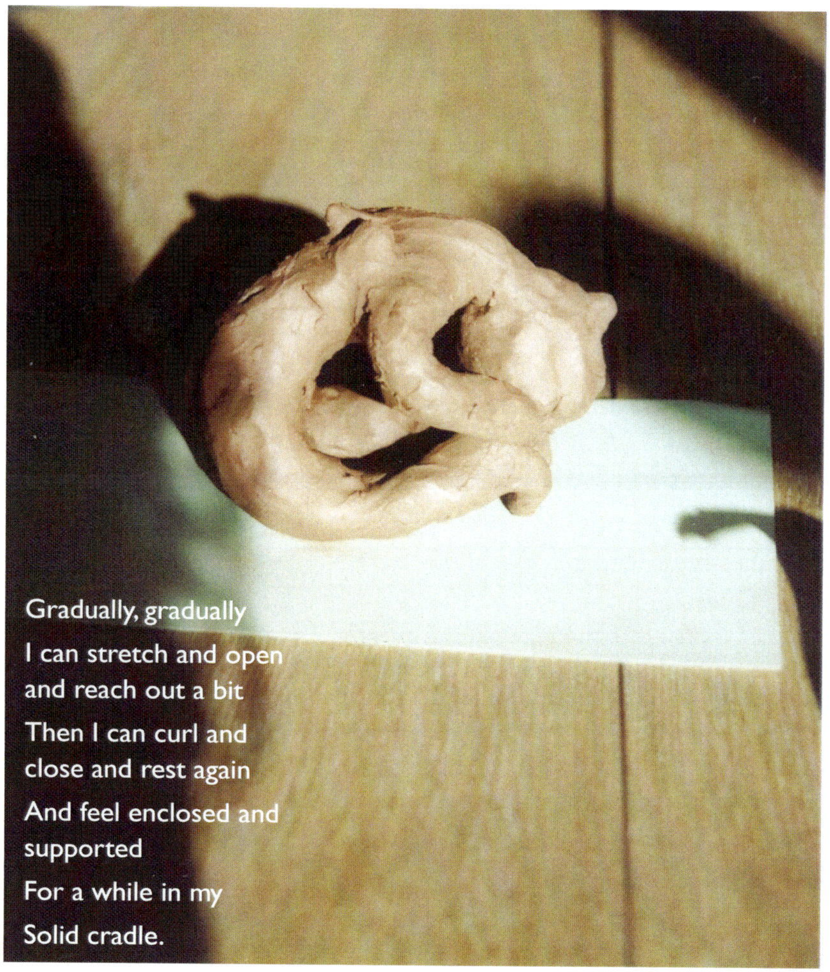
Gradually, gradually
I can stretch and open
and reach out a bit
Then I can curl and
close and rest again
And feel enclosed and
supported
For a while in my
Solid cradle.

This poem was written by a woman with a long-term illness after moving and working with clay. Learning to relax, rest and not fight her illness was an important step in managing day to day.

[6] Relaxing and sensing the body can also bring up fears and vulnerabilities. Some studies report that for 4% of the population relaxation aggravates rather than eases symptoms.

W had a car accident which had left her with permanent pain in her legs and suffering from depression after retirement. 'I sit still now with my eyes closed and listen to music, I have started to do this on a regular basis since the sessions and I really find it very relaxing.'

K retired after two heart attacks. He specifically came for relaxation. 'It's the opening up of spaces in your joints – it really does affect the weight of your body. I did once go to sleep during the session.'

Too often in our fast-paced world, driven by targets and specified outcomes, illness or poor health is seen as something that must be quickly overcome. There is pressure to be back on our feet and back to our familiar everyday lives. There is little space or time to reflect, recover and adjust, and there is rarely time for that old fashioned idea of 'convalescence'.

Convalescence *Origin: 15th c. from Latin* convalescere,
From: con *'altogether'* + valescere *'grow strong'*

For most of the people in our groups, returning to how they were was not an option. They sought space and time to explore ways of living more creatively and fully within the constraints of their situation. Many people found they could relax more easily within a group than they could at home alone.

P fractured his pelvis in a fall many years previously, and does not feel he has recovered a sense of equilibrium in his spine. He says his back is 'completely unstable and liable to go out at any time'. He moves restlessly throughout the session. Constant movement is the only way he feels he can maintain himself. Even at night he says he has to get up and walk about. He suffers from blinding headaches and at times even his vision is affected. His face is gaunt with pain; he says he suffers from depression and reiterates throughout that 'nothing helps.

During a relaxation, P panics and says his back has 'gone out'; he says only his wife can help with this. I go over and ask permission to touch and give support to his spine. I place a hand gently front and back of his upper torso. I breathe and wait for a sense of connection between P's sternum and spine that may help him settle and find stability. Gradually P begins to breathe more evenly and his body relaxes into the support of my hands. He seems calmer, more expanded. He comments that his back is 'back in' again. Later he takes colours and draws a bridge with a river going under – this is a familiar place he loves to visit, 'A place that is always there, that has banks to hold it in – yet is always flowing, moving on.' Naming these qualities of the river seemed to help P find a different quality for himself in his body.

Making: trusting the process

Man is most himself when he is at play

Friedrich Schiller

We always brought a wide selection of materials to each session – we thought of this as a well-stocked larder or kitchen where ingredients needed to be appetising. It was important to invest in materials of good quality so that people could feel their making was valued. We brought art materials: paints, charcoal, pastels, varieties of paper, string, glue, wool, clay, as well as natural materials such as stones, moss, shells or wood. With carefully chosen, sensuous ingredients people were inspired to set out in their making. The aim was 'to make' moment by moment – as in spontaneous cooking – adding, mixing and reducing ingredients, always exploring, till something emerged.

Making a place
Choose a stone from the scattered pile.
Like a child choosing a sweet in a shop, allow yourself to be drawn to particular quality… size, shape, texture, colour.
Describe it to a partner ..what does it evoke, remind you of? Imagine the stone has a voice…what might it say? Now choose a spot in the room to place it… how does it feel? Then gather other materials to ***make a place for the stone***
What emerges? …landscape…weather…season…people…animals… presences? Take time to look and share with another the imagined stories of this place Move in response to the place … Write.. the story of this place

A 'neutral' task such as the above allowed each person's imagination to go where needed.

J took early retirement after a 'nervous breakdown'. He suffered from acute stress and was initially very nervous about coming to a group.

After moving, he chose a marble from among a collection of stones as an image to convey something of his previous moving. Cupping the marble gently in his hand he said he suffered from obsessive compulsive disorder and could not tolerate any untidiness – he commented on the smooth perfection of the marble: 'No rough edges'. Continuing to look, he remarked on 'the flame of the candle reflecting like a heart in its glass. And the windows and the whole room,' he laughed, 'the whole world is in there.'

J was smiling, something important for him was being communicated and shared. Next session he returned and said he had slept well after the session and that the image of the marble had been with him all week. 'It is inside me here,' he said, tapping his chest, his face bright with delight, 'I feel over the moon.'

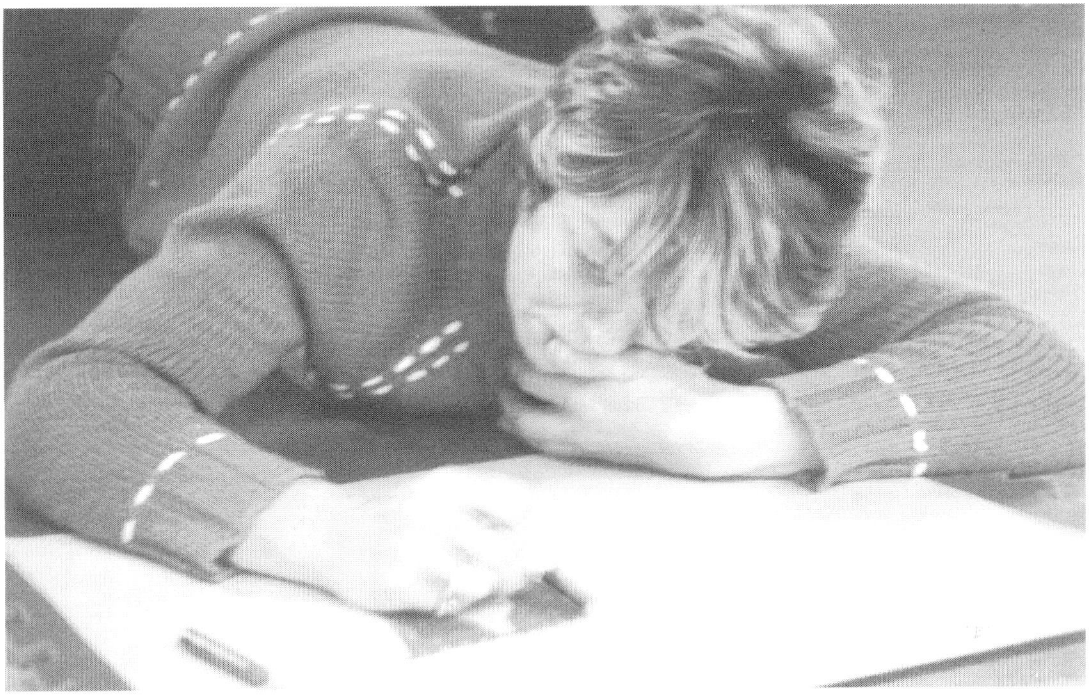

Improvisation as process – the unforeseen

We encouraged people to let go of plans or deliberate intentions and work spontaneously with a sense of movement in whatever they did, allowing moment-by-moment choices to shape their process. People worked slowly with great attention to details and qualities, trusting the creative process itself to bring forth the landscapes and stories that mattered to them, landscapes – that often surprised people with associations as forgotten memories surfaced – were shared and communicated with others. These 'makings' created worlds where a person could indirectly explore aspects of their lives. The metaphors and images they found as they played and created were a means of feeling a way towards new understanding.

> **Lucy**: 'When you first said about making something I thought ... Oh no ... as I am not clever at making things and I thought it would have to be right – everybody seemed as though they were really getting on and

knew what they were doing and I really didn't know where to start. But then I just put my mind to it and shut everything else out and I really thought about it – and I really enjoyed it ... it was feathers, sheep wool and moss – a safe place – I liked that because I used to like making things when I was young – it brought my childhood back a bit ... feeling a safe place, to rest in. I did really like making that. I completely switched off from everything... I think if there had been a fire I would still have kept going... Everybody was so quiet when they were doing it – no one was speaking – people were completely concentrating on what they were doing... and their thoughts – and that must be good mustn't it...? You could actually tell people's feelings from what they made – you could see how that person was feeling – and there wasn't a word spoken.'

Clay Making

Clay making – Marie spent a long time writing this piece, totally engrossed in it

Perhaps my stone-age self
Sat like this one frosty morning
Making with cold clay, a useful bowl, a water-carrier.
But as the clay grew under her stiff fingers
A pattern emerged, thumb printed,
And the decorative edge became lop-sided
So water would trickle out.
And then the clay became for her like my pelvis,
Useful bone-bearer, carrier of emotions,
But sacred, too, a holy grail,
Not the chalice, long sought for,
But a platter to hold the less salubrious aspects of my being. For I, too,
was created out of clay,
Like the original Adam,
Not from his bone to be his companion,
My purpose to share his sorrows
And comfort his distress.
My purpose is to have joy,
To live for my own creativity.

Moulded and moulding
The cold clay became warm,
Its shadows sun-reflecting
To lie perhaps on a sunny hillside
Until in centuries future
The archaeologists will realise
We may set out to make a useful pot
But end up with the sacredness of our own being.

Seeking: a language of expression

Creating with others generates a slipstream – people are carried along within a group energy, and as time goes on there is an increasing sense of safety, of belonging alongside others. For each person this allows a deep immersion in whatever they are creatively engaged with – be it movement, paint, words or other materials. Art making, like dreaming, can totally absorb and refresh our perception as something new, or as yet unknown, emerges into form.

The medicine of art lies in it taking what is buried and invisible inside of us and puts it outside in a way that it can be looked at and shared; creating a place of conversation, a

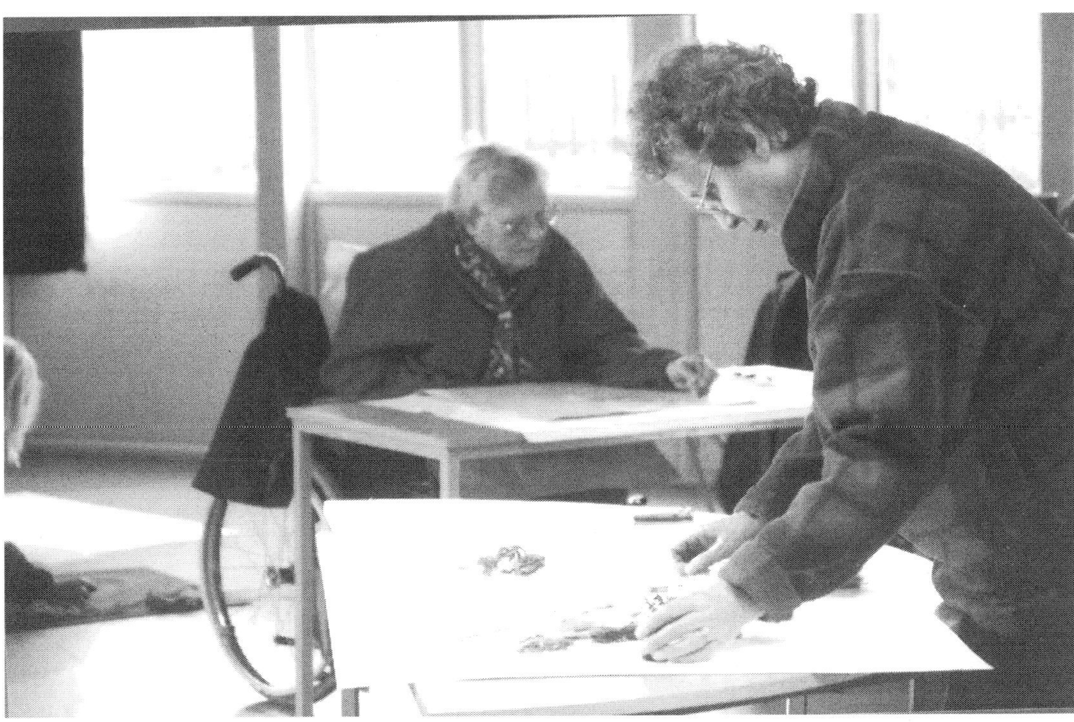

moving out of monologue into a place of shared experience. The stories, metaphors and images that emerged as people made, wrote or moved were personal and vivid ways of expressing what they felt, communicating the complex and layered nature of their experience. Metaphor and story allow surprising and often contradictory feelings to be felt and expressed.

> **Keith**: 'I think the other thing is that when you are working with limited materials its almost another way of living your life because that's what you do with your life, you work with limited materials, and they may not look very promising. You have to look at them in a different way – turn them upside down – turn them sideways and make the best of what you've got in the old-fashioned tradition... You not only amaze yourself with what you are doing, but you are amazed with your results – things do change!'

Finding words

> Poetry is a life-cherishing force, for poems are not words, after all, but fires for the coal, ropes let down to the lost, something as necessary as bread for the hungry.
>
> Mary Oliver[7]

Many of us find it hard to find words for what we feel, but we encouraged people to write in the wake of moving or making. Movement awakens a person's sensory landscape to textures, colours, qualities, which gives rise to a refreshed palette of words and phrases that evoke the feel of a person's experiences. One word calls up another and each word draws in its wake other words, voices, associations that gradually begin to form a poem or story. These writings are like small spells – they make visible the uniqueness of each person's life world.

Robert: writing after working with clay

> A piece of driftwood shaped by waves that smooth the curves and
> soften sharpness.
> An uncertain creature stretching neck and arms in a struggle to

[7] Mary Oliver, *A Poetry Handbook: A Prose Guide to Understanding and Writing Poetry.*

emerge into its own shape, becoming itself.

A shattered cornucopia, dribbling its last contents. Cornucopia with a scorpion's tail. Steep path ending with a door into summer – or into darkness?

A barking dragon propped on its elbows, lifting its face to the sun.

Fingers shaping.

Joan's story

A young woman arrived in our group. On her first day she was tense, her voice barely audible. Throughout the session she sat alone, seemed not to engage, her body held rigid – yet towards the end of the session she began to mould a piece of clay, smoothing and rounding it endlessly. Afterwards as others engaged in writing, another participant came up and asked if he could read her something he had written – a response to what she had made. She nodded mutely. These were his words:

Sleep little pod
Sleep as long as you need.
Wake up little pod.
When you are ready.

Joan did not seem to respond, but the following week she returned and began to join in, painting a tree with branches full of colour and life. Over the following weeks we discovered she suffered from depression. After living abroad for many years and having a fulfilling career she had became increasingly isolated after the birth of her two children. Her husband worked long hours and she was increasingly alone. Eventually she returned to England with her children whilst her husband continued to work abroad. Yet Joan had become so ill that her husband had given up his job, and returned home to look after the children. She had recently made a serious suicide attempt, nor was that her first attempt. Joan felt she had to get to the bottom of her depression. As a girl she had an eating disorder and felt beset with emotional problems and feeling now that she had to get to the source in order to survive. 'I have to have time for me. I have to find out who I am.'

Over the weeks that followed Joan seemed to blossom, became more communicative even taking a lead in sessions. It made us realise just how potent the 'right' word or image can be; to feel seen and accepted for who you are is in itself life affirming and healing.

Reflecting together

After people had finished making, we asked them to get together in pairs to share and reflect on each other's work. This gave each person a chance to look in more depth, and explore what had emerged. A partner offered a fresh eye, noticing details or qualities that enriched the maker's sense of what was there. This quiet talking together was an important part of the whole process of sharing and discovering new and often surprising narratives embedded in whatever had been made. These imaginative narratives enriched people's language and revealed new perspectives on their lives and circumstances.

Looking together enabled a sharing of stories and insights. This process also shifted the focus away from us as leaders and encouraged conversations to go where each person needed. Sharing around creative work offers a unique view into another's lifeworld, it created deep loyalties as people discovered their strengths and the value of their own contributions to others.

Opening up the 'stories': A key aspect of this phase was bring an open mind to the particulars of what a person had made, and not try to explain, interpret or judge. We all have a tendency to dismiss or diminish what we have created. But there is never only one perspective or story. Looking and sharing with a partner helped people let go of their initial assumptions and sift through details to see more of what was there and what it spoke to.

With a partner alongside we can explore the associations and landscapes of what we are doing with less fear of getting lost or overwhelmed. Listening with another, pondering the images, noticing, questioning and together filling out details until a deeper sense of meaning becomes clear. And we discover a world that is shared, no longer simply 'inside me', but coming alive and growing between us.

> A true poem ends in a clarification of life – not necessarily a great clarification such as sects or cults are founded on – but a momentary stay against confusion.
>
> Robert Frost

Our well being is strengthened when there is time to communicate, to feel valued and to explore outside the confines of our situation. An arts practice infuses new content into our lives, creating a context for communication, where there is time for a person to listen and be listened to on many levels and supported in their creative expression. To feel recognised and known as a person rather than a focus on illness or diagnosis is in itself strengthening. An artist working within these fragile communities is companion and guide – able to meet, explore and play alongside without overwhelming, a role which depends utterly on sensitivity to another's fears and vulnerabilities.

'Making' in any medium springs from a need within all of us to communicate and to share with others. Without expression our sense of self shrinks and diminishes. What we create always in some way speaks into being a part of ourselves which is as yet unvoiced and unseen. The presence of a partner or companion who goes with us in our journeys of imagination, making alongside of us, watching, looking and sharing in what we have made, enables us to get to know the 'life' and significance of our images more deeply. What we make, or do, or say, grows and comes more alive for us as it is heard and received by another.[8]

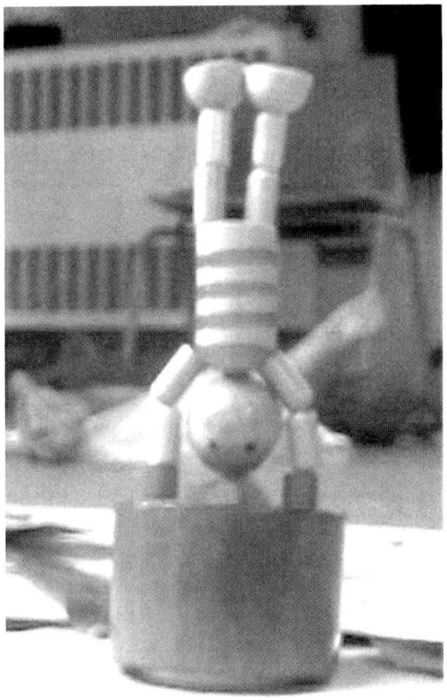

Jim: 'This little bloke I see as myself in another aspect ... and he was my mate when I did a castaway island in that corner. I think it is the best position for viewing life (upside down) ... I really like him ... I did quite surprise myself – I am no way an artist but two or three of my pictures came out quite well and considering it is 55 years since I attempted it pictorially it is quite an achievement in my life. I think when we were given a choice of pieces, shells, stones, I made myself a cosy little corner, like a fellow on a desert island, like a castaway – I was quite happy with that – with various things on my mat – it was all very different....

'What this image said to me is: "won't you step into it and make it complete" ... I called it Cosmos – I am a cosmos – not a big one – just a micro-cosmos really – probably very like you as well – where do I live? in the actual centre of the world – my world ... I am responsible for myself and of course the cosmos too – it is all me really – I float and rotate you know – you could say I live in a world where there is hardly time for anything – so cycling round checkpoints is the best way of covering the world – come to think of it I'd better get on my bike now to meet you in your cosmos!'

[8] See 'Looking at what you have made' in Tufnell & Crickmay, *A Widening Field*

Amy: 'I painted this scarecrow... I had quite a good body when I was younger and before surgery – and the things I dressed up in as a child were quite amazing – I am a tramp in one [photograph] I put on a black bin liner with a tube sticking out and said I was a hoover – in another one I am absolutely unrecognisable – but in the best one I am a scarecrow and I had this broomstick through my arms and straw sticking out the ends – I remember knocking everybody over – I couldn't have a drink – someone had to help me – and 'making' today brought it all back – I've always had very little self image of myself and would never have dreamt of dressing up till now – Last words I wrote were "Be ... be who I am ... no more ... no less" and that is what I have learnt ... to be who I am NOW.'

I wrote down:

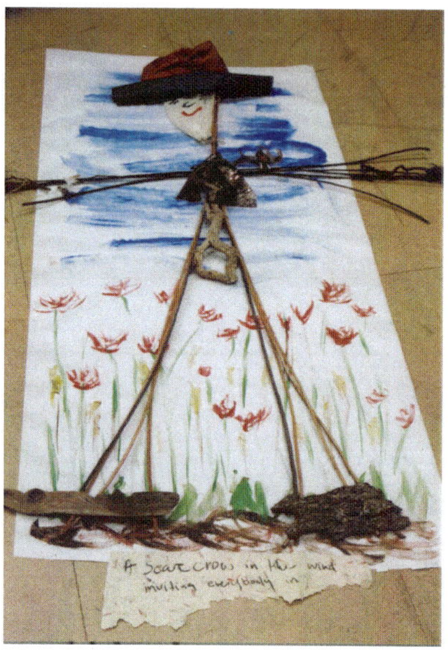

A Scarecrow in the Wind

A scarecrow in the wind
Inviting everyone in.
A robin on my shoulder
Forever growing bolder.
I am not a pretty sight
But neither am I a fright.

I've got my place among the flowers.
I'm supposed to have preventative powers,
But that is not who I am,
That is just a scam.
All I want to do
Is dancing in the wind
And this is my way in.

After moving and making we shared lunch. Eating together created an informal opportunity to exchange, talk and get to know each other or rest. The hour-long space of a lunch break helped people pace themselves – particularly important for people with ME or MS, or those in chronic pain.

Then we re-gathered in a circle. People read aloud what they had written, or spoke about what they had made and feelings that had emerged. There was no pressure to speak but most people enjoyed sharing their insights, thoughts and feelings.

We referred to this final phase of our sessions as 'harvesting'. The word harvest conveyed the sense of gathering up from all that had happened in the session; that there was always something valuable to be shared and gleaned from each other; a ripening and deepening of conversations within the group.

Reflections on the project

Participant responses

Keith 'I am a lot happier with the new me I didn't think I could ever do it Family & friends have commented repeatedly that I have cheered up and become much more "outgoing", which I think means more agreeable and lively. They must have noticed so it must be right. At 79, nearly, that isn't bad! The pills I'm on have been reduced to their weakest strength (Losec, Citalozian). I could probably do without the latter now... Walking much better and further despite an injured right leg. Starting to sleep better. I feel younger! ... at the time I started attending the classes I really was "in the depths" for various reasons, including bereavement. But not now!'

Joan: 'It has gone from being a really difficult thing for me walking through the door – to thinking, "Great its Tuesday, fantastic!" It makes me feel comforted, looked after, I feel I am amongst friends. I can speak. The movement is so relaxing – These last two weeks between the breath and the movement I have really got in touch with a very peaceful side of me ... and it has made me very aware of when I am away from here of my breath – taking thoughts on the in breath and releasing them on the out breath in movement – it has been so lovely.'

Amy: 'I feel the sessions have given me back a sense of my own life, made me feel creative again after the cancer and surgery. They give me a chance to express fears and anxieties of the past and hopes for the future … give me a recipe, a way forward, of mindfully living through physical and mental problems.'

Marie: 'This course has helped me tremendously to start feeling alive again rather than just living. I realise I had been creatively 'dead' for quite a few years while cancer was taking hold and after surgery and subsequent treatment of chemotherapy and radiotherapy. This has given me hope for a brighter future.'

Laura: 'Since I have been coming to this group and coming feeling really crap, I can go home quite bright. It's amazing – everybody's got their amazing different points and it's like you take them home with you. Nobody can shut me up on a Tuesday night – it does me the world of good.'

A doctor's response

'Patients with enduring health problems construct psychological mechanisms around their self-image in an attempt to make sense of their 'unfair' experience. These constructs can be of immense value in terms of allowing limited function without interference from more realistic enduring emotional distress. However like most psychological solutions, they can also form barriers to improvements in function; especially when the conditions may be variable, improvements however temporary, may not be taken advantage of.

'Patients' external lives may become restricted due to their disability but also due to a diminishment in the opportunities for self-expression. Lack of self-expression leads to lack of experience of the self and loss of self leads to further diminishment.

'Interrupting this cycle is one of the main tasks of a general practitioner caring for people with enduring health problems but it is extremely difficult; these patterns of behaviour become established over years of pain and disappointment.

'This programme allowed patients to explore these issues at a concrete level. By using artistic metaphors their psychological constructs are externalised, examined and may therefore be available for change. It is my experience that the patients who have attended this programme have reconnected with core values, become more open to suggestion, rediscovered their personal initiative and have also benefited from the positive experience of meeting others with enduring health problems.'

Dr Gavin Young, former GP at Temple Sowerby Medical Centre:
'I feel the project has been about enabling people who are limited within their body, not able to do or act or be in the way that they would like to be, to find a way of overcoming some of their limitations and perhaps discovering they are not as limited as they had thought.'

Endings

Over the three years of the project we felt that our approaches were finally shaping themselves appropriately; the work was becoming embedded within the Eden Valley community and we had finally located the appropriate spaces to work in. Health services were referring and patients seeking out the sessions. And we ourselves were heartened and delighted by the changes people experienced as they explored creatively, their sense of their own resources strengthened immeasurably. People reported sleeping better, reducing medication, getting out more and generally feeling more confident and invigorated. Our goal had been to work long enough for people within the groups to develop the confidence and leadership skills to enable them to continue in small groups (4-5 members) after our own input was ended. But our groups ceased to run before this was possible. As so often with these projects, lack of funding closed us down prematurely. For a while members continued to meet informally but they commented sadly that without a strong creative focus/input, they tended to slip back into social exchanges which kept them stuck in their familiar illness narrative, and did not bring out the wit and depth of their creative adventures.

Afterword

When the project failed to gain further funding I was devastated and, convinced that eventually we would find support, I continued to run sessions. The success of such projects depend utterly on trust. My fourteen years of working within Dr Gavin's surgery had laid the foundations and enabled me to learn in depth about the impact of illness on an individual and on their families and friends – and the profound need at such times for approaches that might help a person recover hope and a capacity for well being.

Of all the projects and teaching I have engaged with over my forty years as a dance artist this project demonstrated the life-enhancing potency of creativity. Among the widely diverse members of our groups I witnessed such imaginative originality, kindness, generosity of spirit, humour and wit that creating together brought about.

Throughout the country, dance artists and others have been creating projects in support of the wider issues of health. In supporting people to listen to and care for their bodies through the medium of dance they bring a particular quality of listening, a vitality that awakens heart and soul. My dream is that every surgery, every hospital has dancers and artists in their team to support the health, happiness and well being of those in their care.

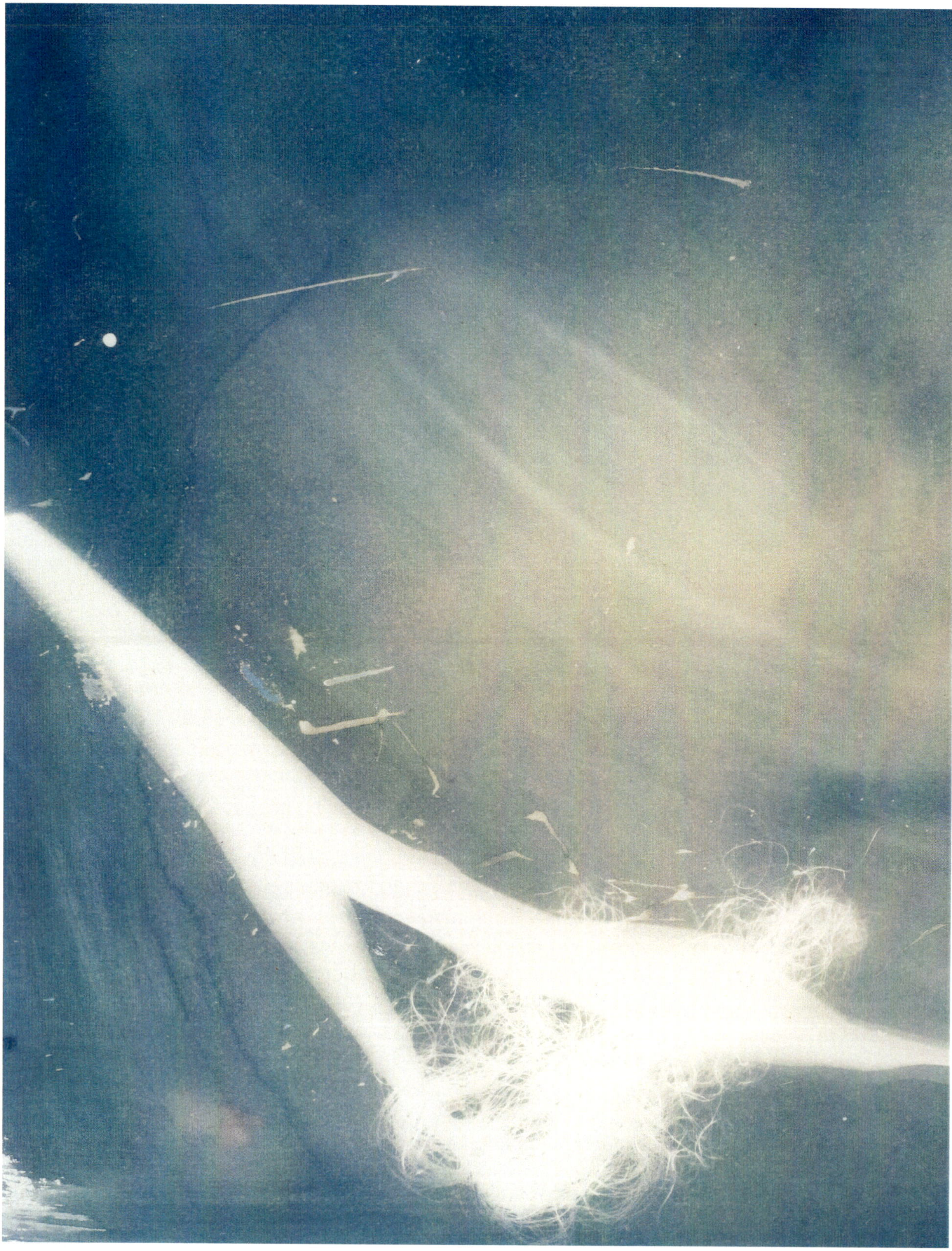

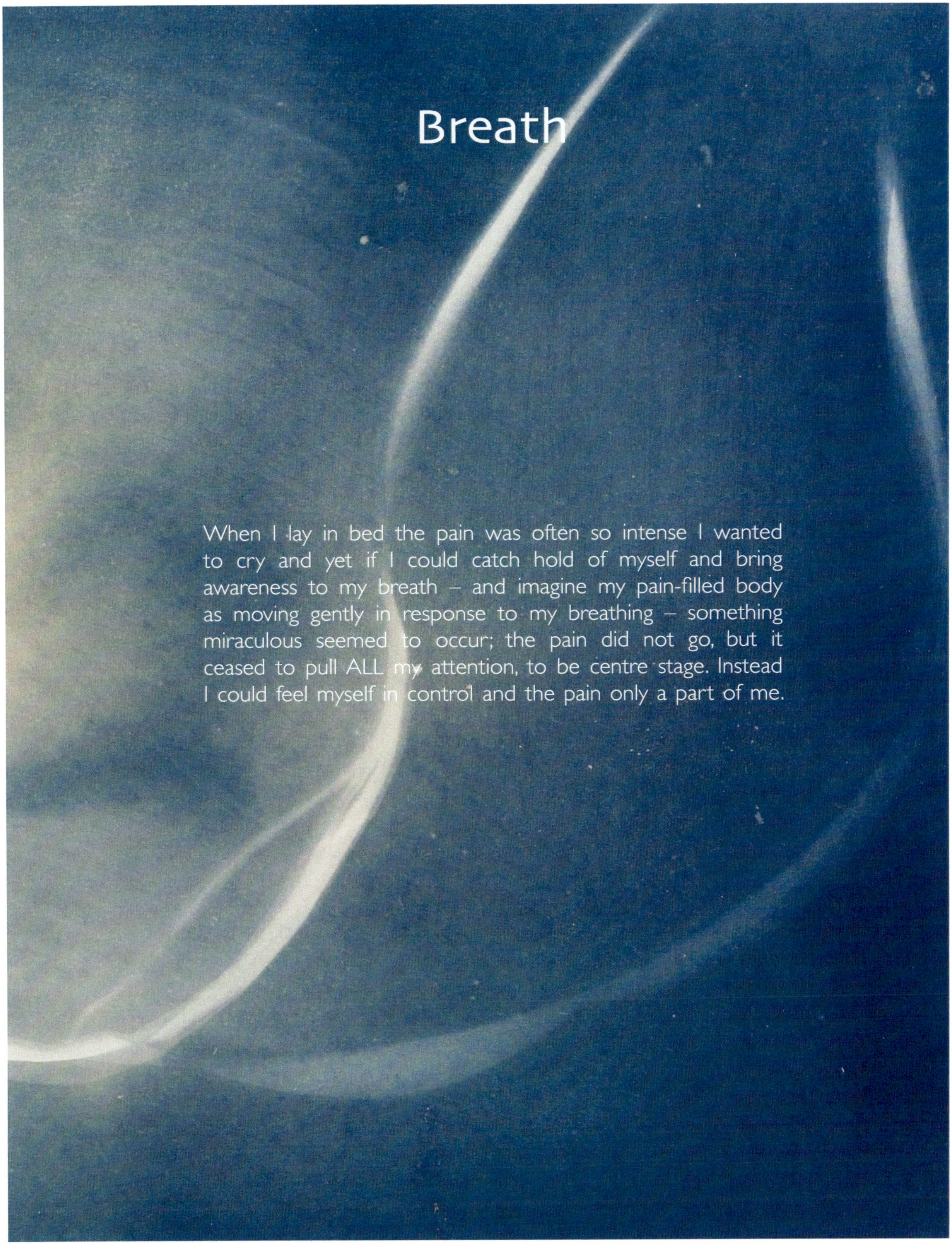

Breath

When I lay in bed the pain was often so intense I wanted to cry and yet if I could catch hold of myself and bring awareness to my breath – and imagine my pain-filled body as moving gently in response to my breathing – something miraculous seemed to occur; the pain did not go, but it ceased to pull ALL my attention, to be centre stage. Instead I could feel myself in control and the pain only a part of me.

Creating space... movement... inside

Breath is the gateway into movement, and nothing so swiftly alters how we feel than how we breathe. Slowly, softly, like a rising tide, our breathing creates movement, rhythm and connection throughout the body. Inhalation and exhalation may be barely perceptible, yet they set the tone within our bodies and affect every aspect of our daily functioning. All of our tissues – blood, muscle, bone, organ, nerve and connective tissue – all the 75 trillion cells which form the constellation of our bodies, rely on this life-giving exchange of carbon dioxide for oxygen. Without sufficient breath,[1] our bodies (and our lives) quickly feel blocked, airless and out of touch; even a few minutes without renewing oxygen damages our tissues.

Stop the breath
Briefly... hold your breath
Notice what happens in your body... how you feel?
Let in the breath again... what do you notice?
Share with another

Breath creates a sense of space inside us, opening up pathways between the many parts of ourselves. And as we take time to feel the movement of breath coming and going in our bodies we may awaken to sensation and feeling. Gradually, as we drop more deeply into the rhythms of breath, memory and association begin to appear. Breath is more than a mechanical event – it is a literal and metaphorical doorway into change and healing. Nothing so richly awakens the unique stories of a person's life as deepening awareness of breath.

All the chemistries of our bodies are affected by how we breathe, or fail to breathe. Oxygen is the fuel that releases energy from glucose in our cells. From the lungs, life-giving oxygen is absorbed, bound onto the haemoglobin of red blood cells and, through the powerful action of the heart and diaphragm, transported throughout our bodies.

[1]We breathe on average 12-15 times a minute, at least 17,000 times a day. At rest, each inhalation draws in half a litre of air into the lungs, 7-8 litres per minute, we can increase this five-fold during strenuous exercise.

Simply listening and resting in the moment-by-moment movement of breath, without expectation or trying to change anything, is a first step in quietening the mind's anxieties and bringing awareness to our bodies. As we slow down and follow the subtle movements of inhalation and exhalation, attention begins to shift from the general to the finer detail of sensation within the body and then outwards to the wider field of the whole body and our surroundings. (This can be a first step in bringing relief from pain.)

> My days are taken up with listening and touching, listening to words, to voices, and to breathing. My business is the nature of breath and liquid, the effects of liquid and dryness on human sound. I am trained. I keep my hearing in good order. I avoid loud noises and loud music. I live in a quiet street. I am attuned to sound. My ears are a listening bell. I can hear illness.
>
> Kay Syrad, *Send* (Cinnamon Press, 2015)

'I usually begin a session with the breath. I invite each person to take time to listen to their breath – and imagine making slow exhalations into different areas of their body, visualising the space between the joints expanding as the breath enters. After a while I invite people to form pairs: one of them is to close their eyes and drop into their breath, whilst the other (whose eyes are open) simply watches and tunes into their partner's moving breath. Then I suggest that the partner with eyes closed begins to find simple physical movements to 'speak 'the breath and express its rhythm and pattern. Their partner is tasked to mirror these movements, following and joining each detail. After a short while their movements synchronise, the support of the partner palpably sensed. As this shared dancing continues, the movement becomes finer, the detail clearer, and gestures more confident. This is a subtle exercise and it never fails to astonish me how powerful it is simply to have your breath witnessed and held.'

Lucinda Jarrett, Rosettalife, on her work in hospice

Finding breath

Settle

Every day... take time to settle... feel comfortable... spacious... find stillness
Feel the contact of your pelvis with floor or chair...
Sense your weight...yielding ... giving way to gravity
Breathe... let your belly soften... and your face
Imagine... all the molecules of your body slowly coming to rest
Gentle... as snow falling... gentle as rain
Sense the rise and fall of your breath... entering... leaving your body

Find rhythm

Sense... breath filling ... and emptying ...moments of stillness
At the top of the in breath... at the bottom of the out breath
Take time... to let body feel and receive the movement and passage of each breath
Now deep... now shallow
Softening... opening... making space... inside
Let the liquid weight of the brain soften... spread out
Let the mind... quieten
Listen... follow the changing tide... inward and returning outward
Each breath a different pace... story

Sensing movement inside

Take a deep breath... follow it inward.
Imagine the breath... as a stream... travelling into... penetrating every crevice
Imagine space opening inside... valleys... pathways... caverns
Give way... into streams... ripples... eddies...

Opening outwards

Sense the air around you
Open the windows of the senses... scent... sound... taste... touch
What do you notice... feel... hear
Let breath move... and flow... as the tide... as wind over water
Listen... breathe... follow the breath out from the body... into what is around you
Let the body welcome... say YES to each breath... following wherever it moves

Afterwards

Open your eyes... write, draw and share with another... what has emerged

We breathe air, air breathes and buoys us. Breathing involves a continual oscillation between exhaling and inhaling, offering ourselves to the world at one moment and drawing the world into ourselves at the next.

David Abram, *Becoming Animal: An earthly cosmology*

A breath story

M is in her early fifties. A series of whiplash injuries have almost crippled her. Her face looks bruised, she is exhausted with pain, and both legs are very swollen. M has almost no flexion or mobility in her hips. Walking is dragging herself along with the support of a frame on wheels; she must sit down after a few 'steps' to rest. It takes her almost half an hour to get from her car into the village hall where we work, yet she is willing to try anything and we were touched that she came to our sessions.

Once arrived it was difficult for M to get comfortable, pain kept her restless and shifting constantly. She could not lie down. To try and give her support in sitting we experimented with various cushions till a modicum of comfort was achieved.

After a visualisation focused on the movement of breath, M chose a range of colours and drew – sometimes with her eyes open, sometimes with them closed – a sweeping river of colours that covered the entire surface of a large sheet of paper. Looking at it, it seemed to be an evocation, a song on paper of her feelings about her life and breath. The freedom and flow of her drawing contrasted poignantly with the painful immobility of her body. She spoke of the pleasure she found in drawing and all it conjured up for her – losing herself in the sense of wind and water, and a memory of earlier, happier times, when she used to go sailing. She said she felt she was breathing more fully, felt herself expand, softer, with a sense of movement inside herself. She took the drawing home with great care and pinned it on her wall. The following week, she commented that looking at it each day reminded her to connect her painful daily movements to her breathing. It also gave her heart to remember – an affirmation and reminder of resources still present within her.

The journey of breath

Air enters the body through the nose or mouth. The ethmoid bone which forms the upper regions of the nose is a delicate, thin-walled bone lying between the eyes, and honeycombed with air sinuses. Its curved passages spiral the incoming air so that it comes into contact with the nasal linings of mucous membrane, thereby moistening, warming and cleaning the air. Many of the bones of the face and skull have connecting sinuses which also moisten and filter the air as it comes into our bodies. The olfactory bulb, which gives us our sense of smell, sits on top of the ethmoid and drops millions of tiny ciliated nerve fibres down into the membranes below, which read the air for scent.

Air travels down the pharynx, which divides into trachea in front (for air) and oesophagus behind (for food). Millions of tiny filaments or cilia, on cells that line the trachea, clean the air of particles as it passes down towards the bronchi.

As the air travels down, it passes through our vocal cords and larynx (this gives us the ability to speak and make sounds). The trachea (windpipe) branches into the two bronchial 'trees' which lead down into the lungs where they divide and subdivide into ever smaller twig-like tubules which become tiny delicate air sacs or alveoli.

The lungs are formed of over 300 million tiny alveoli which create a vast surface of exchange to keep all our cells supplied with oxygen. As the leaves of a tree receive and photosynthesise from the atmosphere, so the fragile membranes of our alveoli allow a constant diffusion of oxygen for carbon dioxide (their surface area equivalent to that of a 20–30 year old oak tree or a tennis court). The subtle balancing of this gas exchange plays a crucial role in maintaining the pH or acid/alkaline balance of our bodies. Each lung can take in a gallon or two of air. It takes about three breath cycles for blood to travel through the body and return to the heart for reoxygenation.

Normal breathing occurs without conscious control through neurological and chemical feedback from receptors in the brainstem, pons and brain itself, which monitor and respond to oxygen/carbon dioxide levels in our blood and brain. These messages stimulate the diaphragm to contract. As the dome of the diaphragm flattens and moves down on inhalation, air is drawn into the lungs. The movement of the diaphragm is global in its

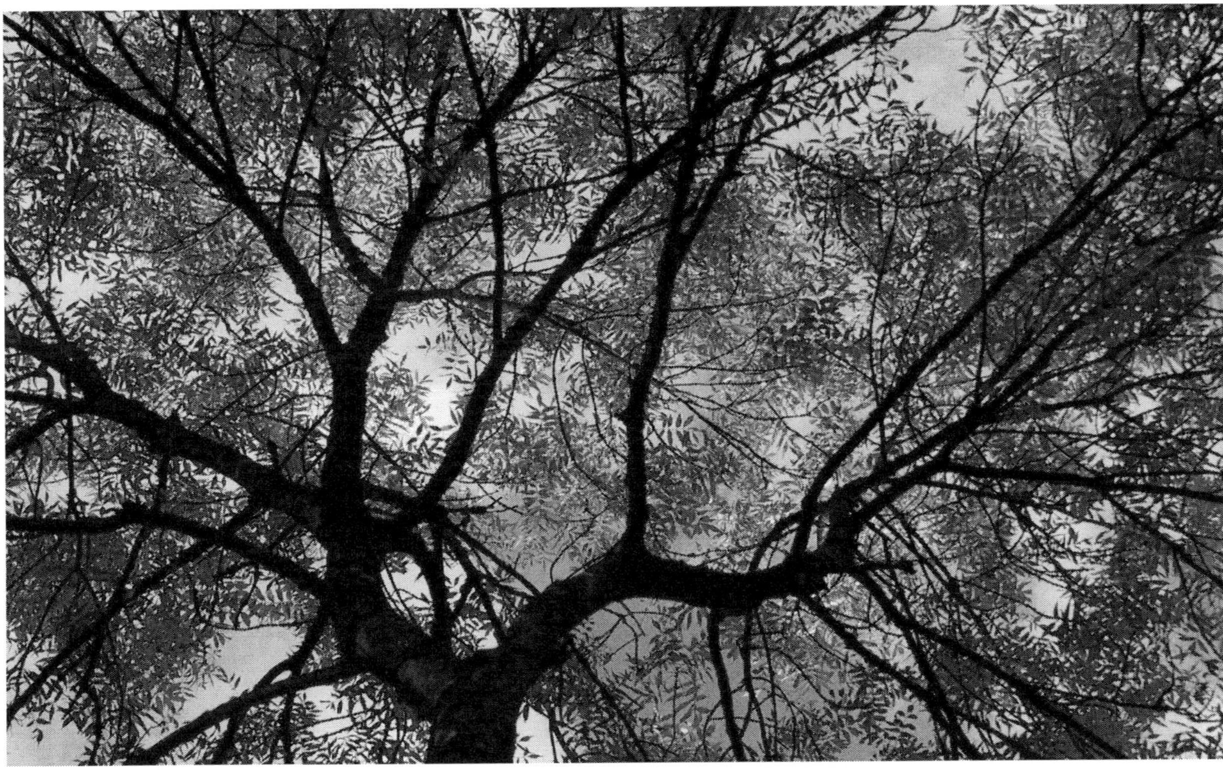

impact. It is the biggest muscle of the body and is in direct contact with almost all the organs. When it moves freely, it massages these organs and stimulates the movement of blood, lymph, food and nerve impulses throughout. Its movement affects spine, sacrum and ribs, to which it is connected. It intermingles with the psoas, pleura of the lungs, and pericardium of the heart; gut, aorta and vena cava all pass through it. The 'pumping' action of the diaphragm thus aids the return of blood to the heart and also affects the movement of digestion.

Poor posture inevitably has a damaging impact on our breathing. Stress, depression, emotions, lack of body awareness all affect how we breathe. The entire respiratory system (trachea, larynx, bronchial tubes, lungs) hangs directly from the base of the skull and so is profoundly influenced by the flexibility and length of the spine which elevates the head. Tension dramatically affects the free movement of ribs and lungs; without strain patterns, breathing and movement aid each other.

Setting the breath free ... three blockades

There are three main areas where we tend to restrict the free flow of breath into and out from our bodies:

face, jaw and throat

shoulders and arms

ribs and diaphragm

Creating space

(Breathe…imagine... lengthening... opening... space between head and pelvis
The spine is many separate bones... let each breathe
Imagine spaces... cushions of air... between vertebrae

Notice the rise of the ribs... as the diaphragm descends...
Sense how ribcage/basket... changes shape
Imagine…breath moving inside your body… as colour… as sound… as weather
Travelling... between... throat and shoulder... between hip and knee
Brightening... nourishing... every cell
Sense liquid spaces... between bones... each joint breathing
Sense depth and volume... front to back... left side through to right
Let your edges soften … let the space you occupy change... expand... as your breathe

How far... does each breath travel?
Move... and become the breath
Allow images/memories/stories... to drift into your mind...
***Write, paint, move** and **share** with another*

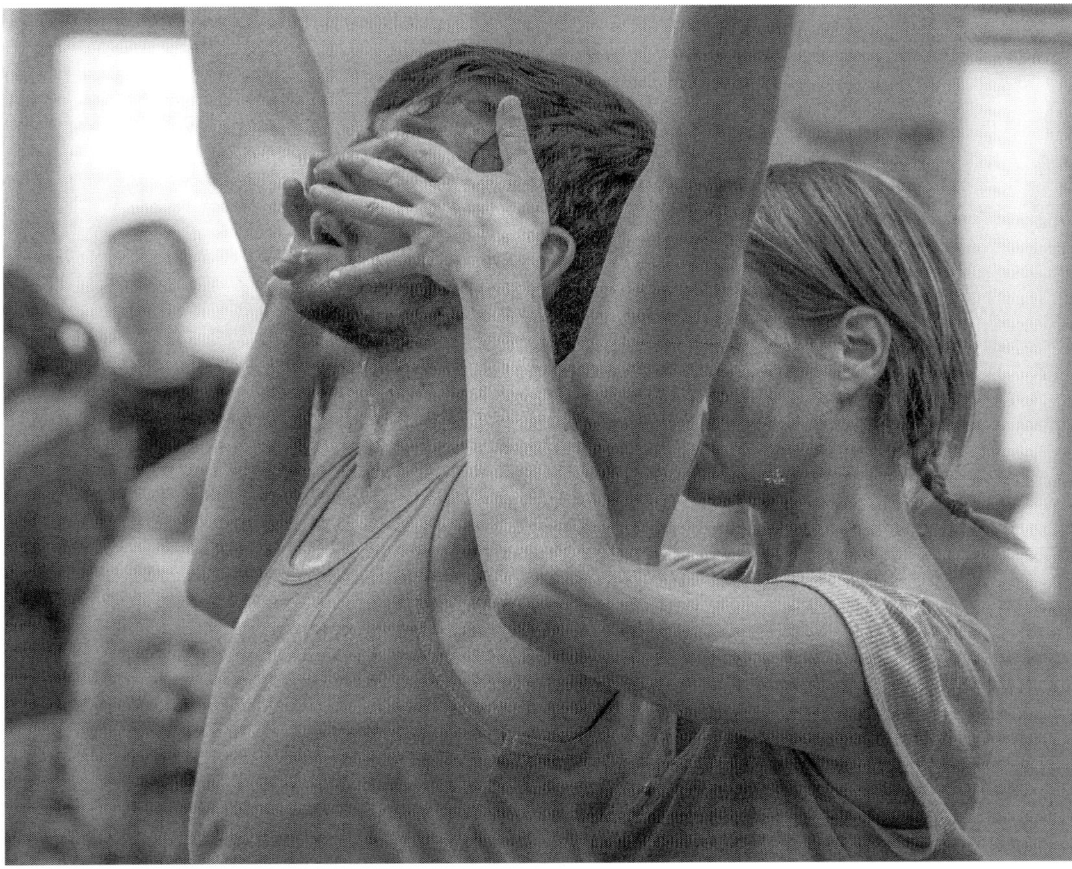

Freeing the face and jaw

The jaw and throat often hold tension. Our faces are formed of fourteen bones. Most of these are hollowed out with sinuses, which lightens the face with all its subtleties of movement. The number of bones and their mutual movement reduces the impact of the jaw's activity on the brain. The jaw is the most mobile bone of the head. 38% of neurological input to the brain comes from the face, mouth and jaw. We smile, chatter, bite, clench our teeth, cry and don't cry. To a significant degree, the 136 muscles above and below the pivot of the jaw set the pattern of our posture – how we hold ourselves. Freeing the face and jaw has a profound impact on how we breathe and feel. Relaxing the face helps integrate the whole body. Yawning, laughing, smiling can all bring a sense of ease. We speak by means of the breath.

Freeing the face

Get comfortable...
Exhale... bring your two hands to your face... let them rest across its surface
Let your fingers gently map... feel out
The delicate structures...landscape... of face and throat
Imagine... the face behind your face
Feel... the qualities of each bone
Inhale... let air sift through the inside of your face ... softening... opening
Feel out the strong hoop of your jaw
Imagine... sense... the inner spaces of the mouth
Sense... soft palate at the back... hard dome of the roof of the mouth
Yawn... let the mouth stretch wide... opening the passage of throat downward
Explore sounding the exhalation... gust...sigh (this helps slow and focus attention)
Feel ... the sounds of breath... resonating through face and throat
Opening inside passages... chambers...dissolving expression

Let the mouth change shape ... spread wide... close up small
Breathe... hum... hiss... blow... blow... whistle ...murmur
Let sound... and imagined sound... begin to awaken... movement
Shifting the balance of head... of neck
Let the rest of the body support... follow
Listen... let the face... lead the spine... lead the body

Write... or take paint, or clay, to draw or mould... what appears? share with another

Face Dances

Remy Charlip invited peopled to explore making the face dance, alternately as wide, as narrow, as long and as short... as possible.

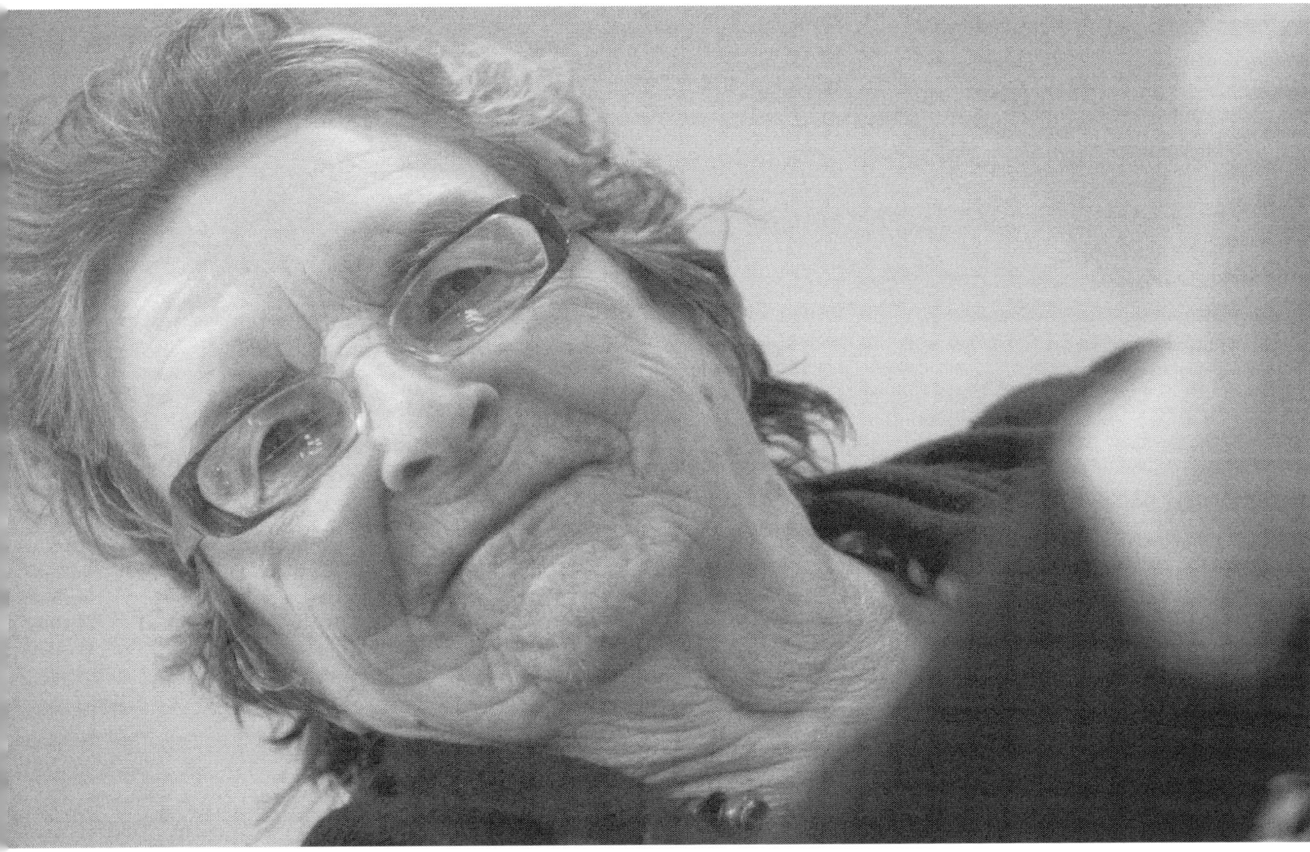

Smiling is one of the most important elements of our movement sessions. When I take someone's hands and look into their eyes, I feel in my body their relief that they, finally, are being seen. Almost invisibly and immediately, their breathing sifts into a gentler, calmer breath. Being touched, being seen, visible and valued, a smile breaks through. A smiling face is like meeting a new person altogether. "Ah, there you are. Here I am. Time to begin.'"

Filipa Pereira-Stubbs, *Dancing in Hospital*

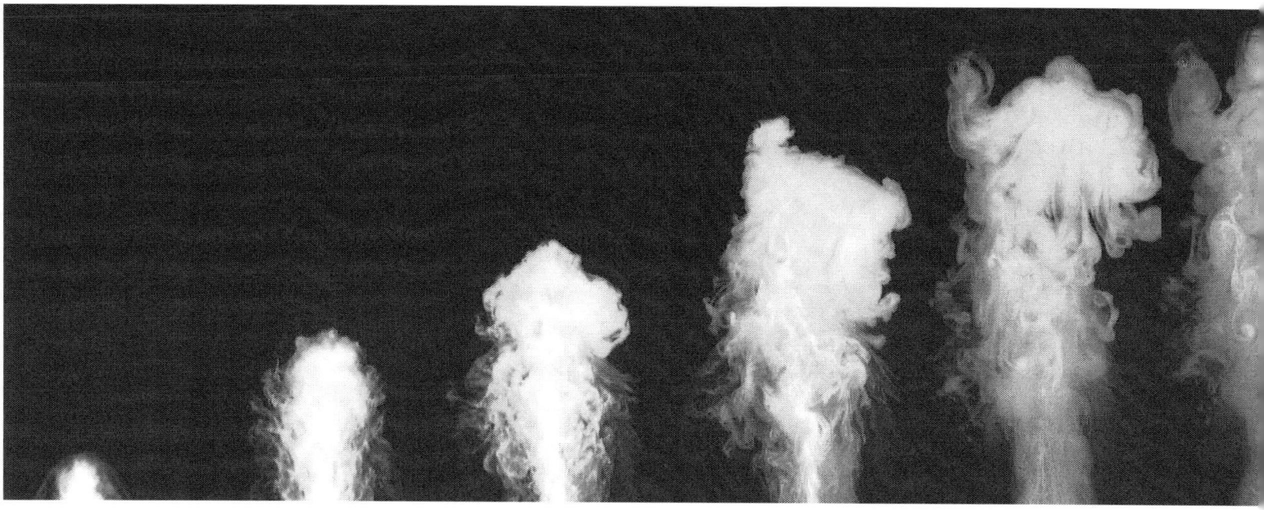

Sounding breath ... inner sound to outer world ... *from Katherine Zeterson*

Find your most comfortable position.
Close your eyes.
Breathe as you are. Settle.

Start to focus your listening.
Seek to hear the sounds outside the room.
Silently acknowledge the familiar and the unfamiliar...
Draw your listening closer into the room...
You might hear other people, the creaking of furniture, the humming of heating systems... Hear what you hear and know that you hear it.

Then move your listening into your self. Hear your breath enter your body. Imagine yourself riding on the air as it enters your body and listen to the air travelling through the miraculous passages to the alveoli, and then listen to the air as it passes back through the body and out through the nose or the mouth... listen to your blood in your veins and your heart pumping...

And from this place of simple sound allow that next breath to vibrate the vocal cords. Notice the sound and the feeling of the sound.
As each exhale follows the next, allow the sound to extend and release, dancing and shaping in the air.
See in your mind's eye the colour and the texture of each sound as it comes, and the patterns your sounded breath paints in the air.
Notice the difference in the feeling and the sound of long and short breaths, the light and the strong breaths.

As you sound your breath allow your body to join in the sonic dance. A hand may wish to rise and fall with a sounded breath. Your feet may wish to step, your torso may wish to turn or lift. Allow your limbs to be led by your free, sounded breath.

If there are others in the room your sounded breath may seek harmony, dissonance, dialogue with the sounds of others...

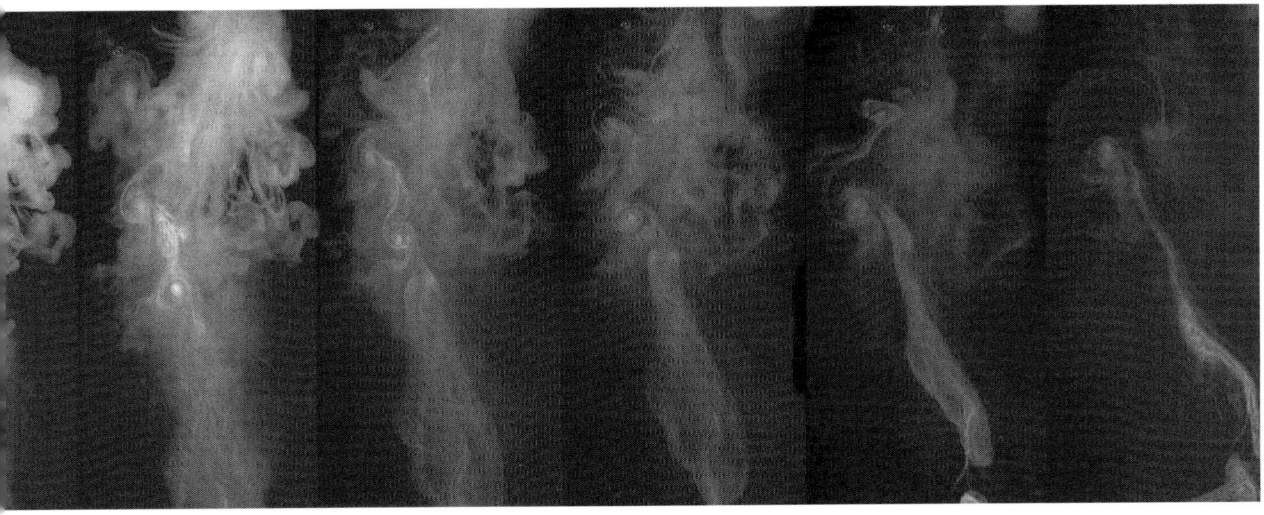

Keep listening, keep feeling and allow your body to follow your sound.

Sound your breath through your voice until you wish to hear again the sound of your breath itself. As you return to the quiet of almost-silent breath, continue to allow your body to be as it wishes, in movement or in stillness.

When all is again barely perceptible to the ear, then allow your eyes to open.
Into that ringing silence you may wish to share with one another through words in sounded breath as spoken voice... or just through collective stillness...

Our bodies are infinitely wise. Breath leads us to sound and silence, to movement and stillness. Sounding our breath into voice releases our inner sense to the outer world..

***Sounding breath** (as a group) from Eva Karczag*

Begin in a circle...
One by one, each sound the first letter of your name e.g. Mmmm... Cccc... etc. Listen.
On the second round, sound until breath runs out.
On the third and fourth rounds, join the previous sound before it ends. Two or even 3 or 4 sounds mingle as each sounder's breath runs out and more sounds join.
On the fifth round, make the sound short, and join immediately the previous sounder is done.

It's fun to do this a few times because a round happens so fast ... at times it almost seems like speaking in a new language. Then, open it up to anyone sounding the first syllable of their name, at any time, for as long or as short as they wish.

Take into walking... play with others making sound... are you close or distant from other sounders? Are you making short or long sounds? When does your sound enter? When does it end?

Gather... disperse... let sound and movement create clusters... groupings... allow happenings... Surprises. Eventually add gestures and movement in response to sound.

The many expressions of breath

*speeches ... chants ... songs ... lamentations ... riddles ... yarns ...
hoots ... whoops ... pantings ... whispers ... hissings ... beseechings ... praises ...
pleadings ... yawns ... prayers ... roars ... shouts ... gasps ... murmurs ... whistlings*

Arms and shoulders

Upper-body tension can play havoc with our breathing. If the muscles of the neck and shoulder are tense, this prevents the free movement of lungs and ribs. Moving the arms and freeing up through the shoulders can swiftly free the breath through this area.

The shoulder girdle is formed of a loose yoke of four bones that open the arm out to the edge of the body so that the wide-ranging action of the arm does not impact on the vital functioning of heart and lungs. The shoulder blade is like a floating raft connecting the arm into the entire length of the spine from head to pelvis.

There are many blood vessels travelling through the shoulder girdle and neck to and from the heart, brain and arms. A complex array of muscles connects and balances head and shoulder. As blood moves from the heart to brain and arm, it has to journey through areas that are easily contracted with tension.

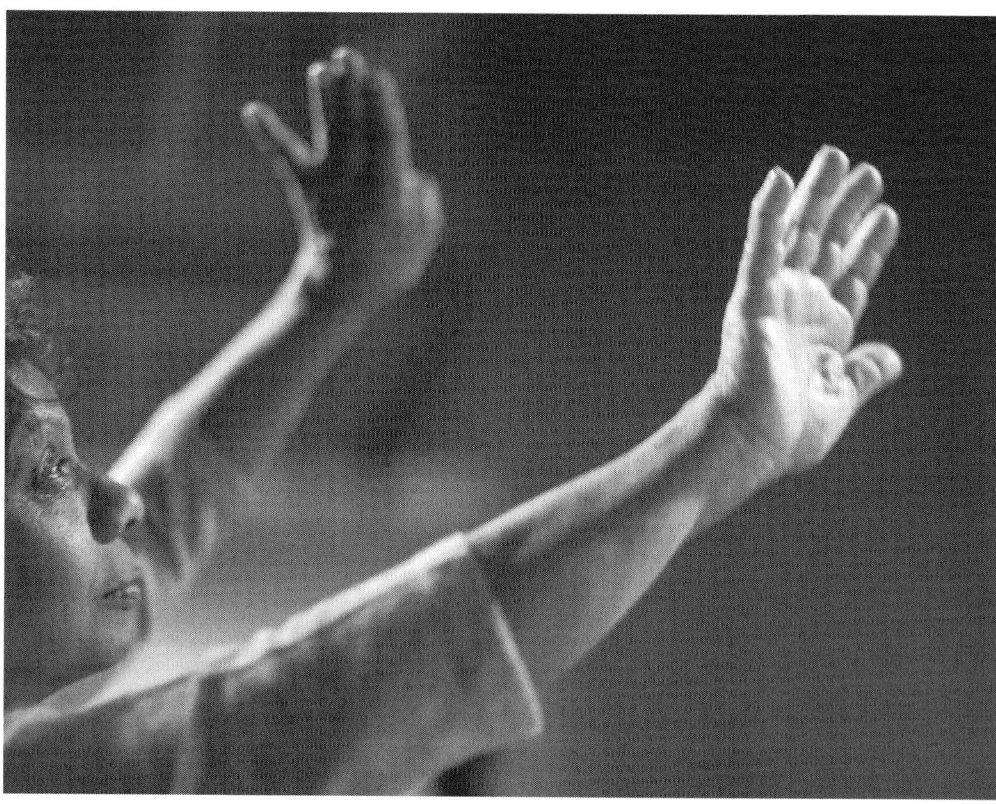

Arm dances

Sense your breath
Sense the depth of your shoulders front to back
Let them melt... downwards... outwards on the movement of your breath
Sense and move each shoulder... each elbow... wrist and the small bones of the hand
Let these many parts... each have a voice... move...
Fold and unfold... reach... far and near... cradle
Make pathways through the air... as wings... as fins
Right arm is different to left... imagine a conversation

Other possibilities
Meet another hand-to-hand
Press... push... pull... agree... disagree
Wake up the whole field of the shoulders and arms
Free the breath and the passage of blood

B was awaiting heart surgery. She tended to sit hunched, with arms tightly crossed, and quickly tired with any movement. But she spoke of her love of sailing and of the boats which went around the Scottish Isles, something that she had not been able to do for many years. Following this brief sharing, her arms opened and were flung high as she moved her story.

Diaphragm and ribs

As we breathe in, the diaphragm descends and the ribs lift – and then fall.Diaphragmatic breathing – with a long, slow exhale – is key to stimulating the vagus nerve[2], steadying heart rate and lowering blood pressure. The diaphragm is in direct contact with all major organs of our body. When it moves freely it moves the heart itself. Conversely, when the diaphragm is restricted, poor breathing results, affecting heart, digestion, blood flow – as well as blocking the flow of emotions.

Feeling overwhelmed, helpless, unstable and losing control are all symptoms of stress and hypertension (when we may also hyperventilate and feel dizzy with excessive oxygen). A first step in bringing back a sense of control is focusing on exhalation, and on a physical sense of the body weight and mass, feeling feet, bones and the ground. The body can lead the mind (as much as the mind leads the body). As the diaphragm descends on inhalation, it moves the heart which releases hormones to the frontal cortex to calm.

The ribcage protects heart and lungs and is formed of 24 ribs which are held together by cartilage in front and jointed to the spine in back. The lungs have no muscle – they are inflated and deflated by movements of the ribcage and diaphragm to which they are attached.

With a partner or alone:
Place two hands on the ribcage... breathe... listen
Follow the movement of the ribs as they rise and fall
Sense how ribcage/basket... changes shape
Sense movement in neck... in chest...
Between shoulder blades... as they float in back... opening out from the spine.
Sense depth... between sternum and spine
Follow movement as it arises... let the rest of the body support... and follow

[2] Vagus nerve (vagus, Latin 'wandering') originates in the medulla oblongata (a part of the brain stem) and extends all the way down from the brain stem to the colon. It sends fibres to the pharynx (throat), larynx (voice box), trachea (windpipe), lungs, heart, oesophagus, and intestinal tract, as far as the transverse portion of the colon. It brings sensory information back to the brain from the ear, tongue, pharynx, and larynx. It helps to regulate the heartbeat, control muscle movement, keeps a person breathing, and transmits a variety of chemicals through the body. It is also responsible for keeping the digestive tract in working order, contracting the muscles of the stomach and intestines to help process food, and sending back information about what is being digested and what the body is getting out of it.

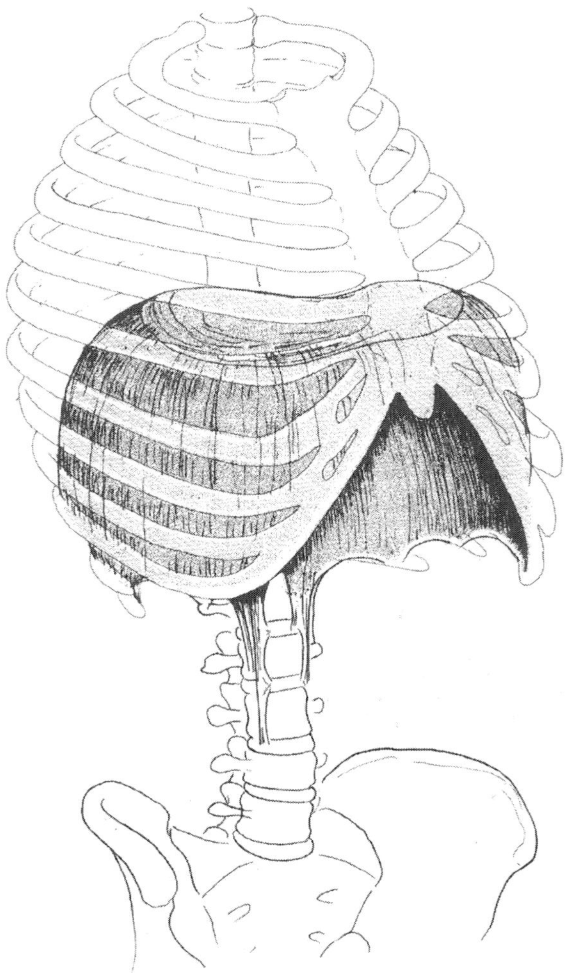

J suffers from chronic obstructive pulmonary disease. His body is thin, frail and his breathing is laboured. He told us how often he became more ill when he returns from visiting his daughter down in the South. He felt that the pressure of more people down there makes him feel 'choked up' and even less able to breathe – an indicator of how susceptible his body is to any extra stress. He constantly invented movements for himself that helped him breathe more easily, arching, leaning and stretching his ribs and spine – and surprised us all as he flung himself to the floor in his chosen pantomime character – the wolf in Red Riding Hood!

Working with others ... breath to breath

All spiritual and healing traditions begin with the breath as a way of getting in tune with the rhythms of another; it is a gentle yet powerful way of beginning, particularly when a person is fragile or in pain. Listening to the breath brings about a shared rhythm and pace, awakening receptivity, a coming to rest in the moment that also brings awareness of an inward sense of movement that connects all parts and aspects of a person, body and soul.

Taking time to sense beneath the surface to anatomical structures, sensing the form of a part – and the moving relationship of a part to the whole – helps tune us to the subtle movements present throughout a person's body. Listening to the breath of another can engage many levels of attention, to structure, to tissue movement and to the dream body. As we drop deeper into the rhythms of breath, stories and memories arise. Many creation myths begin with breath – listening to breath awakens each person's unique life world.

> 'We begin sessions by taking time to shift our bodies in chairs and wheelchairs. We talk about how useful being supported can be. We mustn't entirely hate being chair-bound. We uncross legs, ankles. We push our slippered or socked feet into the ground, tentatively twinkling toes, sensing movement far below. Our hips shift back into the back of the chair, spines pushing into the support of the back. I watch as sternums lift, heads lift, gazes emerge, hunched backs straighten, torsos lift, and space is made for the organs. The gentle piano music helps us relax into more fluid breathing. Within minutes our tense and broken group of bodies has moved into a sense of lightness, openness and possibility.'
>
> Filipa Pereira-Stubbs, *Dancing in Hospital*

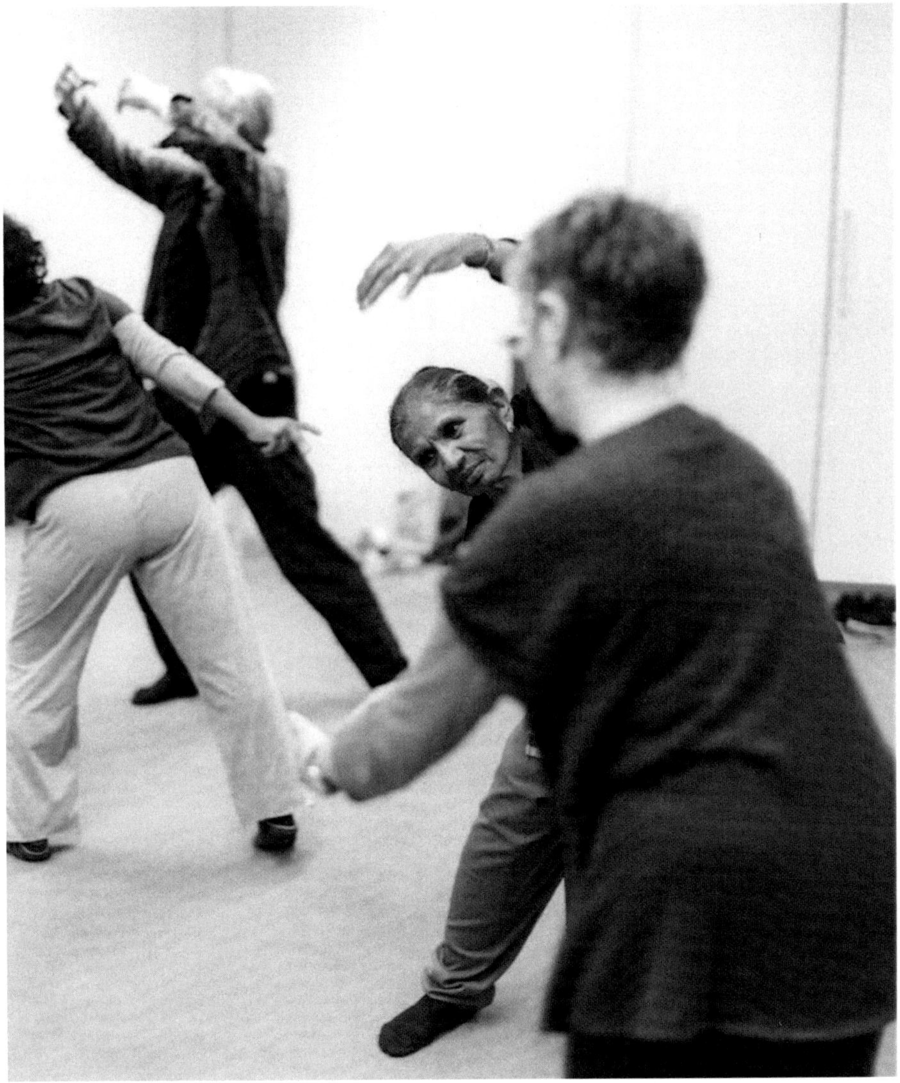

W has Multiple Sclerosis. She has limited mobility and numbness in limbs. Hand to hand we share and follow a 'breath' dance, listening palm to palm – arms become wings, moments of glide, of suspension, tiny, fragile finger movements. Afterwards, W draws. An image of an owl emerges. She speaks of how she loves owls; the spread of their wings; the silent glide of flight is for her an image that evokes a soft, widening aspect of the breath. She says the image returned to her throughout the following week and reminded her to breathe and move inside.

The imagination of breath

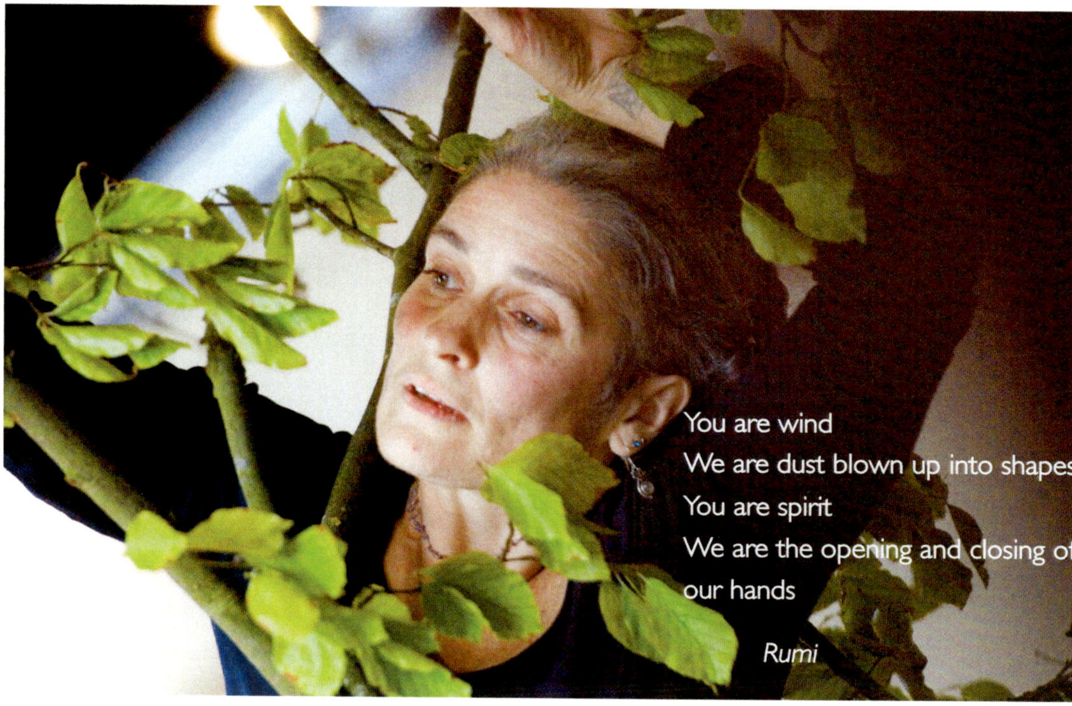
You are wind
We are dust blown up into shapes,
You are spirit
We are the opening and closing of
our hands
Rumi

Pneuma Greek ... breath, wind, spirit ... that which is breathed or blown

At birth the cry of a newborn child signals a change in state from fluid to air – the foramen ovale between the two upper chambers of the heart closes – and our lungs begin to function.

Everything that lives on land needs oxygen from the air. As fish live and depend on water so air is the dynamic yet invisible medium in which we live. The Earth's atmosphere is around 40–50 miles thick and was created by the photosynthetic action of plants over millions of years. This atmospheric mantle of air surrounding Earth makes life possible.

> 'Watching the animals come and go, feeling the land swell up to meet them and then feeling it grow still at their departure, I came to think of the migrations as breath, as the land breathing. In spring the great inhalation of light and animals. The long-bated breath of summer. And the exhalation that propelled them all south in the fall.'
>
> Barry Lopez, *Arctic Dreams: Imagination and Desire in a Northern Landscape*, p.162

We humans can only live in the lower levels 5 kilometres deep. Air is moved around the globe by weather and belts of wind carrying scents, sound waves, water molecules. Inside our bodies, life-renewing oxygen is carried to every cell through 65,000 miles of capillary, 'blown' by the beat of our heart, the pumping action of diaphragm and muscles, and by a gentle, trickling diffusion of fluids through membranes.

Air has many changing qualities and alters its density according to prevailing conditions, contracting and expanding in response to minute shifts in temperature. There is mountain air, sea air, bog air, city air, moving belts of high and low pressure. Birds flying on their great migrations around the earth are linked through the elasticity of air – the aerial form of their flight echoes the expanding and contracting processes of air – in flight they become as one body. Each bird rides on the wave of air created by the beating wings of the leader; the individual birds united in the moving field of air. So breath, when it is unimpeded by tension or injury, unites the whole body in a symphony of movements. The elasticity of lungs and chest are expressions of this property of air.

gusts ... breezes ... whirlwinds ... eddies ... storm fronts ... cross-currents ... gales ...
whiffs ... blasts ... breaths

Indigenous cultures all acknowledge the sacred power of wind, air and breath as the vital yet unknowable medium on which all life on earth depends and is connected. Conception is perceived as the 'meeting' of different Winds: there is a Dawn Wind, a Yellow Wind, a Wind of Darkness, a Father of Winds and a creator or Master of Breath; it is these Winds that give life, movement, awareness and speech to all living things. The ever-present influence and passage of winds through the body is reflected in the spiralling whorls on the tips of fingers, toes and crown of the head.[3]

'I am a feather on every wind'
Leontes. Shakespeare, *The Winter's Tale*

A place to breathe
Where do you go for a breath of fresh air?
Remember a place where you breathed easily.
Close your eyes and imagine into whatever appears,
Then make, move or write to explore ... a place to breathe

[3] Drawn from David Abram's *Spell of the Sensuous.*

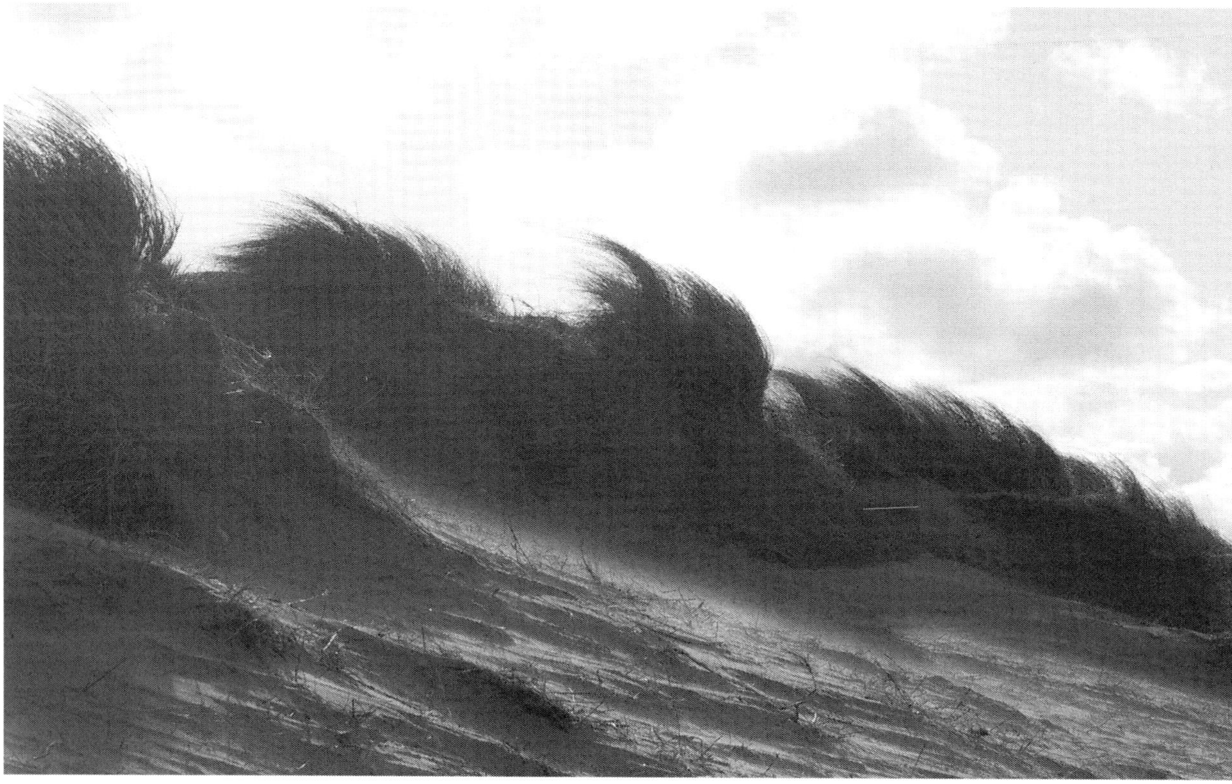

A breath of fresh air
Open the window... open the door... go outside...
Sense the movement of air outdoors – listen...
Let the air refresh... blow away... whatever feels stuck
Let your edges soften – become permeable
Let the air pass through you
Imagine becoming the wind
breeze ... tornado ... zephyr ... hurricane ... gust ... sigh ... whisper ... puff

Take large sheets of paper, paint and water
Allow the hands... weightedness... and lightness
Let your hands map the moving air inside and out
***Write** as the air*
Let in... voices... words... images... stories... memories
Share with another

Other possibilities
Shape the paper... tear... fold... mould... till the paper becomes a 3D landscape.
Gather two or three other materials to this 'place'.
Notice what is emerging... a landscape... a scene... a person
Move or Write *to find the gestures or words that emerge. Share with another*

Aramaic distinguishes different phases of breath – breath as the free air all around us, breath as it begins to enter and fill the body, breath that remains trapped inside and fails to come out, whereby we fall out of contact with life around us.

Breath portrait
Take a huge sheet of paper, paint, charcoal, graphite, pastel, a small bowl of water
Lie... or sit... rest some part of your body on the smooth surface of paper
Take time to sense your breathing body against the surface of paper
Listen... let breath come and go throughout your body
Sense its shifting nuance... here and there
As a wind over a field of long grass

Feel the air around your fingers... wrists
Let your hands move... to express the movement of breath
When you are ready, take colour... charcoal, paint
Let your hands 'speak' the breath with each mark
Work mark by mark... marks that glide... dash... hesitate... scratch... whisper
Add water
Follow rhythms... qualities... textures...
What forms... patterns... begin to appear?
Let each breath leave its trace

A gift
Move, paint or write... to find and explore
What gift the wind, your breath, the air might bring

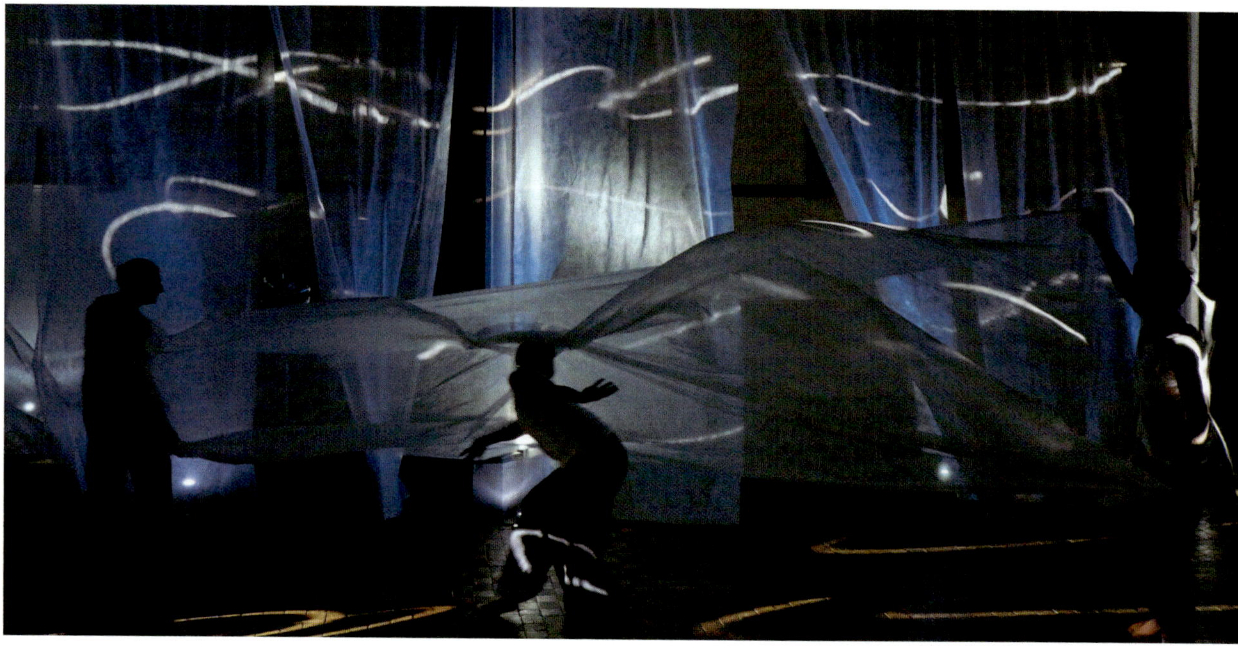

Many folk tales involve the hero/heroine travelling to the Four Winds in order to recover something lost.

'From the bedroom to the bathroom,
passing white owls in flight'
Sue Field

'In early 2010 I worked as a musician with Sue Field, an artist living with motor neurone disease. At that time she was unable to walk but could use a computer slowly and could talk with some difficulty. She was supported on either side by dancers and her long-standing friend and carer. I played a folk harp to accompany her movement. Initially we all took our cue from Sue's breath, following the ebb and flow. I would make phrases which corresponded with her breathing rhythm, which she then took as inspiration to move, rising up on an in-breath and sinking back on an out-breath. The music was therefore a 'bio-feedback' process, amplifying and reflecting her own breath cycles back to her. After several minutes, once we were comfortably synchronised, and taking care to monitor her energy level, I would begin to extend the phrase length, adding a few more notes, or reaching the arch of my phrases late, which she would then follow, deepening her breath, taking in more air and moving further in her own breath dance. Eventually she indicated that she wished to move to a standing position, and it was as if the music lifted her up, and the phrasing was such that the air seemed to move right through her body. Still supported by her helpers, she thrust herself forward as if flying like a bird. Later she read one of her poems aloud, and I would catch words and sing them back to her with the harp, again amplifying and reflecting, allowing some words to dwell on the same notes that she was speaking on, or making words longer, or repeating them. She responded to this and we duetted on an equal footing. It is my belief that the breath and the music enabled Sue to move in a way that would not otherwise have been possible for her at that time. She seemed to be able to transcend the physical boundaries of her condition and literally rise above them.'[4]

Sylvia Hallett, musician

[4] This became a performance devised by Sue Field and Ann Shepherd, with Lucinda Jarrett (Rosetta Life) and Kate Willis; music by Sylvia Hallett.

somewhere i have never travelled, gladly beyond

somewhere i have never travelled, gladly beyond
any experience, your eyes have their silence:
in your most frail gesture are things which enclose me,
or which i cannot touch because they are too near

your slightest look easily will unclose me
though i have closed myself as fingers,
you open always petal by petal myself as Spring opens
(touching skilfully, mysteriously) her first rose

or if your wish be to close me, i and
my life will shut very beautifully, suddenly,
as when the heart of this flower imagines
the snow carefully everywhere descending;

nothing which we are to perceive in this world equals
the power of your intense fragility: whose texture
compels me with the color of its countries,
rendering death and forever with each breathing

(i do not know what it is about you that closes
and opens; only something in me understands
the voice of your eyes is deeper than all roses)
nobody, not even the rain, has such small hands

e.e. cummings, *100 selected poems*

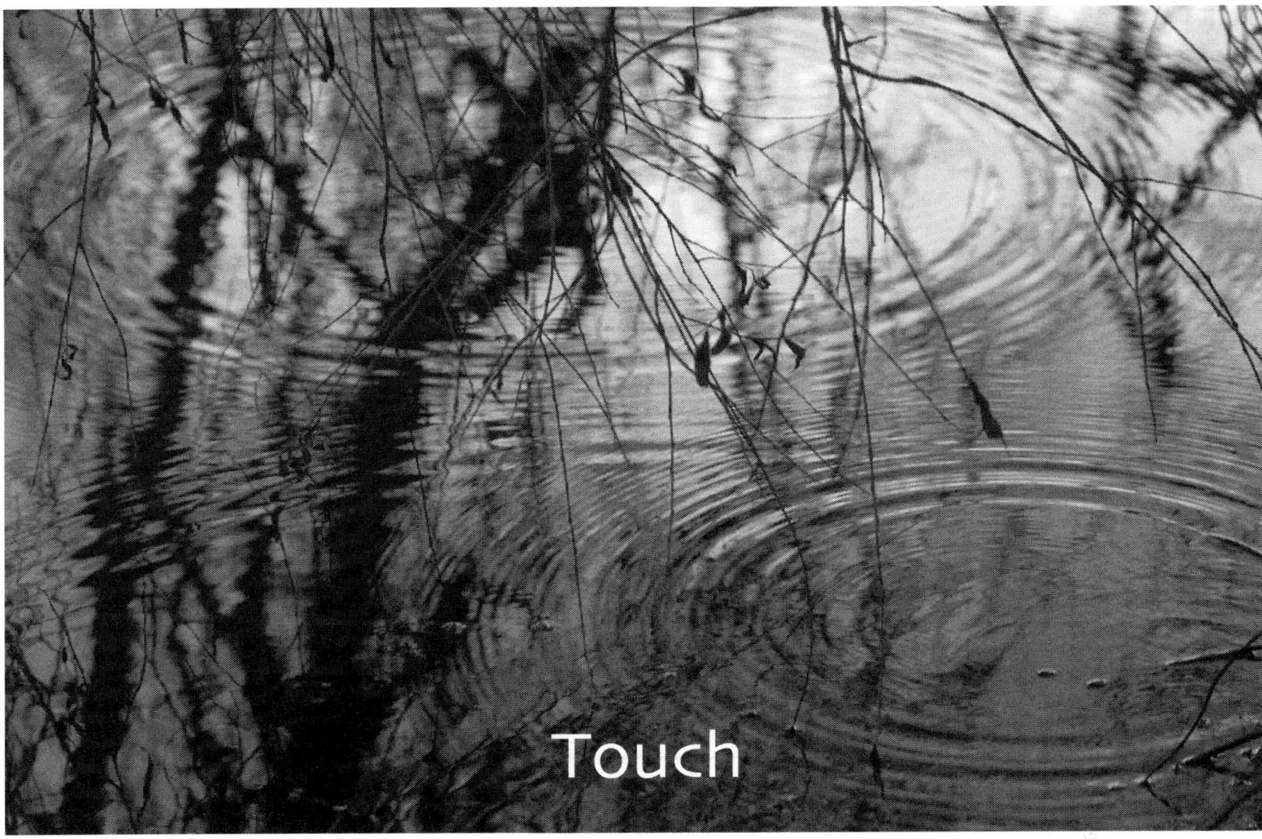

Touch

The greatest sense of our bodies is our touch sense. It is probably the chief sense in the processes of sleeping and waking; it gives us knowledge of depth, thickness and form; we feel, we love and hate, are touchy and are touched, through the touch corpuscles of our skin.

J. Lionel Taylor, *The Stages of Life* (1921) quoted in Montagu, *Touching: The human significance of skin*

We are formed out of touch. Moment by moment the world touches me – the feel of grass or of pebbles under my feet, the feel of light and of air on my skin – all touch and shape this moment of how I feel. And from the flow of blood in my heart to the tone of my skin, my body responds. The sense of touch forms the basis for all other sensory functioning.

Touch has been called 'the mother of the senses'. It is the first sensory system to evolve in all animal life forms. Even the most primitive single-celled organisms respond to touch. Our other senses – sight, hearing, taste, smell, and our kinaesthetic sense – are sensitisations of neural cells to particular kinds of touch: compressions of air on the eardrum, photons on the retina, chemicals on the nasal membrane etc. At six weeks, the human embryo responds to pressure waves and rhythmical movements of the heart, its skin sensitive and responsive before either eyes or ears.

In the underdeveloped newborn cortex, the area devoted to integrating tactile and kinaesthetic stimulation is the only part to be metabolically active at birth, which gives further indication of the importance of physical contact for the developing nervous system. Tactile experience is vital to cortical growth, stimulating the growth of myelin (insulating material around nerves) as well as boosting hormone secretions, which affect growth and physiological organisation. Touch (physical contact) is vital to an infant's ability to thrive and for their nervous system to develop. Without the stimulus and sensory feedback of touch, an infant's nervous system cannot locate and operate crucial muscles or activate the autonomic reflexes.

Skin and brain arise from the same embryological layer, the ectoderm; this connectedness explains something of why even a light touch on our skin can bring about profound changes throughout our body. There is a swift information highway from skin to brain which in turn responds and regulates our chemistries. From the soles of our feet to the crown of our head, the skin is threaded by over half a million sensory fibres that register the smallest changes in temperature, pain, pressure. Waking and sleeping information (sensation) from the skin communicates with the central nervous system which in turn assesses and responds.

The language of touch

> When I begin on the ward filled with elderly men and women, I always begin by offering my hand, introducing myself in a clear voice and with a steady handshake. How do you do, I say. How are you today Mr Jones... Mrs Smith... Mrs Brown... This familiar etiquette of introducing oneself properly never fails to stir a response. My hand is taken, and attention is brought to this first interaction. How do you do, they say... and then, What do you do?
>
> Filipa Pereira-Stubbs, *Dancing in Hospital*

Our sense of touch underlies how we perceive and communicate with others, it lays the foundations for our feelings of safety and belonging. It gives us a clear sense of how we are in our physical bodies, whilst also giving us a vital sense of our boundaries and of containment. Sensory feedback from the skin and senses is crucial for a coherent sense of ourselves and our surroundings. The sensory isolation of solitary confinement is known to be one of the harshest forms of punishment.

As infants' touch (and movement) are the primary means through which we learn and develop our nervous system. Young children are impelled to touch whatever is around them, exploring through their bodies the qualities and properties of their surroundings. And throughout life, touch and movement shape and affect how we perceive and communicate. Helen Keller, deaf and blind from infancy, was taught to speak through touch.

In our everyday lives we use many different kinds of touch. We touch to greet, to console, to steady or reassure, we touch to wake up, to protect and to warn, and we may also touch or be touched to punish or control. The language of touch is not uniform, it is rich, subtle and varied – and holds a multiplicity of possibilities. Touch is often a way in which we begin to connect with another who is frail, in pain, or has lost the capacity to move independently. Simple touch, like a greeting, acknowledges a person and, as in a conversation, initiates communication.

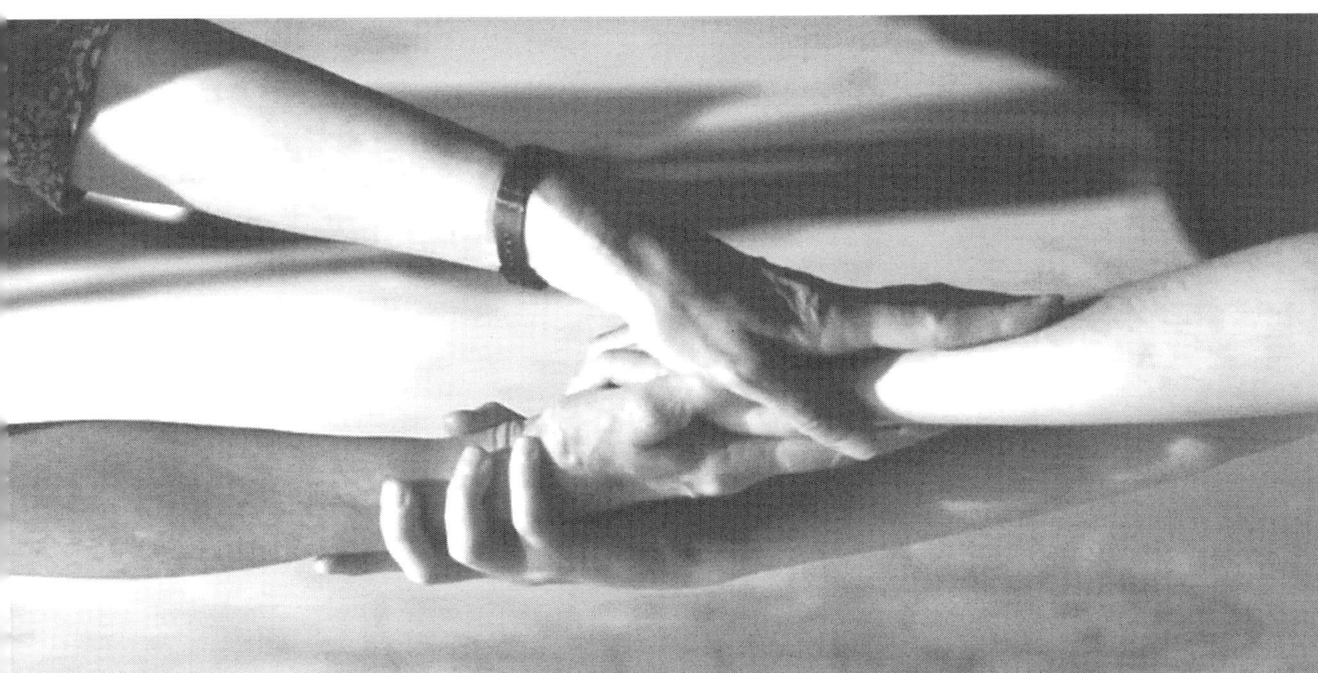

Dancing hand to hand

When we dance with others, touch, moving hand to hand, is often the way we communicate in the flow of movement, from the swift hand clasps of capoeira, to elaborate lifts and duets of ballet, from the intimate and varying contact of waltz, jive and tango, to the linked hands of circle dances in Greece and the Balkans. In the dances of Aboriginal peoples, movement and touch are inextricably linked to prayers for healing. As we move, touch is the means by which we keep in step, in rhythm together.

Touch has the longest entry in the OED (six pages) – an indicator of how deeply the sense of touch shapes our language and construction of meaning. We describe ourselves as touched, in and out of touch, of losing touch, of feeling touchy or touched up, someone is touchy-feely, another seems untouchable. Our language is awash with words that reflect the vital tactility of our experience.

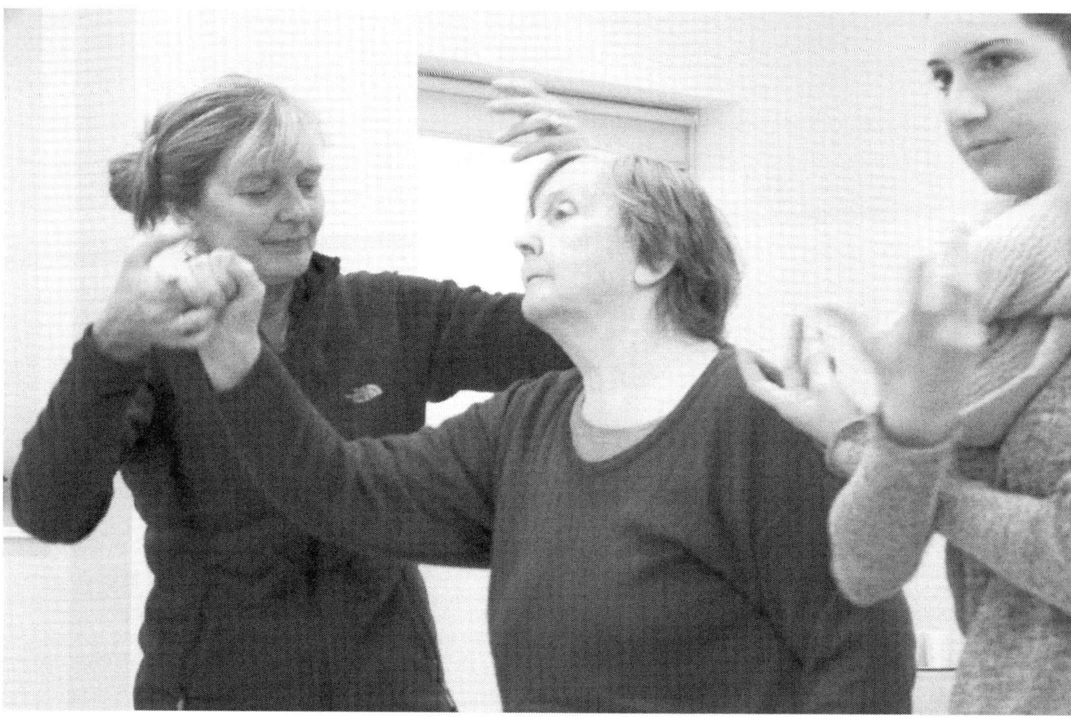

Touchdown ... touchstone ... touchline ... touching ... a touch of flu ... touch base ... touch a chord

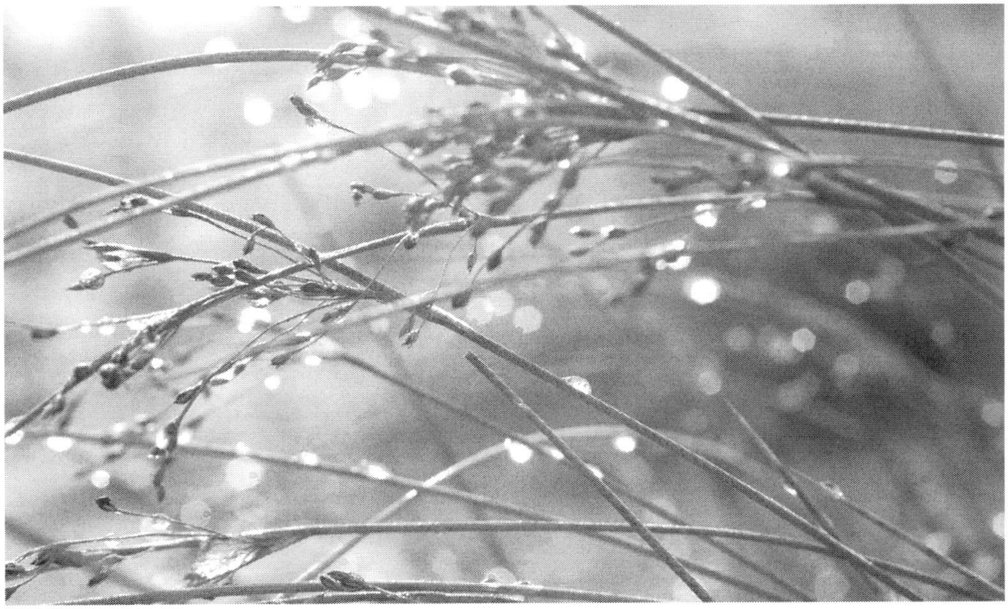

"**Tapping like raindrops**" Susanna Recchia, account from working at Richard House Children's Hospice – a project with Rosetta Life

'This is how the dance begins. My dance companion is a child who at first lies passively on a beanbag. His carer has been trying to engage with him through touch as she observes other dancers doing. The child doesn't seem to respond and the carer steps back slightly confused.

There is music playing; it has an underlying pulse and, as I approach the child, I begin to lightly brush and tap his arms in sync with the music.

I wait for a signal that seems to imply a YES, I will come with you.

My touch seems welcomed and his face opens into a smile. My fingertips follow the music with gentle, repetitive strokes along his arms and hands. My dancing companion cannot see and his movement is very limited, so I begin to make sounds as I continue tracing the length of his lower legs. Again his face responds: smiling and turning his head from side to side to join this touch dance. At times his head slightly tilts back when a smile appears.

We continue with our rhythmical dance. I notice that his legs are restless and perhaps uncomfortable. I take a piece of soft fabric; as I sense the fresh temperature and the silky texture of the cloth in my hands, I try to share these sensations with my little companion by resting the light, falling weight of the cloth onto his limbs. It is my suggestion to help him connect or feel some easing. His delight is unmistakeable, his face still shining with smiles together with small turns and tilts of the head. His whole body responds to stroking, to tapping, to sounds and music. I am there in this dance, I am offering suggestions, he responds with fuller breaths, softer legs and big smiles.'

Lack of touch – untouched

Our tactile needs do not diminish with age – if anything they seem to increase. For older people, research reveals a correlation between lack of touch and senile traits such as irritability, forgetfulness, careless grooming, and eating habits.

> The elderly in particular are condemned to living long days without touch, without contact. Critical then to take time to offer the companionship of supporting hands, the comfort of warm hands on aching bones, tense shoulders. With permission, myself, staff and volunteers use our hands to guide perception of sensation, to awaken minute shifts and changes in proprioception. In a sense, our aim is to help people re-map their awareness of their body landscapes. Where does that breaking spine meet a too-heavy head? How does the paralysed frozen arm hinge on a bony shoulder? Body responds to warmth, to touch – sometimes the movement is so small it can barely be seen. But to the mover, concentrating with eyes closed, an area is coming alive and is being invited to participate – and unlocking is happening.
>
> Filipa Pereira-Stubbs, *Dancing in Hospital*

Lack of touch is known to cause many of the symptoms of malnutrition. Children who lack touch grow more slowly, have depressed immune responses, are more emotionally distressed, less curious, less lively, and less active problem-solvers. Children who are undernourished by touch tend to withdraw into themselves or conversely to exhibit unruly behaviour, perhaps in an attempt to secure attention. Such children tend to become adults who have a muted capacity for self-awareness, self-regulation, personal intimacy and general maladaptive responses to the conditions of their lives – they seem what we might term 'out of touch'. Lack of touch and lack of self-awareness often go hand in hand, resulting in pain, alienation and lack of empathy. Our physical, emotional and mental health and resilience depends in many ways on receiving enough nourishing touch.[1]

Studies on violent crime all connect harsh and isolated childhoods with antisocial behaviour. Dr Prescott, a developmental neurophysiologist at the National Institute of Child Health and Human Development, writes: 'I believe that deprivation of body touch, contact and movement are the basic causes of a number of emotional disturbances including depressive and autistic behaviours, hyperactivity, sexual aberrations, drug abuse, violence and aggression.'[2]

[1] Drawn from Deane Juhan, *Touched by the Goddess: The physical, psychological and spiritual powers of bodywork.*

[2] *ibid.*

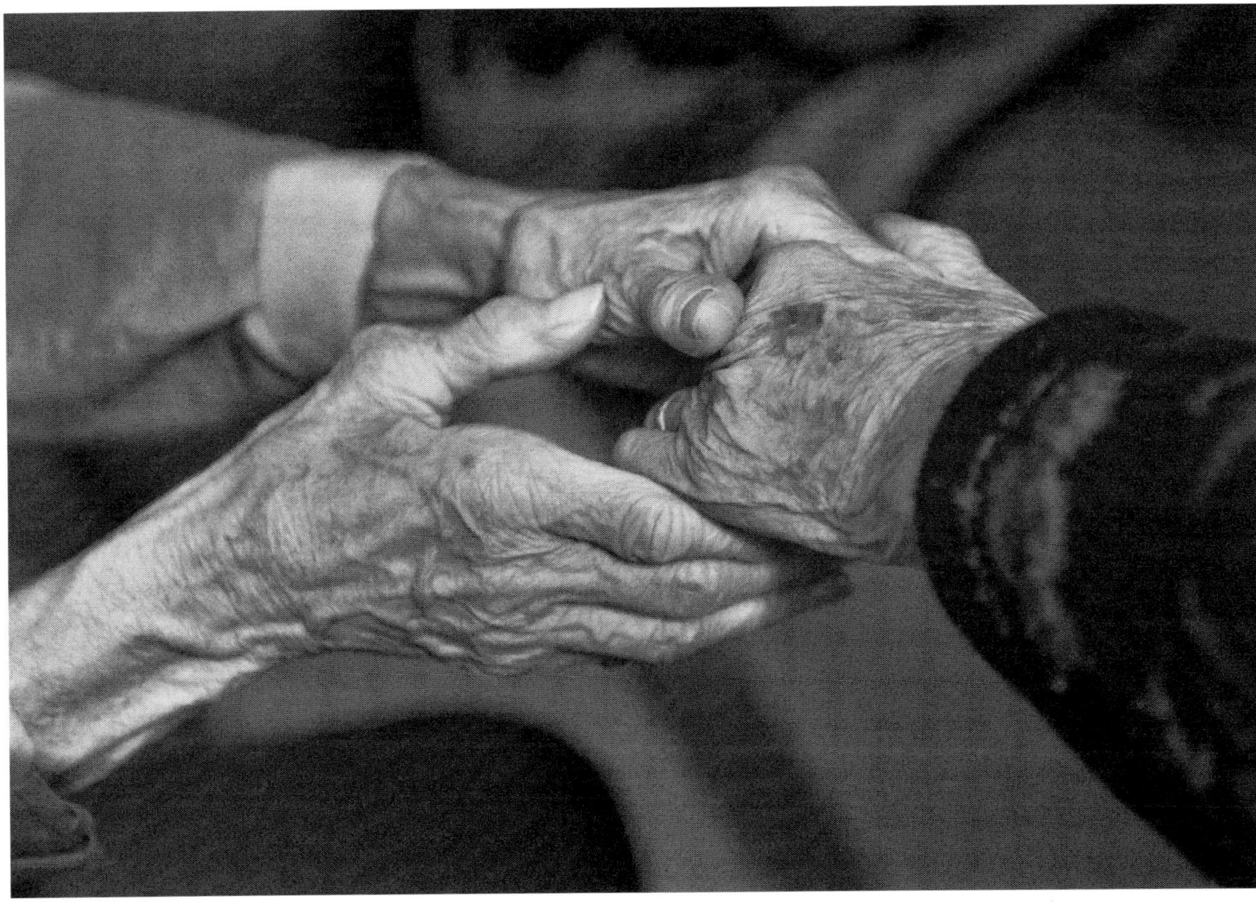

In 2001, the *Independent* newspaper reported estimates that in the UK 300,000 children were currently living with serious domestic violence. Each year 100,000 children run away from home.

In the early 20th century, the 90–98% mortality rate of young children in American orphanages and foundling homes provoked concern. Despite adequate food, children wasted away and died within a year. Yet this dire situation was dramatically reversed as severe understaffing was relieved by volunteers who took time to physically handle and play with the children. In more recent times, the world was shocked by images from Romanian orphanages where children suffered from severely stunted growth and mental retardation; they too were physically isolated and untouched in their cots.

In 1981 an American hospital reported a story of premature infants carefully monitored and protected in incubators. These tiny creatures were so small it was thought 'unsafe to touch' and so touch was strictly forbidden. Despite careful regulation of temperature, food etc., these fragile infants did not thrive. Yet in one week, despite no changes in protocol, some of these little ones began to develop and put on weight. Investigation revealed a new night nurse who, unable to bear the cries of these 'little shrimps', had opened the incubators and gently stroked to calm them. Results were almost instantaneous; further evidence that touch is a biological and developmental need.[3]

Touching (notes for practice)

A conversation

E: What do you want from touch? What do you get?

R: Things become clearer, in the sense of clearing, and also clearer in my head about what my body is doing. Sometimes parts of my body feel like one mass, as opposed to differentiated parts. It doesn't feel like I have muscles or blood vessels, and touch brings back for me that I have muscles and they go this way and that way...

E: So directions, different substances, structures...

R: Yes, and sometimes when body parts feel cloudy, touch clears out the cloudiness.

I still haven't figured out how touch works with pain because sometimes it alleviates it a lot, sometimes a little, sometimes it just changes the type of pain, and other times the pain just stays there but everything is clearer and easier around it. Occasionally it can intensify the pain, but that also helps me enter it differently.

Sometimes the touch on my swollen foot feels like there's a water pillow under my skin, and although the touch is at the surface, it feels like perhaps there are receptors deeper, under the liquid.

E: When your foot is swollen and I touch it, it feels like there's a static, unmoving quality, and my touch begins to bring a little movement into it, and once movement is there, your body can take over more.

Eva Karczag, in conversation

3 Drawn from Dr David Servan-Schreiber, *Healing Without Freud or Prozac*

A listening touch ... the invitation to move

Skilful, attuned touch is a highly developed form of human communication. The human hand can receive, discriminate and convey an extraordinary amount of information, giving the body precise and intelligent feedback about itself.

Touch is often a crucial and everyday part of a dancer's toolkit. On days when we feel trapped by inertia or where for reason of ill health we cannot move, touch can be a gentle yet powerful stimulus to kindle a sense of movement and a shift from passive into active engagement. Touch is a language, offering a means of communication when words fail.

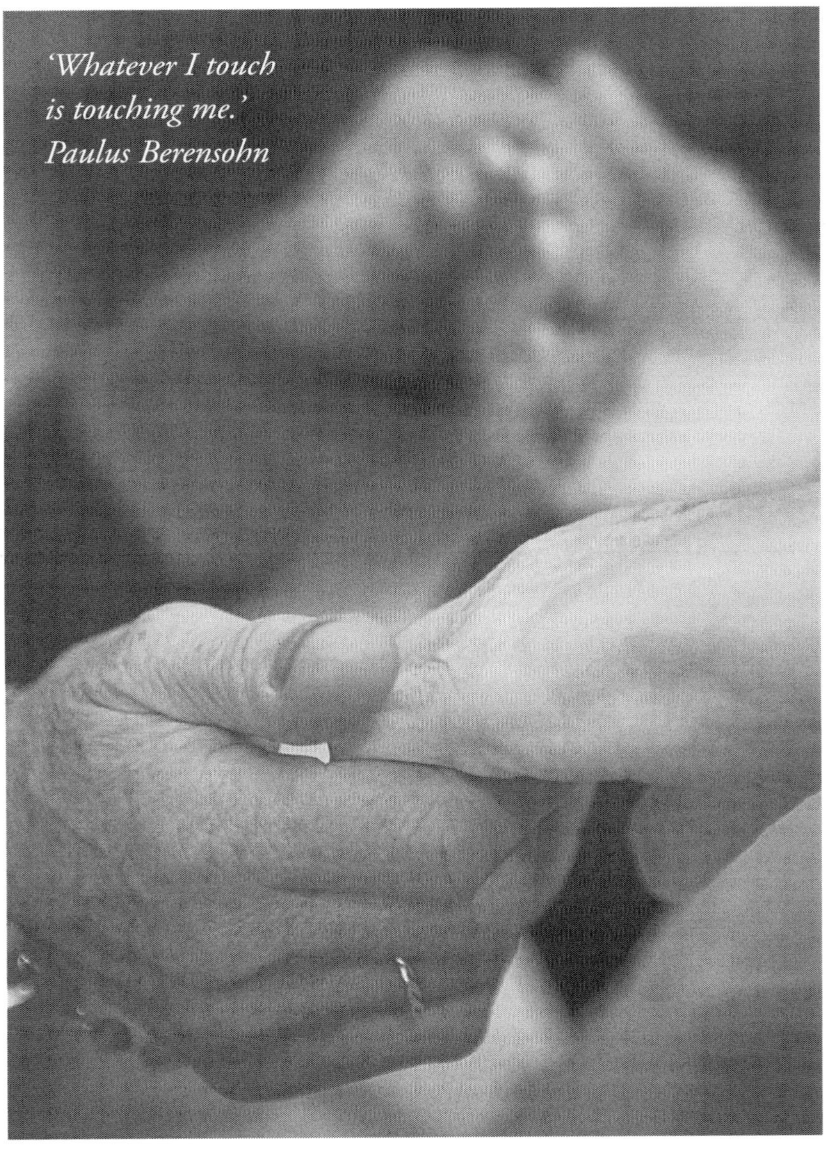

Two dances through touch in a children's hospice

Susanna Recchia, dance artist

'I arrive at the children's hospice in the playroom and meet a boy. He has a heavy cold, nose running, dark circles under his eyes. I help him out of the chair onto the floor. My desire is to tune in with his physicality. There is no verbal communication involved in our encounter. My first reaction is to mirror his positions and place my whole body like his; I try to physically understand how his legs, arms, torso and head are organised in relation to gravity and grasp something of his mobility. His hands can push but his legs drag. By observing and repeating exactly the actions he is doing, I can begin to feel what is mobile and what is unable to move. He seems to enjoy travelling around, dragging himself to visit other children in the room. I follow his actions, not waiting for a reaction or a direct response. I notice he is holding his feet. On impulse, I offer him mine. He responds straight away by squeezing and playing with my feet. I can sense his strength and I respond by pushing into his hands. I receive a clear push back which becomes resistance; here we meet. I feel a sense of deep satisfaction in this human encounter; I meet him not just by mirroring, but by engaging his attention, his strength and his ability to encounter another human being on an active physical level through movement. I meet him equally, through a physical exchange, not through pity. He then begins falling forward with his torso – putting his head on the floor. I copy him, at times making direct contact with his head and spine, which he seems to enjoy. He doesn't retreat; he stays with the touch. I feel his body soften under my hands. Suddenly I realise he is fast asleep, a small curled-up child on the floor breathing and resting.'

'My second dance is with a young girl. She is in a wheelchair. She rocks back and forth while biting a towel that she is holding in her right hand. I imagine that without the towel she would bite herself. I kneel on the floor and place my hands on her knees. I begin to follow her rocking, gradually pushing her knees while staying with the rhythm of her repetitive movement. The quality of her rocking is strong and she seems to put a lot of muscular effort into this action. As I continue to match the rhythm of her rocking as well as her strength, she seems to enjoy the pressure of my hands and arches her back up and away before falling forward again. I constantly bring my attention to her movement, her sense of rhythm, the sounds she makes. I observe and follow her; I observe and respond at the same time, giving slight resistance. The towel she was holding falls on the floor. She starts rubbing her hands vigorously and I put my own hands in between hers to see if she would rub mine. And she does. I receive her touch, I am with her rocking, I am present with her movement and also remain aware of my own breath, my own rhythm. In all this time with her, I feel I am being her edges – I am with her movement whatever it is.

Malcolm Manning once suggested: "Dance the dance you want, not the dance you think your partner wants." I remember this phrase as I see the girl rocking, being strong, forceful and energetic. I meet her as a mover and improviser. I encounter the rocking with the sensation that rocking gives to my own body and field of knowledge that comes from years spent exploring movement – climbing trees, resting my head on my grandmother's lap, gardening with my parents, holding my sister's hand before falling asleep, running to catch a train – as much as from my dance training. We live with and through movement. The rocking could be seen as a sign of malfunctioning, or as a strategy for survival and form of expression. As a dancer, I meet the mover as well as the movement created in our encounter. And even when movement seems non-existent, I remind myself that the heart still beats, the lungs are still increasing and decreasing their volume, blood is still circulating from the heart towards the extremities and back.

Dancing is about planting movement and harvesting self-awareness and the capacity to be in movement when words are not there, when emotions are overwhelming, when pain is unbearable.

Through movement we can connect with others. Whether it is disability, pain, or emotional anguish that seems to block communication, skilful movement interaction can open up avenues of connection where words fail.'

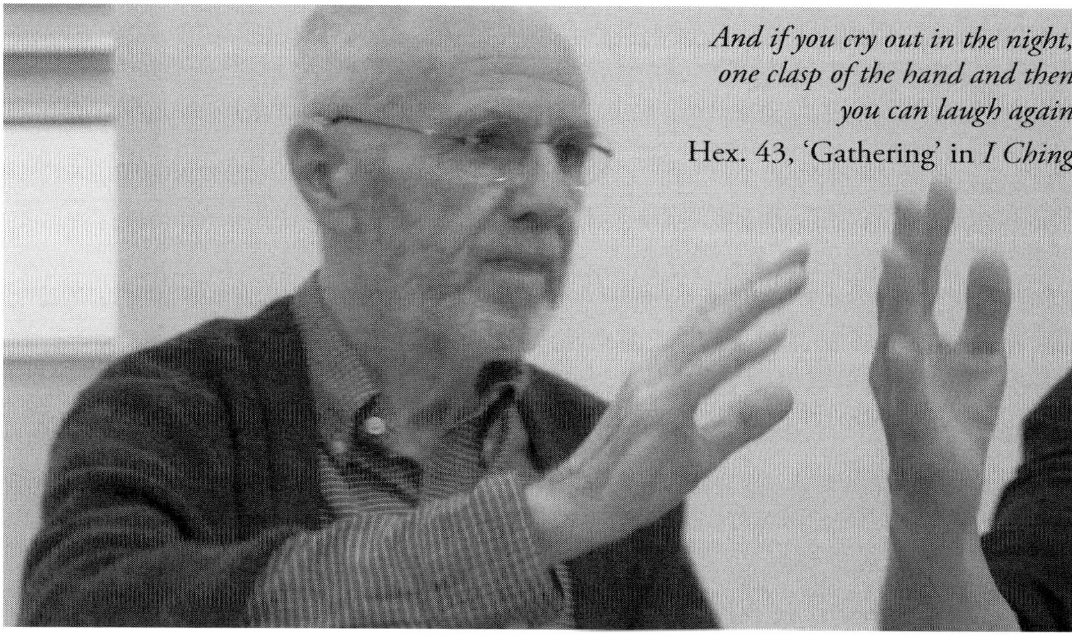
And if you cry out in the night,
one clasp of the hand and then
you can laugh again
Hex. 43, 'Gathering' in *I Ching*

A touch of the hand calms us when we are agitated or distressed. Having a pet to fondle and touch can be as effective in dealing with anxiety and depression as medication.[4] At times a touch or a hug can help us feel better more swiftly than a volume of words. When other senses and functions fail, touch may be the last avenue of communication.

> People who have lost, or are in the process of losing, movement through muscle or motor neurone degeneration, also face speech loss and the inability to communicate with loved ones and friends. Touch-facilitated movement offered a way of being in touch, of communicating with others. As one participant commented: 'I speak and listen with my fingers now. I use this kind of movement to keep in touch with the people I love. I want to keep in touch with my grandson and this is the only way I can.'
>
> Lucinda Jarrett, on her work with people with Motor Neurone disease

A simple contact on a shoulder creates a charge that conveys information throughout the entire body, stimulating awareness and change. The touch of a hand awakens us to particular details of our body that ripple out and connect to the whole unified field of the body. We notice things to which we were previously unaware. When we touch another person, we are also touched ourselves – a bridge of communication opens up between you and me.

[4] Servan-Schreiber, *ibid.*

Touch comes in many shapes and sizes. From a hand resting on a hand or arm, to a back resting against a back breathing together. We are all born knowing experientially the gift of touch. When we give touch, we receive touch in return – an exchange of information from body to body – reciprocity. Touch can draw our attention from deep inside the body to the surface, to skin, and touch can take our attention from skin to depth, addressing and integrating fundamental facets of our being and giving us information about body systems, movement qualities and thought processes, as well as opening spaces for imagination.

Eva Karczag

The touch of a child... of a parent... of a friend... a nurse... a doctor... the surgeon

I always approach the people I touch with respect, and an attitude of listening to their needs rather than mine. When I touch I aim to give a lot of space, both in my hands as well as in my intentions. I know and I don't know, the not knowing probably being even more important than the knowing.

Lisa Dowler

When people are fragile or ill they are infinitely more sensitive to feeling pushed, pressured or controlled in any way. It takes time and patience when working creatively through touch to establish a mutuality – a place of meeting – where as in a conversation, each person feels free both to initiate and to follow. Dialogue and connection are a moment-by-moment shared process where invitation follows invitation, and response follows response.

Within a hospital context touch is not always appropriate, but when it is, I find non-directive touch establishes for me and the other person who we are as individuals i.e. where our being begins and ends. It also illuminates the place where we can meet. I find it the most powerful of the senses when working with another person. When working with Laura, I found that underneath my touch her muscles responded by softening, releasing her joints and allowing her to move more freely with a smoother quality, which isn't characteristic of someone with hypertonic cerebral palsy.

Lisa Dowler

The need for resistance (defining boundary)

J, who suffers from schizophrenia, arrives to a session. She speaks fast and non-stop. The rest of the group seem to withdraw, overwhelmed by this relentless flood of chatter. J seems unaware of this and on an impulse I offer her my hand and ask her to meet it and push back. Swiftly we are engaged in a 50/50 play of weight. Gradually we use other parts of the body, shoulder to shoulder, elbow to back, head to shoulder. J is absorbed in what is becoming a body mapping. She is breathing more fully, and is quiet, no longer talking incessantly. Later she says: 'I feel like me now'.

Lucinda Jarrett, Rosetta Life, on her work in end of life care:

Mr T referred himself to work with me. He was living with Progressive Supra Nuclear Palsy (PSP) a rare life-limiting neurodegenerative condition that affects movement, control of walking and balance, speech, swallowing, vision, mood and behaviour, and thinking. I visited him at his home ten times between June and October 2009. During the months we worked together Mr T was at a stage of his illness when he could no longer stand unaided or use his hands. He was also losing his sight and his speech had become indistinct and slurred.

I offered light touch or massage to connect with his sensory awareness. 'What part of your body would you like to move from?' I would ask him and he nearly always replied, 'My heart'. I would then quietly place my

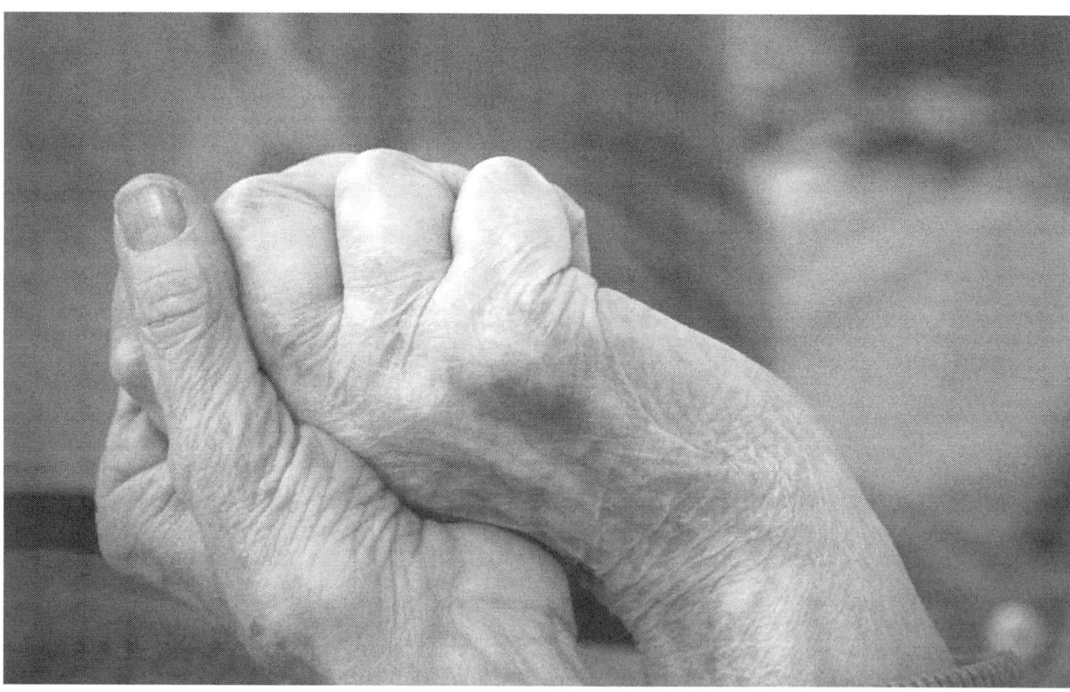

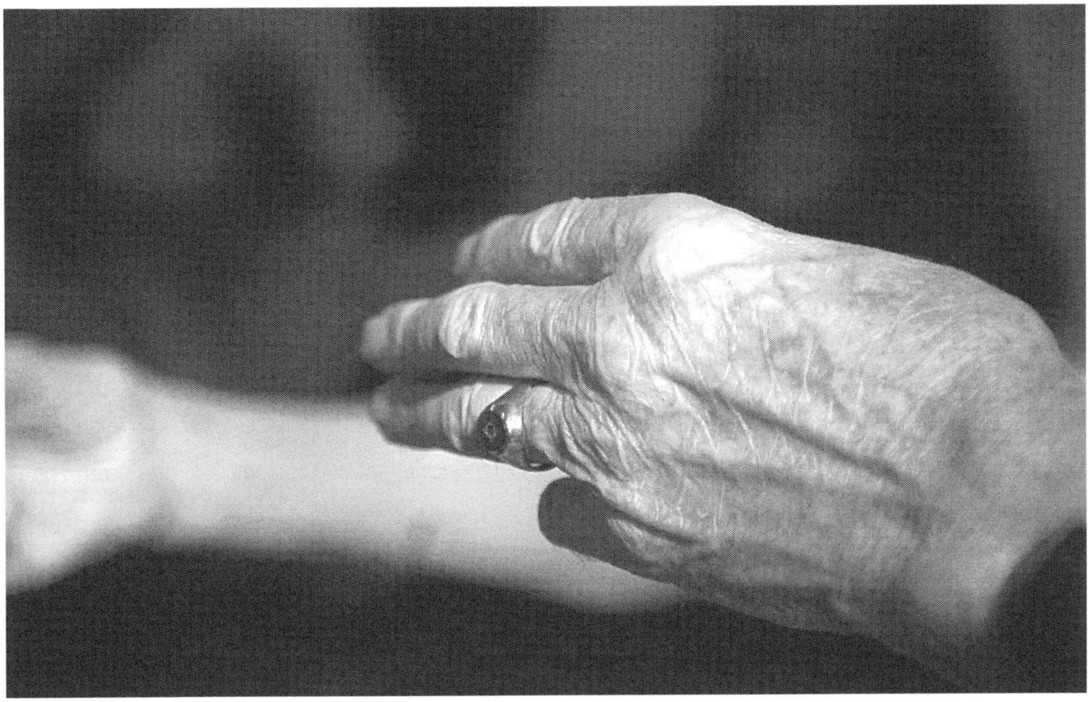

hand upon his heart, and he would exhale – almost vocalising – a long out breath, as if releasing tension or pain. This began a serpentine 'dance' which moved outwards from his chest, to his shoulder and arms, a flowing touch-facilitated river of movements.

Touch is intimate. When speech abandons us, touch becomes a vital channel of communication. In Mr T's words, '*I want to keep talking*', '*We talk through our fingers*'. At one point I became worried that our relationship had too few boundaries and invited a colleague, an Alexander practitioner, to witness a session and help me understand the complexity of the relationship. She introduced movement games that balanced the softness of my movement with strength and resistance, enabling Mr T to pull and push, to take leadership of our nascent choreography. I found that I could help him structure a movement sequence aesthetically, which we subsequently filmed.

touch

Different cultures ... different needs

A quiet touch can be a life-affirming support to someone who is isolated and alone, or for those with very restricted movement – yet it is vital that artists or dancers, familiar with touch, are sensitive to how varying people's need for boundary or closeness are. What comforts one person may feel intrusive to another. For some the prospect of touch may arouse anxiety and fear – of exposure, of boundary, of invasion; there may also be difficulties in relation to body image. It is important to negotiate contact slowly, step by step. Touch, like movement, is a language shaped by culture and history as much as by physiology; it can soothe, yet it may also call up powerful negative feelings. It takes time to read the signs of what is appropriate for each person. Whenever possible asking permission and offering choice – *where... and how... would you like a hand, a touch?*

Safe touch

We live in a time when touch has become a 'touchy subject', and in many fields of work increasingly taboo. There is currently a concept of 'safe touch'; in many contexts dancers and artists are challenged as to whether their work is safe, and questions raised as to how to touch safely. Touch, the sense most vital to our growth, health and well being has, in the public eye, become tainted by sexual innuendo and fear of abuse. Artists need to be articulate on behalf of touch – to be sensitive to these fears and also able to convey something of the profound importance of touch.

In healthcare settings:

'Working in healthcare settings, there will always be a staff member aware that you are doing a session. Ensure that you are not working in a closed room where your work cannot be seen. Be visible. Communicate what you are doing to other staff, whether on a busy bay, by a patient's bedside, or in the day room with a group. If you are responsible for any other staff members (or volunteers or family) be sure to lead and be firm in your guidance – at the very least, have them experience touch themselves, show them what you mean, and make sure they understand the intention of the touch work. At the same time, reassure them that using touch to connect and communicate with another human is a wonderful and effective practice.' Filipa Pereira-Stubbs

In primary schools:

'Children automatically run up and want to hug. When distressed or anxious they often seek out contact with an adult. We have clear guidance on how to keep safe whilst ensuring we do not reject children. We teach children about personal space, to ask for hugs and for staff to give them in view of other adults and always side-to-side. Staff are skilled at responding to children who bear hug them, quickly and gently manoeuvring a child so they are sideways on with a hand maintaining contact with the child. Younger children have personalised plans that may include receiving a hug, for example, in the morning on arrival at school. This is written and signed by carers, teachers and a senior member of staff, clearly outlining how this happens and always in view of a second adult.'

Karen Adcock Doyle

Getting in touch

Let a hand come to rest on your partner... an ear listening
Let your hand soften... to receive
Soften... your wrist... and the length of your forearm
Open... the length of your spine... open your shoulders
(Wherever there is tension in your own body it transmits to your partner)
Wait... listen as your partner breathes...
Watch... as a presence seems to come alive... movement eddies under your hand...
A meeting... a fish rising to the surface of water
As in a conversation... listen and follow...
Varying contact... from skin to deeper within... to bone
Float... support... invite... pause
Let the rhythm of your shared breath guide
Let your hands... your body... sense... respond... follow whatever is emerging

Touch protocol

Stay alert to any clues as to how a person is experiencing touch, checking in verbally, sensing changes in breath, skin tone and other bodily clues, that participants are at ease with what is happening, where possible offering choice. When we touch another person they are also touching us; notice your own responses. Touch can soothe, but it may also open a Pandora's box of memory and emotion; anger, feelings of helplessness, shame, loss or grief may be stimulated through a touch that is experienced as insensitive.

If possible and appropriate, ask permission: Can we touch? Where would you like a hand?

Check in: How does that feel?

Like the story of the Three Bears, it is important to offer choice:

Is this touch... too close... too light... too deep... too slow... too fast... just right?

Negotiating touch … Diane Amans dance artist

'Although it is now considered essential in health and care settings to tell someone what you are going to do before you touch them: "I'm just going to listen to your breathing, Jessie" – or preferably ask their permission: "Is it all right if I just move your legs?" – I sometimes prefer to negotiate the contact non-verbally. If I'm working with someone who has advanced dementia and struggles to understand verbal communication, I think it's more effective if I tune into their body language and observe carefully how they respond to my attempts to initiate contact.

'Here's an example from a hospital ward for adults in dementia care. I often use a prop such as a large balloon or a scarf and move with it – watching for any signs of engagement (eye contact, postural shift, changes in breathing). If I see a smile, an encouraging glance, I'll move a bit closer. If the person stretches a hand, I'll bring the prop within reach and we have contact through a scarf or balloon. From here I'm negotiating a relationship that might develop to include touch. All this is without speech. I haven't followed protocol but in my own way I've asked permission. I've also managed to work in a spontaneous way which, I believe, allows me to be more person-centred.

'I think this issue of listening for bodily clues is very important. I express my feelings physically – and enjoy hugging people – but I'm aware that, with some people, I wouldn't initiate a hug. I can think of one person who

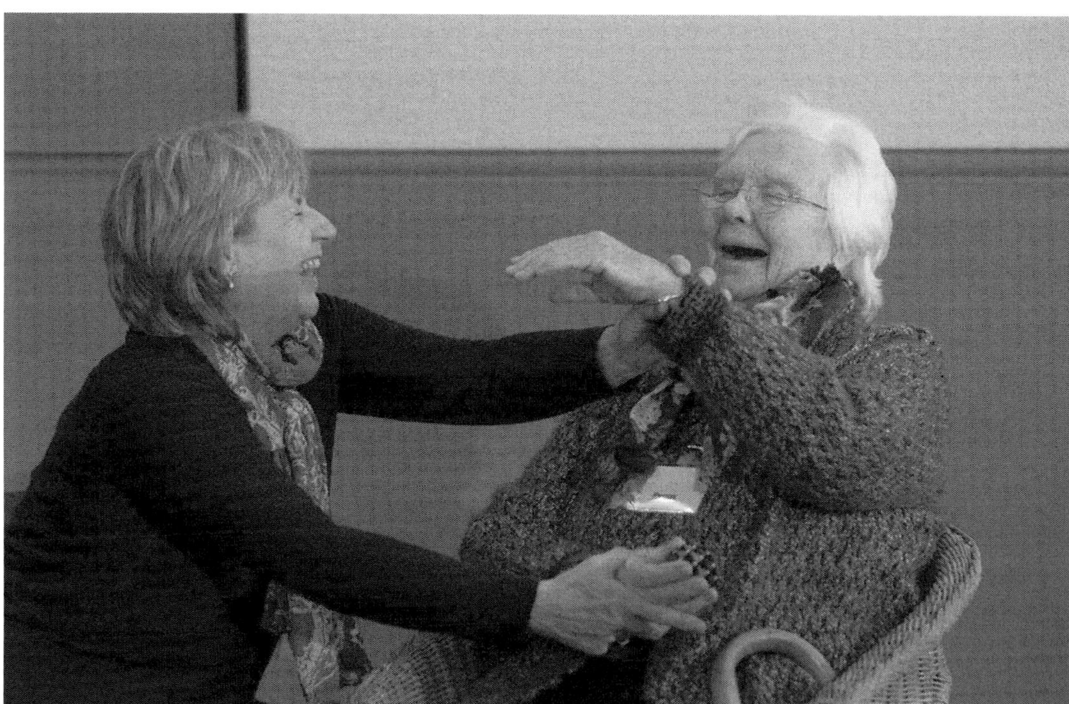

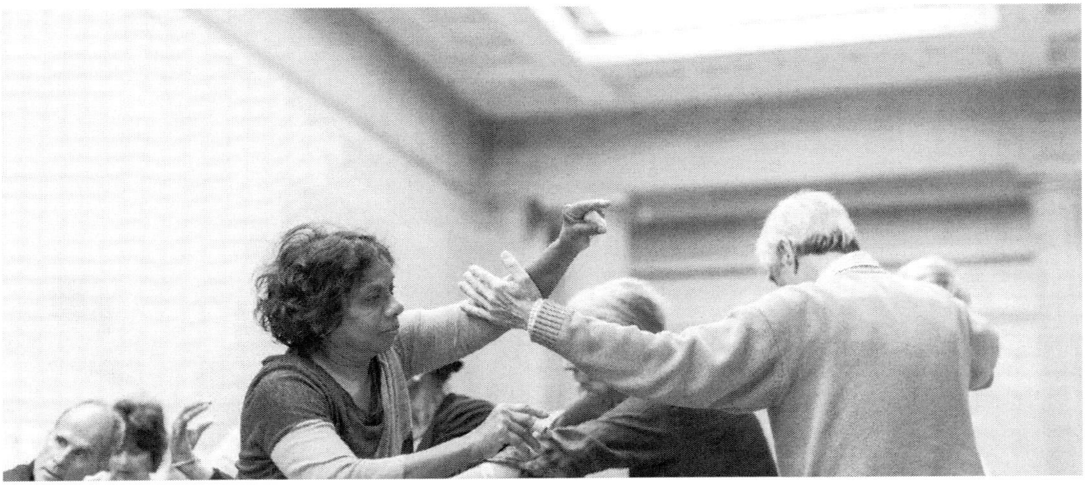

seems to enjoy (or at least meets me halfway with) a hug at Christmas or on her birthday, but not at other times. I haven't talked to her about it; this is based on noticing a slight step back or stiffening when someone has hugged her at other times.'

Explorations with touch

Tell a story with touch on your partner's back (drawn from Chris Thomson)

With the tips of your fingers... walk fingers... slowly along the landscape of shoulder blade... feel into the shape of bone ... touch like slow footsteps as the story unfolds... your partner may begin to move from sensation and story

J's left side burns, it is also numb, painful. We begin breathing together, then with her permission I rest my hands on her shoulder, and begin to walk my fingers slowly along the ridge of her left shoulder blade. With much laughter we map events from her childrens' lives into this painful shoulder - an escape to a tree house, an apple pie made at midnight. This game begins to bring new awareness into J's left side, overlaying the painful memories layered in her tissues .

YES…NO …PERHAPS
Lightly… place a hand on a shoulder or arm of a partner
Partner closes their eyes. Listen.
What do you notice? what qualities, textures, movements do you sense?

Moving gradually from passive to active
Allow the stimulation of touch to awaken movement – coming to meet the touch
Explore giving a direction in space to the touch
Choose: to go with... or against... Resistance can offer as much as compliance/ acceptance...

Alternate between... going with... doing nothing... pushing back
Imagine...yourself as support to your partner
Explore the range of touch from just a hand to a fuller contact.
Write or make from this

Reflex ...jump *(a wake-up game)*
Offer a touch to a partner – partner responds – vary the quality of stimulus... of response... allow your response to surprise yourself and the other person
Some of the options when touched:
Echo... follow... counter... give way... take over
Resist... go against... refuse movement –
Be passive / go flop / allow –
Go with / follow / cooperate –
Initiate / take the lead

Blind sight - from Lucia Walker
In pairs: one closes their eyes and lays hands on another
Partner with eyes open... slowly begin to move
Partner with eyes closed... follow with touch
Let your hands: float... find... rest... be carried... inquire

There is a surprising beauty when the one who is touching simply follows the mover, their hands riding, floating, on the movement, listening, following wherever it is going – and the sudden freedom for the mover, feeling heard, followed.

Two stories : movement and touch in hospital from Filipa Pereira-Stubbs

C, a young nineteen year old, had lost ability to feel, to control muscles and ligaments. We met on the neurorehabilitation ward. No one knew how his disease had begun, what was happening or what would happen next. He was in limbo; he and his family were stunned.

'When I first met him, he flopped torso and limbs into motion, with very little control and much frustration.

We have been working together for over five weeks. Accompanying his physiotherapy regime is the weekly dance session. Having initially vigorously denied any interest in music and movement, he is now the first to turn up in his wheelchair, giving himself over fully to the session and eagerly putting in music requests for the following week.

The magic for C happened when he realised I wasn't going to tell him what to do. Instead, I have asked him how he wanted to move. I have fitted my fingers and hands to the tiny and tentative shapes and movements he could make. Maintaining a steady and calm energetic focus, I consistently and repeatedly reminded him that I could feel his movement under my fingers, and he, in turn, eventually would be able to feel my fingers.

We found ways of clasping wrists and forearms so that together we could use the music to enter into swinging and swaying torso movements. We found that guitar-solo sounds could propel arms into windmill movements – and with time, we enjoyed more and more that the lifting of arms could be slower, deliberate, shaping the space around us – expressing our delight in brash dance anthems.

In our latest sessions, C's fingertips have indeed begun to respond to mine – flutterings of feeling and sensation – enough for us to trace the melodies and rhythms of the songs together. Enough for us to coordinate torso with limbs. Enough for us to be delighting in dancing together.

J has left hospital, but comes to the movement sessions, inspired by C's progress. Having lived for ten years with a paralysed side, thinking she must have suffered a stroke of some kind or another, she was finally informed that, in fact, she had been living with a brain tumour which caused her paralysis. At the age of 80, having opted for an extensive operation to remove the tumour, she now finds herself not only recovering from the operation, but having to restore her body to movement.

Her daughter is vigilant and determined to help her mother find her way back to movement. J comes to the sessions, joins in, but always seemed clouded by exhaustion and aching pain. Despite my invitation for her to slow down and find a softer pace of movement, she kept forcing herself. Finally, last week, during one of our more meditative movement tasks, I asked her to close her eyes whilst I cradled her head with my hands. I held her jaw and top of the neck/spine lightly. I asked her to let me hold her head *for* her, and for her to give her tight shoulders permission to let go – I would look after her head for her.

Under the touch of the tips of my fingers, I felt her gradually yield and release tension. She began to sway her head softly and slowly side to side, tipping weight one way and another. Really listening. I reminded her to move slowly and really feel the sensation of weight shifting. Her breath became fuller, and her whole body settled into itself as she brought her focus to her head. After just a couple of minutes, her head was moving with fluidity and softness – the first time I had experienced her move naturally – unforced, unlaboured. She found ease. She found connection. When the song came to an end, I sat down next to her. She looked at me with wide eyes, pain-free, shining. The rest of the group sat very quietly, sensing the clear shift of potential in this little old lady.

The practice of saying 'yes' ... Eva Karczag

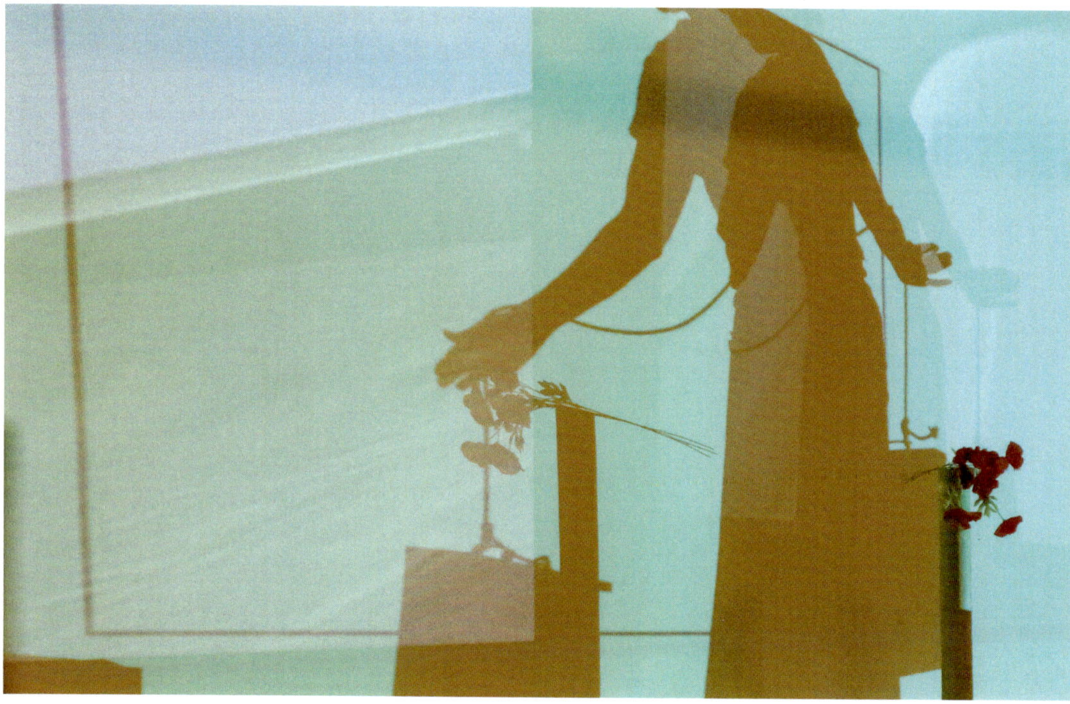

When I was 6 my parents said yes to the unknown. During a time of political upheaval and revolution, they left family, friends, language, culture, the life they had known, and travelled halfway round the world to begin life anew. In the new country, faced with a new culture and a new language, I watched them say yes to any and all possibilities that came their way, in order to create a safe and secure life for us. We internalise experiences and this helps shape the course of our lives.

The skull balances on top of the atlas (the topmost vertebra of the curved and lengthening spine), on two small feet, the occipital condyles. The skull's two feet settle into two indentations that receive them, creating a joint, a place of movement. This relationship of head and atlas gives rise to the movement of head rocking delicately forward and backward, the tiniest nodding action, the yes, that frees head and neck, and leads the body into movement.

consider emptiness — being open, available, willing
consider fullness — being full of possibility, full of movement.

empty ... and ... full
full ... and ... empty

this is the practice of saying 'yes' to any possibility that presents itself

When I was in my early 20s, I said yes to the unknown. During a time of questioning, of searching for the kind of dancing that allowed me to feel well in my body, right in myself, I left the forms of dancing I knew, and began a long process of un-learning. I was undoing the patterns I had learned and practiced in order to be able to discover how to embody my own body and moving. Whenever I have said 'no' to ways of working that did not sit well with me, I have also said 'yes' to practices that gave me more space, more freedom, more possibilities to explore and inhabit more fully who I am.

The atlas rests on the axis, the second vertebra. It slips down onto the small upwardly projecting bony shaft of the axis, surrounding it like a ring. At this joint, the movement turns from side to side, a no. In the body, yes lies above no, no below yes.

consider weight and generosity in giving, and say yes to weight
consider breath and generosity in taking and returning, and say yes to breathing
consider energy and abundance, and say yes to energy

consider having arrived and say 'yes' to generosity in presence and availability

this is the practice of saying 'yes' to any possibility that presents itself

As I began to explore and understand my own body, how it is intimately connected to my thinking, feeling and imaginative self, I found my breathing expanding and deepening.

Twenty-four finely curved ribs form the flexible, moving basket that contains our lungs and heart. On each breath, each finger-like rib articulates at the joint where it connects to the spine, and moves, expanding upward and outward on the in-breath, emptying and softly floating downward on the out-breath, to hang like branches of pine trees moving in the wind.

this is an expanded, expansive state, where movement is a given
any kind of movement ... small/large ... fast/slow ... tight/loose ... hard/soft
energetic/languid ... on the floor/ in the air ... in one spot/ covering a lot of space

this is the practice of saying 'yes' to any possibility that presents itself

As I continued searching and exploring the practices I encountered, I began to discover clarity in my direction. I could inhabit my love of creating work and performing, and I could engage with my curiosity about the miracle of the body, and through deepening my understanding hone it to become responsive, articulate and expressive. I could go this way ... and this way ... different interests feeding each other and fuelling my passion for moving.

The hip joint is the meeting and settling of the round ball head of the thigh bone into the deep cup, container of the hip socket. Here torso and legs connect. When torso is free to follow the upward direction of the head, this way, legs can be free to hang downward, this way, to become hanging supports. Hip joint can then become a spacious and open place, allowing for free movement of limbs and torso, and opening multidirectional possibilities for the whole moving body.

yes — I'll try going this way — yes
yes — I'll find out what this feels like — yes
yes — I'll explore this even though I don't yet know what it is — yes

this is the practice of saying 'yes' to any movement — whatever it might be
yes — this is the practice of expanding horizons
and of saying 'yes' to any possibility that presents itself

My work involves travel, moving around the world, living in many cultures, meeting many people. In order to not feel uprooted and ungrounded, I need to find my roots anywhere and everywhere I happen to find myself. There was a time when I began to realise that home is my body. When I can place my feet firmly on the ground, I know I have arrived.

The twenty-six delicate bones of the foot form an exquisitely articulated structure that makes moving on uneven terrain as possible as moving on flat ground. The arches of each foot ensure that strength and flexibility are available to us each time we take a step.

this is a place where there is no judgment — no thinking about should or can't
this is a place where moving is
this is a place where body is doing the speaking,
where body finds its eloquence
a place of 'kinaesthetic delight'

this is the practice of saying 'yes' to any possibility that presents itself

as you begin to think of moving,
let this be the practice of saying 'yes' to any and all possibilities that present themselves.

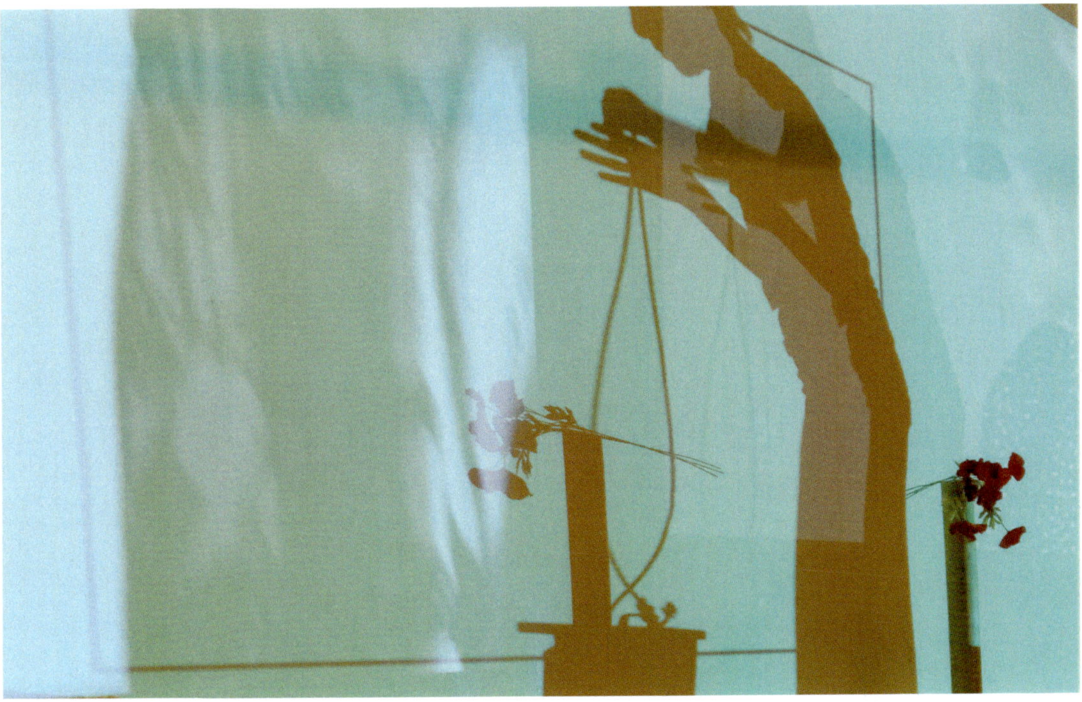

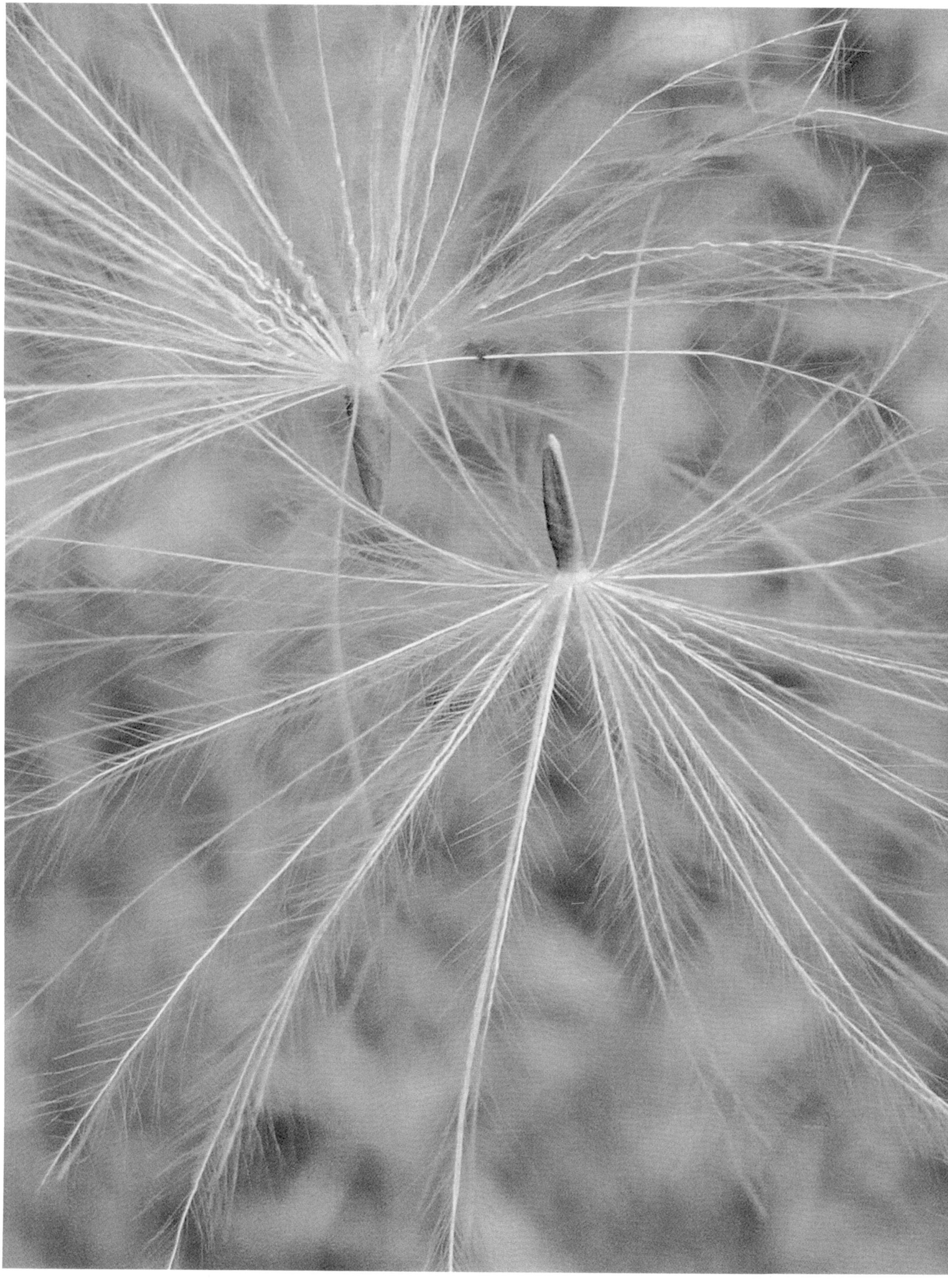

Between you and me ... working one-to-one

He returns to Lilian. He bends over her once more, his hand touching her skin. He listens with his stethoscope one more time. He listens with every fibre of his being, he listens to what he imagines Lilian is telling him: there are registers and nuances, he is taking into himself what he hears, sound, pulsing, knocking at him, brushing him. He listens with and without the stethoscope. He taps. What he hears, he touches; he observes a rhythm that is not sound but movement, a great throb of movement, two hearts beating here in this body – or three, his own joining. He is overwhelmed by the heartbeats; he is taking the combat of each beat into his own, his heart is swollen, he will burst. But what he wants more than anything is to suspend this moment, to keep this moment from evolving, to stay with these three hearts beating, patiently, sounding as regularly as bells. He and Lilian: a listening pair.

From the novella *Send* by Kay Syrad

The work in this chapter outlines something of the potency of relationship in strengthening a person's resources. Regaining confidence in one's body can help a person feel more able to cope and manage their circumstances. An artists' multi-dimensional, improvisatory approach supports communication, play and relaxation which helps reduce the fear and aloneness experienced by many when faced by the unpredictability of illness. An empathic and creative relationship strengthens each of us (and is perhaps the basis of the long recognised power of placebo).

Creating connection

"Welcome to the island of small things
where every movement becomes a dance
where transformation and learning is individual
where both action and rest have the same value"
Susanna Recchia, dance artist

Small Things Dance Collective is a Dance in Health initiative formed by Cath Hawkins and Lisa Dowler. For over nine years they have been working a day a week with children at Alder Hey Hospital, Liverpool. In the financially pressured climate the sustained nature of this project is a small miracle. It is also a tribute to the dedication of the artists and the trust the hospital health team feel for their work and its contribution to the wellbeing of children in their care. Lisa and Cath work across three hospital wards. In Cardiac and Orthopaedic they work with children and young people both before and in the days following their surgery. They also work in Neuromedical where patients are undergoing rehabilitation for neurological conditions such as acquired brain injury or complex and multiple learning disabilities. These patients can be long-term – they may work with children for over six months.

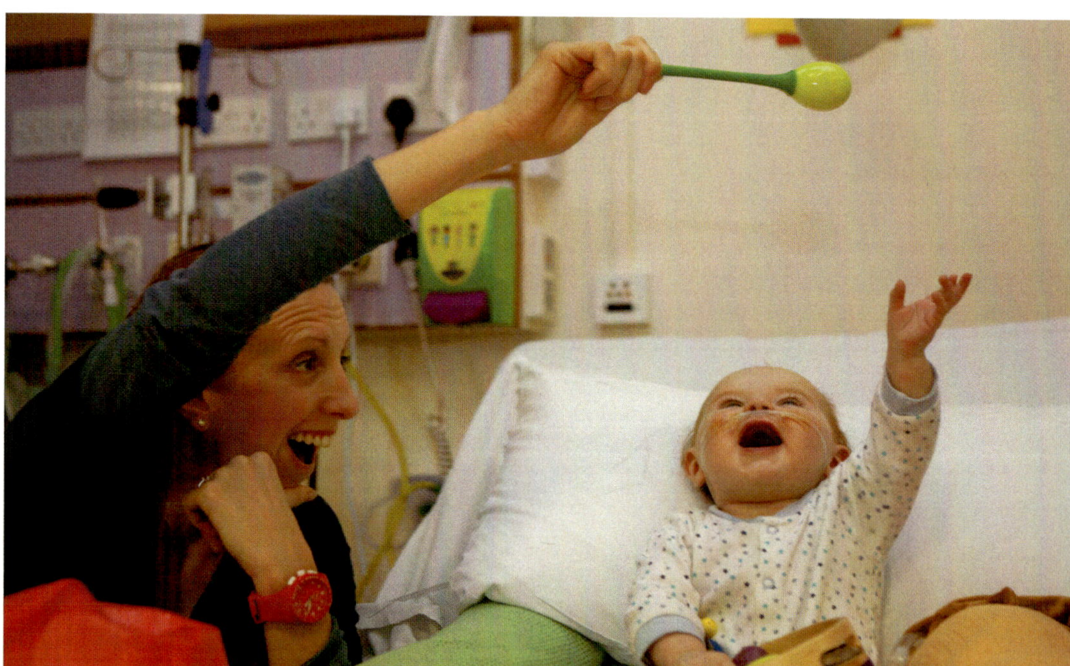

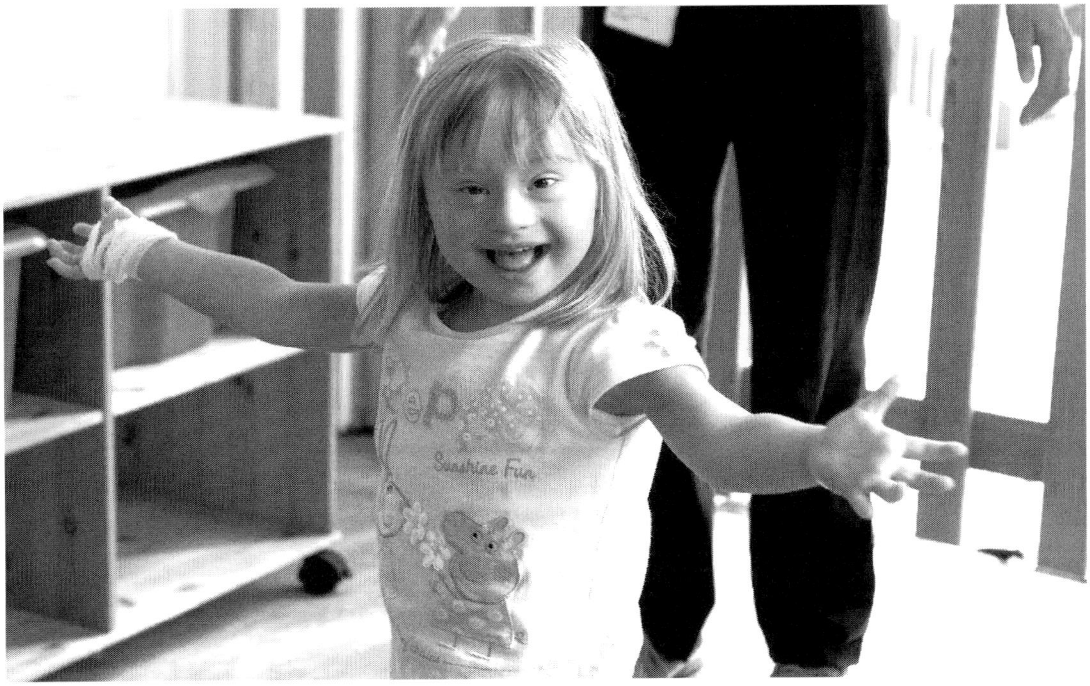

The name of their company, 'Small Things', perfectly reflects an approach of engaging through the small, fragile, often barely perceptible movements that give expression to a child's world. In a target-driven culture where bland and often grandiose slogans have become the norm, it is a relief to witness work that is unassuming and tender – work which listens respectfully and creatively to the children in hospital and can bring about profound shifts in their well being.

Arriving with Cath and Lisa in the morning there are requests from staff on different wards to go to patients the health team feel will benefit. Cath goes to work with a child in pain and awaiting surgery. Seeing the girl later on the ward, she is now cheerful, managing the unfamiliar environment and has recovered enough resilience and confidence to initiate games with Cath, Lisa and another child awaiting heart surgery.

A story: listening for movement

Lisa visits a young boy with an acquired brain injury following a road traffic accident. The boy is in isolation due to a stomach infection. His grandmother is present, attending him most days since the accident. Lisa greets the boy gently but warmly. He is lying somewhat awkwardly in a wheelchair. There is a slight flicker of response in his eyes. He has a code – closing his left hand for No, a blink for Yes. Lisa chats quietly to both the boy and his grandmother, then puts on some music and gently places her hands on his left leg. Her hands are quiet, respectful, listening. They mould to his calf and ankle. She asks how it feels, and waits for the blink that gives permission to go on. Her hands move, touching and sometimes gently moving his limbs. Her contact is quiet and though her hands seem still, they are listening and following micro movements – movements invisible to the eye but palpable to the trained hand. Colour seems to brighten the boy's pale face, his breathing deepens as he relaxes. Then his left leg becomes active – small jerks and jumps that signal this habitually inert leg may be regaining nerve impulse and connection. Later in conversation Lisa ponders how it might be if this boy could receive listening touch every day – might it speed recovery. (see another account of this in Harry's story part 4)

A story: working with pain

There is another request for Lisa and Cath to visit a child in palliative care. E is wary and in great pain. Her eyes are dark and watchful. She is not sure she wants them there and is fearful of yet more pain. Cath's presence is quiet, kind. Her movements are gentle and slowly paced. She lowers herself down beside the bed – so as to not stand over the child – and tells her what they might do and that they will stop immediately if she is uncomfortable. The child can choose moment by moment; this reassures her. Slowly Cath and Lisa roll soft balls along E's legs. The gentle, indirect contact seems to ease E's pain, and she begins to breathe more fully. She then takes a ball and rolls it for herself, enjoying the stimulus. This easing of fear and anxiety must seem to an anxious parent like a small miracle; to witness their child regain ease and confidence. In E's case, there is a bubbling up of words, of reaching out to the dancers with questions, suggestions of more movements, and sharing of other experiences – games played at home, that link this child back to her familiar world.

Staff comment on how much Lisa and Cath's work relieves pain[1]. This is not their specific intention, but comes about indirectly through the way their work encourages breath and subtle movement. They often begin with light touch, which relaxes and brings a sense of being listened to. Tissues held tight with pain and apprehension begin to yield, soften. In hospital a child is inevitably subjected to the pushings and proddings of medical procedures. The non-invasive, non-directive touch that Lisa and Cath use, opens the door back into feeling and play, a dialogue without words that offers choice and helps restore a child's sense of autonomy.

[1] With support from the hospital's Research Department, the Pain Service and Play Specialists, they devised a mixed method study across the three wards. Using validated pain assessment tools appropriate to the patients' ability to communicate, an assessment of patient's pain was made before and after the somatic dance session by a third party. 92% experienced a reduction in pain and for 80% this was more than a 50% reduction.

Qualities of presence

Spacious flexible curious comfortable sensitive grounded responsive creative compassionate playful interested

Lisa and Cath are unhurried and infinitely patient in their work. There is no sense of needing to achieve something. They embody a quiet spaciousness of presence attuning to each child they meet with. Paradoxically, in not trying to achieve specific outcomes – by their very acceptance and availability to the moment of a child's situation – they bring about subtle yet profound changes in a child's state of being. Consultants, play specialists and clinical nurse specialists, from the hospital pain and sedation service, recognise the value of this work in relieving pain, and calming and relaxing their patients.

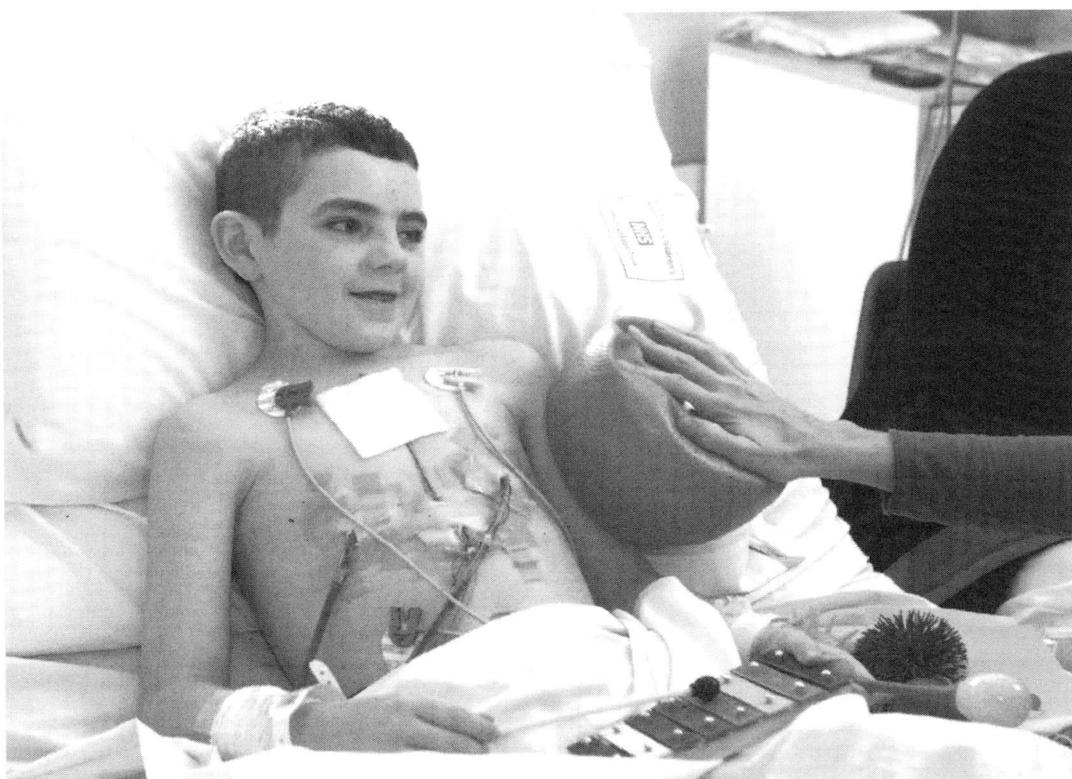

A doctor's response

'Participatory dance in paediatric healthcare settings is unusual. Emotional engagement with the dancers and their use of interesting and colourful props generated a very positive volitional element in infants, children and young people. Movement was achieved in a more relaxed way, with less effort, muscle tension and pain. In children and young people who had increased muscle tone and associated paucity of volitional movement, the environment promoted more spontaneity and relaxation, which in turn increased achievement, and in some instances exceeded results obtained with passive physiotherapy. Even with the use of tailored analgesia informed by the use of paediatric pain scoring tools following surgery, a reluctance to move may be associated with the anticipation that it will be painful. The dance programme was described by patients as something which was fun and provided welcome distraction from clinical routine...

Parents and carers were very keen for their children and young people to be involved in the dance programme because of the benefits they observed. The impact on healthcare staff was threefold. In addition to reduced requirements for analgesia and more rapid mobilisation, they saw how the ward environment was altered in a positive way by the multi-dimensional approach of the dancers.' Dr Jane Radcliffe, Paediatrician

An account from the work of Protein Dance Company

I visited another hospital project: Protein Dance Company was running a six week project in Evelina Children's Hospital, London.

A child is lying huddled in her bed. She is recovering from spinal surgery and has been lying still for a long time, too frightened to move. Parents and health support team are attempting to woo her into action.

A dancer, Jon Beney, is also present. He sits quietly observing, and then begins chat to the child, gradually discovering that she will get a dog when she is out of hospital. They talk about possible names, and he shares his own children's experience of having a pet. Slowly he is sensing and acknowledging her fear through this conversation. He is taking what might seem a sideways approach to gain her trust in him, in order to regain trust in herself. He will lead the way, but first she must trust him. There's a silent message conveyed beneath the words: 'I am listening to you, I hear your anxiety, I am here as a playmate to find a way through this terror'. There is no rush, no direct focus on 'the issue'.

Jon suggests she imagines taking her new puppy out for a walk and begins to initiate a teasing, playful game with ribbons. The ribbons swing by the child and she cannot resist joining in, reaching out to catch these dancing silks. Then she too takes a wand and dances these bright ribbons. Engaged joyfully in play, the child gradually begins to forget her fear. The movement engages her breathing, energising and stimulating the wider supporting networks of muscles that move her arms – a muscle field that includes her whole spine and that gradually enables her, without premeditated thought, to sit up.

Jon is patient, never pushing her in the activity. He uses the utmost delicacy and gentleness to stimulate and reawaken the child's own responses – kindling a playful physicality that connects to the child's whole body – and may enable her to trust moving again.

Jon senses and echoes the child's initial micro-movements in an unspoken, but palpable, 'I am with you' and the child, feeling so subtly supported and recognised, dares to move further. His work encourages small steps, a playful calling out to movement through which the child may feel able to move forward in her recovery.

As she becomes absorbed in this game, the child forgets her fear and moves to the edge of her bed. And Jon, like the Pied Piper, continues, moving fractionally ahead of her, getting up on a chair so he is tall and high above her. Playing with ribbons like a fishing line he invites her to reach up – to be as tall as he is – and she, engaged imaginatively in this game, dares to stand.

Later in the day Jon returns. The child is now moving around the ward, she is playing with a toy dog. Seeing Jon she chases after him.

A story: a dream of wrestling

C is a young boy and another patient in the same hospital. His body seems awkward with discomfort and entirely dependent on the support of his wheelchair. His eyes are great dark pools in a finely boned expressive face. Over the days that they meet, the dancers pick up on his passionate interest in American wrestling and they devise a fight scenario, whereby C becomes an active participant in the 'fight'. His wheelchair is swung and looped in response to the dancers' fight moves. A dancer makes his own body an imaginative extension of C's, so that in this game, C can imagine himself swinging out with blows and punches. It is an extraordinary and generous feat of imagination that the dancers conjure. These dancers are happy to go down to the floor, or to be upside down. They are physical ventriloquists, able to speak in many voices and characters.

C's mother speaks of her happiness on seeing her son's face animated and smiling. She has not seen him smile for five months. She says: 'Because of his condition he is always left out – on the side – you made him the centre.

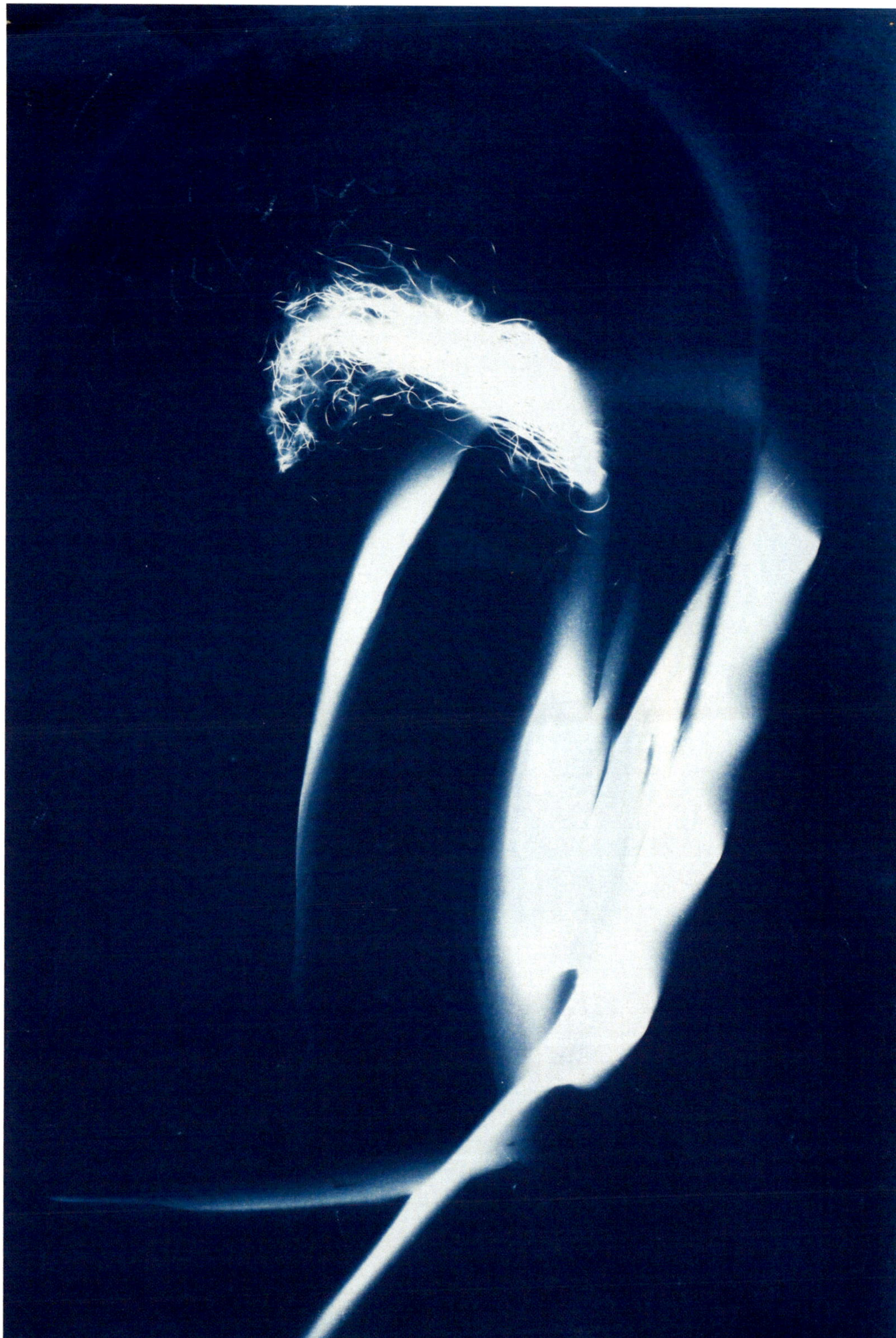

He has so little body movement and yet he was able to follow and repeat the dancer's instructions.' Such comments express the immense value a parent felt in the work.

> It is a very sensitive situation working in a hospital environment, coming in as someone who isn't medically trained. I need to make sure I understand the situation as fully as possible – and understand what the physiotherapist's are wanting to achieve with a child. Wherever possible I talk to the family, to build their trust in what we are doing.... what matters is to find a way to personally engage a child. This work is not so much about 'dance' in the usual sense but always about taking time to connect – sensing what the child wants to do, and following where they lead... It is about being able to enter a child's world, whether their interest is in rugby, wrestling or a particular band.
>
> Summarised from conversations with Jon Beney,
> Protein Dance Company

A listening presence

> Do you have the patience to wait
> Till your mud settles and your waters become clear.
> Can you remain unmoving
> Till the right action arises by itself
>
> Lao Tzu

Time, patience and trust lie at the heart of this work; time to breathe and get in tune with another person, feeling moment-by-moment for a sense of direction, for where communication can grow. It is a delicate and challenging process requiring bodily empathy and every tool in an improviser's toolbox – and the utmost sensitivity to fears and vulnerabilities. Listening for clues as to what might engage a person, going slowly and carefully, listening deeply with every cell of your own body, yet keeping the field of attention wide, gentle, spacious. (Too focused or narrow attention can be claustrophobic) Listening for response in the other person, in whatever form it comes, to guide what is always an emerging process.

Much change occurs in the alchemy of listening; a listening not simply to words but a listening throughout the body; sensing the imaginative feel of another's world. A bodily and imaginative empathy is latent in us all, though often obscured and discounted. In feeling heard and recognized a person can settle, relax, and come home to themselves.

Finding an opening
Listen... for what is familiar, cherished, loved,
A recently viewed film... a story from childhood... a hobby
And above all listen for what feels well, despite pain or illness

Dancers and artists working in the field of health are not seeking to 'cure', but to connect to a person's lifeworld; seeking out the particular and personal and in so doing, strengthening what is well. The work draws on a choreographic sensitivity to the shifting dynamic of relationship and a responsiveness to what may be barely perceptible, nuanced changes in a person – changes in skin tone, brightening of eyes, uncurling of fingers – signals of pleasure or pain. As in a conversation, each encounter unfolds through a moment-by-moment awareness of the subtleties of response; these are co-creative improvisational approaches that seek to engage senses and imagination. It takes the utmost delicacy and gentleness never to push or force an activity – as if blowing gently on the embers of a small fire to kindle trust, delight and curiosity. Artists working within these fragile communities are responsive companion, available to meet and explore alongside – a quality of exchange and reciprocity that is essential to establishing trust. People comment on feeling themselves again, something so easily lost in the challenges of living with illness.

> **Working on oncology** is hugely varied, interesting, challenging and exciting. I have met many different patients, from four-month-old babies to young men and women who have leukaemia, tumours, or are having bone marrow transplants...I'm often asked what I do and I have begun to answer that I listen – and that enables me to offer a response that can include touch, play, movement, creativity, dancing and more. Cancer seems to create distance. I see children and young people distanced from their bodies and, in responding to this, I am lucky enough to watch that disassociation, that gap, close up.
>
> Cath Hawkins, independent dance artist

Curiosity from Latin *curiosus* careful, diligent, curious, akin to *cura* care – a quality related to inquisitive thinking such as exploration, investigation, and learning. Curiosity is associated with all aspects of human development.

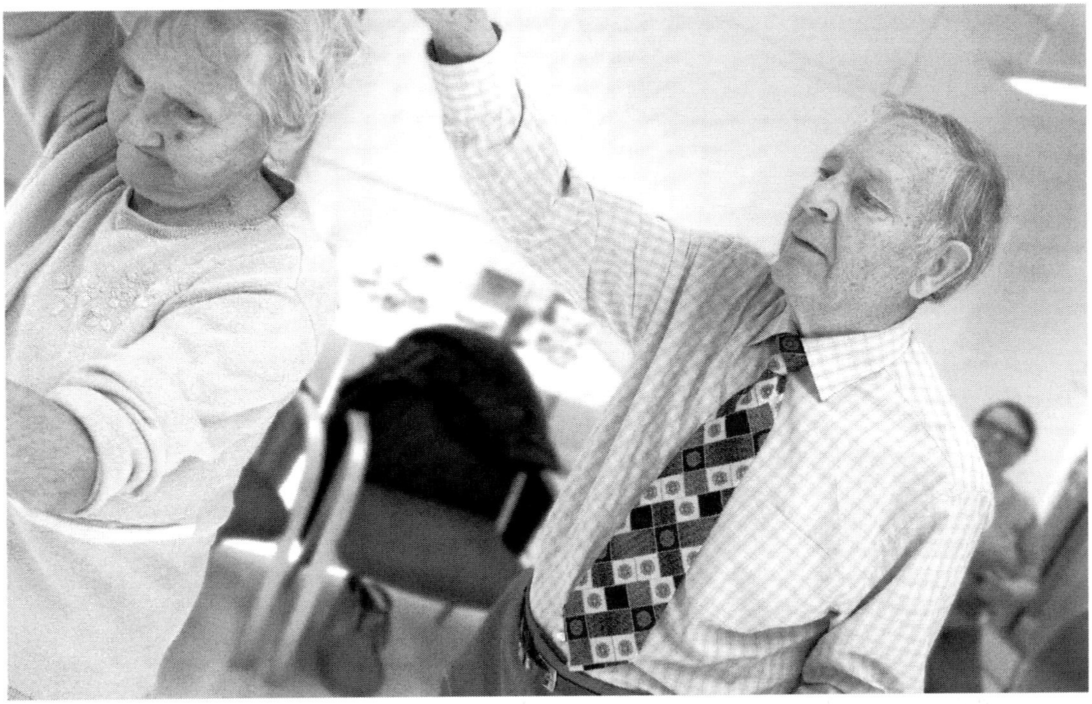

To sense and connect with the silent needs and messages of another's body depends on imaginative and bodily empathy. The living body shimmers with subtle pulsations, barely perceptible movements, shifting qualities and energies. Bodily empathy involves a 'putting on' of the other, an imaginative sympathy for what is conveyed through another's body and a capacity to engage creatively however restricted or compromised their physicality. This is not 'dance' in the conventional sense, but rather communication through movement and the body. Somatic approaches train a bodily listening that is highly sensitive to these bodily movement tones and patterns. Practitioners trained through these approaches listen for micro-movements invisible to the eye yet palpable to touch. Developing a person's awareness of these subtle inner movements relaxes and stimulates blood flow, bringing about a settling and whole body reorganisation – and often an easing of pain. Whatever the situation, being able to go under or beneath illness, reaching for what feels well helps a person reconnect with their resources however buried and obscured.

Sense... underlying form... structure... anatomy
Sense the shape and form of a part
Sense... the relationship of that part... to what is around it... to the whole
Sense... breath... movement... and the space around the body
Imagine your partner as landscape... as weather... as a piece of music.

Presence and the dynamics of attention

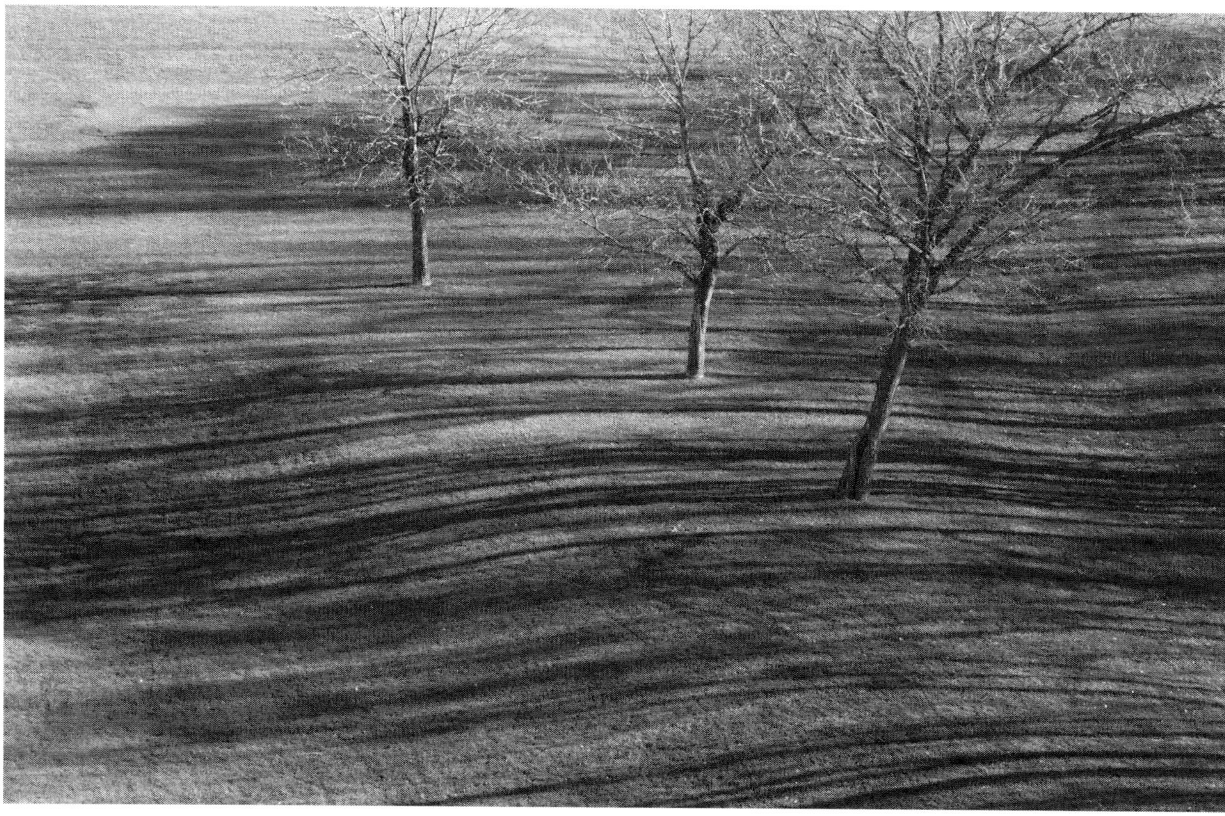

'I who am in the end, a continual dialogue...'
Fernando Pessoa, *Introducing Alvaro de Campos*, poem 445

How effectively we meet and connect creatively with another is determined in a large part by how we are in ourselves and the relational field we create through our presence. The quality and spaciousness of our own presence and attention profoundly affects what happens in a session, so much is communicated simply through resonance. Cultivating self-awareness takes time but is a vital step in being able to perceive the feelings and subtle forces moving through another. Many of us live rushed and crowded lives and it can be difficult to take the necessary time to quieten the mind and get in tune with our own breath and body. Yet this establishes a safe and responsive space when working in contexts where people are fragile and thus easily overwhelmed.

> I sit beside Matt as he struggles to speak about moving. I become very quiet inside and I notice my concern for there to be enough time for him to say what he needs to say. As I become quieter, I have a sense of my ears opening and there is also a moment of orientation as I try to focus on what is being said. This is accompanied by a slight increase of tone in my body, as though I feel I need to become more alert. What if I let go of this? What is happening now? My body, my attention softens and I am aware of the tingling of my skin and it is almost as though I can feel the micro-vibrations as the waves of sound play in my inner ear. The words are barely carried on Matt's breath. I speak them quietly back to him. He remembers waking up after surgery. He continues – but then the effort seems too great.
>
> Kathy Crick, Art Of Touch project

> Switching mind states is hard. This work demands the utmost moment-by-moment focus from me. I notice how busy I am in my everyday life and find it hard to make the switch to the presentness demanded by this work...It is challenging – feeling the moment when things can go forward - when it is right to make suggestions, when to offer something new, or when it is best to simply *be with* a person and wait till they initiate.
>
> Helga Kutter and Susanna Recchia, dancers, Art of Touch Project in hospice with Rosetta Life

Widening the field of attention

Breathe... take time to settle...
Open... the length and axis of your spine... from head to tail

Open... the width and depth of your body... between spine and breastbone
Between left and right shoulder...

Breathe... let there be space... movement... inside

Feel the air... outside your body... feel your edges
Front... back... side... below... above

Notice... what is at the periphery of what you see

Let the field of your attention spread outwards... to the room... and beyond the room... To landscape... to sky... to horizon

Let your attention 'breathe'... expanding outwards... drawing inwards systole... diastole... between horizon... and the inner chambers of your body Notice... in each phase what happens in your body...
In what you notice... feel... around you...

Our attention tends to lock into one modality, often narrow and focused as when we read a book or work on a computer. Yet for creativity to flourish we need to loosen our everyday functional and purposive mind – and let the field of attention 'breathe', widen, be curious. Then, like opening a window and letting in fresh air, our eyes begin to see differently, we discover new possibilities and perspectives.

> I always begin each session with bringing participants in their wheelchairs to the windows and we look out, notice the weather, cloud patterns, qualities of light. This always stimulates discussion and brings people together.
>
> Filipa Pereira-Stubbs

On skills of attention – Lisa Dowler

Important skills for me to enable this work include being able to stay with yourself and your own coordination/process/interest in moving, whilst connecting to others simultaneously. For me, there can be a strong pull to lose touch with myself as I zoom in to another who I perceive to be unwell, in pain or frail, my attention can move towards them and away from myself

Practices from Contact Improvisation have been particularly helpful for me in developing skills in listening to another and allowing myself to be witnessed/listened to at the same time ... we find shared movement and play within the contact

Somatic practices involving refined touch increase our ability to read permission from another, spoken through the body ... that is being sensitive to 'No' or 'Yes' with touch or participation and being able to not 'take it personally', to let your ideas go and give space for something else.

The bodily empathy that underpins this work requires being able to hold dual awareness

– to sense and feel with another, yet also to stay connected to self and surroundings. It involves balancing attention 50-50 between self and other; it is easy to get lost in another person's state of being and lose vital awareness of the space between and around you and another, which can intensify symptoms and overwhelm a person. A spacious lightness of attention enables change and lays the foundation for the safety, groundedness and creative possibility of a session.

Monty Roberts is a horse whisperer, a celebrated and much sought after 'trainer' of horses. He talks of his way of working as 'joining up' with the horse, a process of observing, sensing and connecting with an animal (in direct contrast to the more common practice of 'breaking' a horse).[2] 'Don't look an animal directly in the eye or come at it head on – that challenges a horse. Approach in a relaxed, meandering way. Let your focus drift out to the fence or to other animals. A horse will pick up all your thinking – and if you are anxious or too focused it will run off.'

On preparing and embodiment

from Penny Collinson, course leader, MA Dance & Somatic Wellbeing, University of Central Lancashire:

Before I work with another person I do a number of things to awaken my body and to be receptive and in relationship. This always involves a shift in me from thinking and doing into sensing and being. And from movement which is functional and pedestrian towards movement or actions which emerge out of stillness and intuition. I have to shift my perspective in order to get a clearer 'signal' from my body's antennae. Surprisingly this process of transition can begin with the smallest of things, such as taking a walk which is not purposeful but more about the quality with which my feet meet the ground, the weight of my arms as they swing and the movement of my rib cage caused by my breath.

Dancers and somatic movement practitioners become very practiced at guiding their awareness toward sensory experience – so that in working with others they may pick up on the tiniest of impulses

Whenever I work with a person I *never* know what will happen. I can't possibly know the fullness of what is happening for another, or what I might bring to the encounter. So I listen to the signals in my own body... they tell me... *wait... be still... move closer... touch here... move away... be silent... ask...*

I work one-on-one with people in a small studio space. It's not therapy or dancing, it's body-time. It's dedicated time to listening to what is going on

[2] He is an American, trained the Queen's horses, and though 80 years old, travels worldwide teaching people how to interact more sensitively and effectively with horses (he and his wife Pat have also fostered 47 children along the way).

outside and inside, not to *think* about it but to perceive it through other ways of being. In doing this, there can be a sense of reconnecting to the world around us and to the world within. A part of what I do in practice is to become aware of my own sensations, movements, emotional feeling, images that arise as I attend to another.'

Moving outside the box: art's medicine

'I cannot add years to your life, but can I add life to your years?'
Sandy Crichton, dance artist, *Jabadao*

What is the difference between these approaches and other kinds of therapy, physiotherapy or hands-on healing techniques? I feel the answer lies with intention; an artist seeks to engage creatively with what is well in a person, rather than their illness. Intuition, play and a quality of acceptance lie at the heart of this work and paradoxically are what can initiate change. By not trying to heal, DO, problem solve, or 'make things better' – but through listening and offering a creative and receptive space, a person's own resources are able to surface. This can bring about a profound shift in a person from the passivity of being a patient into artist[3] creatively engaged with the art of being alive, of being well.

Recover: (Thesaurus) get better, get well, convalesce, regain one's strength, regain one's health, get stronger, get back on one's feet, feel oneself again, get back to normal, return to health; be on the mend, be on the road to recovery, pick up, rally, respond to treatment, make progress, improve, heal, take a turn for the better, turn the corner, get out of the woods, get over something, shake something off, pull through, bounce back, revive; pull round; perk up.

[3] I am indebted to Dr Richard Coaten for this phrasing.

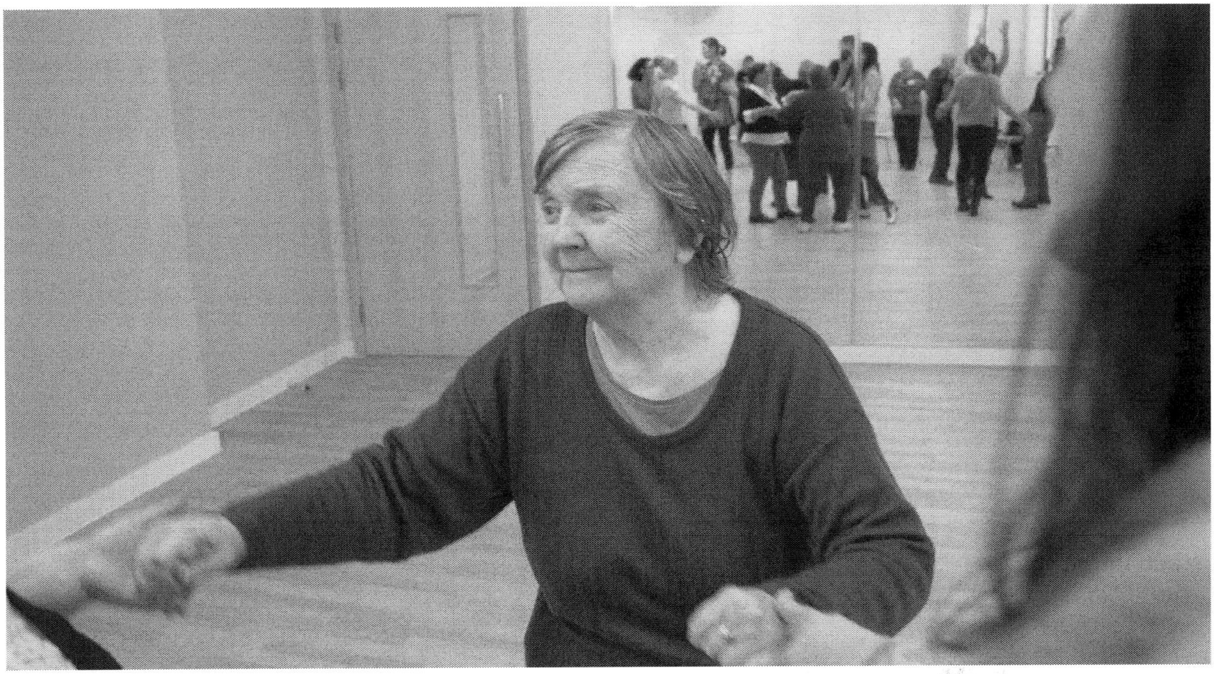

At the centre of our approach is intuition. Sanjani points out that whilst the 'intuitive and empathic practice of improvisation' may often not be considered significant within a world where emotion and practice are held to be inferior to reason and theory, the reality is we exist in a world of uncertainty..... thus for patients existing in a vulnerable place of ambiguity, improvisational practices, whereby they have choice, influence and are listened to, rather than compounding a sense of the unknown, can empower and foster a sense of self in a situation in which it is forces from outside themselves, which affect their future e.g. diagnostics and treatment. As skilled improvisers we are able to work outside of form and allow a session to evolve through intuition and relationship.

Lisa Dowler

Trust and consent: the need for stillness

Working with people with high dependency needs means it is often difficult to understand what a person is feeling. Without voice and, in many instances, without clear cognition, how can we know if we have consent? This is a highly sensitive issue. Being able to slow down, let go of all expectations or desire for outcome or change, establishes the ground for an answering resonance to be perceived. Changes in breath or body tone can signal connection and a willingness to engage. Dancers and artists with a somatic training develop a refined awareness of these fleeting changes in tone that signify pleasure or distress.[4] This depends on cultivating deep stillness and a quietly spacious presence.

> I've witnessed sensitivity in others that is breathtaking in its reach and accuracy. The precondition to sensitivity is stillness. In the same way that a pond on a still day will visibly register the smallest insect alighting on its surface, but on a windy day it won't, our ability to feel the whole is directly proportional to our ability to become still within ourselves.
>
> Phil Shepherd [5]

Keeping safe... the flow of emotion

Emotion: mid-16th c. denoting a public disturbance from French émotion, from émouvoir 'excite', based on Latin emovere, from e- 'out' + movere 'move' – the current sense dates from the early 19th century.

To engage with a creative process involves a letting go into the unknown; we cannot know what memories or vulnerabilities may surface. Emotions are always present in our bodies; grief, fear, anger, feelings we may not want to acknowledge, are often locked away within our tissues. When we engage with movement, the softening and freeing up of muscles and joints often brings emotion to the surface. Steadying awareness in the moment-by-moment physicality of the body and movement (rather than emotions) helps overwhelming feelings to flow and transform. Slowing down, staying connected to surrounding and to the movement of exhalation and inhalation helps transmute strong feelings. Quiet yet firm touch on shoulders or feet can help to ground (firm touch

[4] Thomas Hanna's definition of 'somatic' draws on the Greek soma meaning 'the living body'. Hanna defined 'somatics' as '*the human being experienced by him/herself* from the inside.' This should be distinguished from the medical and anatomical use of the term 'somatic' which relates to 'body' in a purely physical sense, the 'somatic nervous system' for example, relating to our voluntary and reflex muscular action – from a conversation with Gill Clarke.

[5] See Phil Shepherd, *New Self, New World: Recovering Our Senses in the Twenty-First Century.*

connects to bone which brings awareness of support within). Though we tend to suppress or hide tears, they 'break up what may otherwise break us down'.[6] Both tears and laughter increase blood flow and help discharge what may feel overwhelming emotions.

'There are no bad emotions, only stuck emotions.' Candace Pert

Research into heart rate variability shows that when we are stressed, the prefrontal cortex is switched off, the heart begins to race and our capacity to think clearly dissolves. Alan Watkins has described this condition as a 'DIY lobotomy'. Focusing on the exhalation phase of breath, automatically brings the diaphragm into deeper movement (and a steadying in-breath), which affects both gut and heart, and can begin to restore a sense of control, pace and rhythm.

A practical session for social workers from Penny Collinson

Recently, colleagues in Dance and Social Work collaborated on a pilot project teaching embodiment skills to social work students. Our sessions aimed to support students on placement to track their bodily experience as they prepared to meet service users. And afterwards to process, de-stress or re-ground if they felt overwhelmed. One participant spoke of how much empathy and compassion underpins their daily work, much time is spent listening and attending to service users' concerns. Our sessions showed students how to work with their breath, alignment and movement in order to attune to another. To become more perceptually and imaginatively engaged in sensing what was going on. So much of what clients feel and are concerned about never comes into words; sensitivity to body language is thus profoundly important.

We drew on many physical processes to bring a greater sense of orientation to space (in the body and outside of the body) and to rhythm, pace, tone, and flow. We emphasised a living sense of the body and identifying the quality of the relational field at all times.

One participant spoke of how these processes helped her to 'breathe properly' as she engaged with clients, a new skill and a useful resource. Another participant said it had later helped her with her 'anxious' service users to attune her own awareness of how people were in their homes, and how she listens to her body when she is with them. She noted 'being sharper with feelings', her own and her client's, 'being more aware of moods and atmosphere' and generally 'being slightly more switched on'.

Self-preparation is an issue for social workers. One woman described the importance of doing something to tune in prior to meeting the client

[6] Bani Shorter, Jungian analyst, in conversation.

because 'when you knock on people's doors, you don't know what you're going to meet'.[7]

A story: stillness and movement from Susie Tate, dance artist

Mary is the heart and soul of the dance sessions at the hospital. There is dance in every cell of her body: as she moves her eyes twinkle and a little dimple in her right cheek appears and disappears with her endearing smile. Between dancing, she tells stories that go back generations which are at once humorous and delightfully shocking!

Today Mary arrives later than the other participants. We pause to welcome her: she has been on the ward for three months so is a familiar face to many, but nevertheless, welcoming each person to the session where we are a community of people and not patients or staff, is paramount.

Mary rests back in her chair, her legs, which have little movement, are outstretched so her feet, encased in red woolly socks, do not touch the floor – she has not held her weight fully on the ground for many years. I notice her hands begin to dance, an elbow extends, a lift of her arm – but then dropped with a heavy sigh. No dance in her eyes or smile this Monday morning. No stories leading to raucous laughter from the group.

And her legs do not gently rock as they can in response to the motion from her upper body, but just lie with a heavy weighted stillness, which seems to have crept into her whole being. The softness and flow of movement that I know lives within Mary's body is not there today.

Later I asked Mary how she was feeling: 'not so good this morning'. 'I know' I replied. She began to cry.

I moved to her side and rested my hand on hers. We sat together, side by side and slowly I let my hand soften around hers.

As we sat, Mary with eyes now closed, I found myself leafing through my years of training and experiences to see where I could support her stillness, find the dance in her stillness. It lay in the connection of our hands, skin, and all that lies beneath the surface of the skin: water, blood, cells, pulse, breath.

A little lift of her fingers and I replied with a lift of mine, a stretch of hers a stretch of mine, a fold of hers and I envelope mine around. Mary rotates her hand so her palm is now facing upwards and mine is underneath. She turns to look at me, her eyes are lighter, a twinkle. I guide her hand up and there we are reaching high guiding each other with a light touch, pausing when we do, moving when we do.

[7] This text is drawn from work with Tim Lamford, Pat Cox, Dr Julian Manley, students from BA Social Work, and staff and students from Consensus, Preston.

In the hospital Mary is 'immobile'; in the dance sessions, she is still. Paradoxically, stillness is the starting point of all movement. An interest I have in these hospital sessions is in exploring how 'being still' can shift from a state of boredom, lethargy, or sadness to being the start of something else where the body is allowed to unfold if it wishes to, and stillness is given a sense of respect.

It has been said that stillness is the art of movement, but maybe stillness is the secret of movement. In dance, sitting with stillness I find opens space to listen to my body and in turn – in this story – to Mary's body and the quiet dances within.

There may have been chaos within Mary, upset or hurt that Monday. I do not know; I am not there to know but to be where she is and, if moving seems right, we will move, if not, we will find the gentle movement that lies within stillness.

Mary's dance today may have been a fleeting light in an otherwise grey morning, or not. But it was a small journey from a still point where a connection was made and where words were not needed, but by listening a meeting point was found.

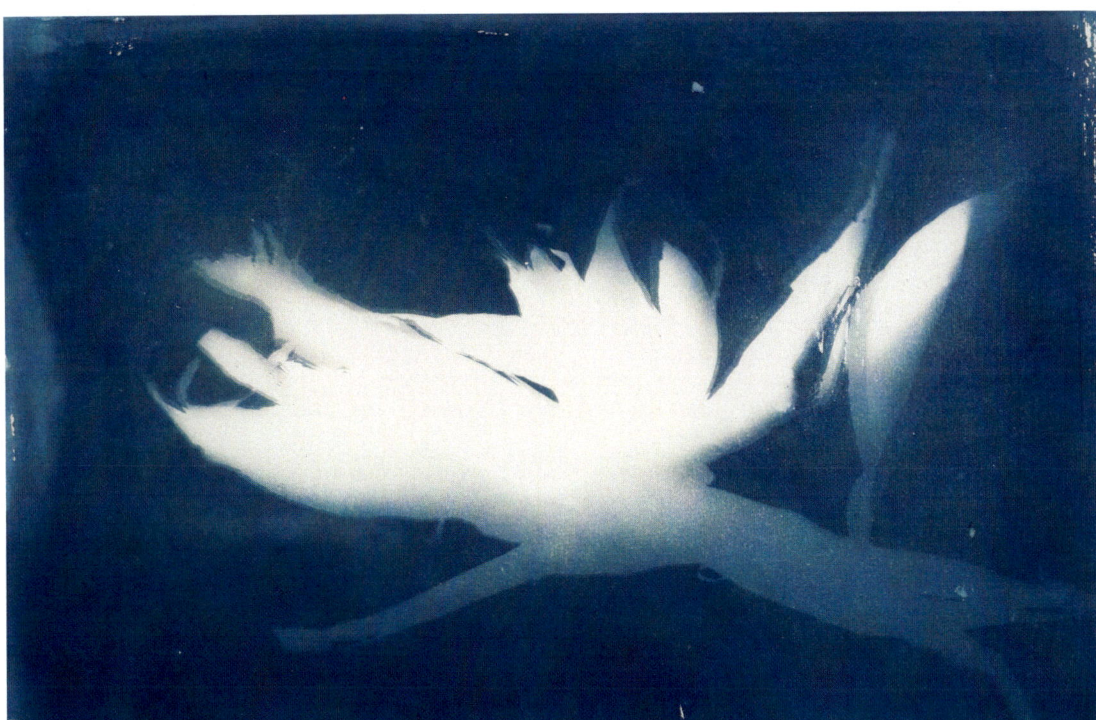

Self-care in times of chaos and violence …
Michal Shahak

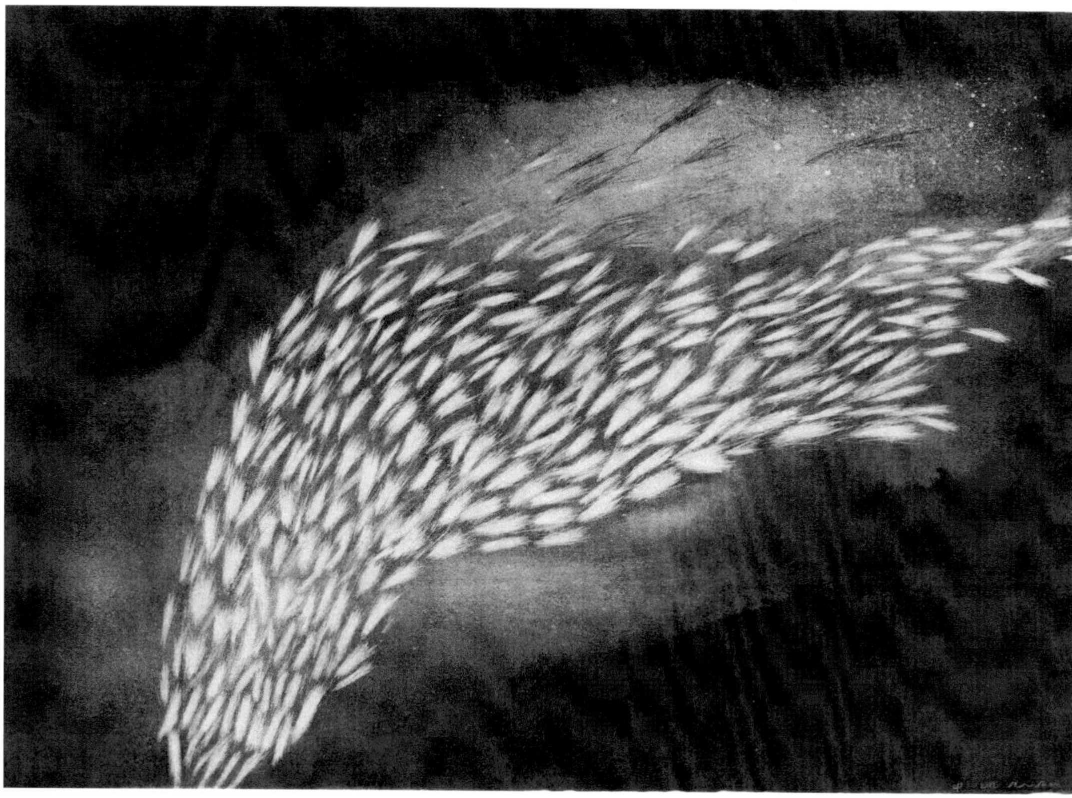

Trauma is in the air we breath
The outside isn't left outside
Air enters our lungs and becomes internal – 'us'. Breath is life.
Our breath – our life
The air we breathe becomes us
Oxygen is mixed with fear and tension
Strain is present in the individual and in the collective body-mind

High arousal and activation is a norm – a way of being in the collective system I am part of. I feel it in my own body – the global high tone and reactivity is present in the way we interact, drive, speak, cut into each other's sentences, in the way we perceive the environment and react. High-intensity survival states are prevalent even when there is no threat present. Survival responses have become ingrained in our collective ways of being. Our responses are reactions – fast, intense and highly charged. One could say that collectively the level of arousal is constantly high. It is as if a whole society is on a flight or fight mode.

I enter the studio.

My body and whole being begins to steady. Quieten.
I'm embraced by the space. My attention can go inward and a sense of restoring equilibrium is evolving from within. I'm in my haven. I root to the ground, notice my breath, and sense the presence of my body in this space.

The studio where I have my clinical practice has become a refuge. The place where I support clients to balance body and mind is also my own support – a vital resource where I can restore the natural internal ebb and flow, the self-regulation of my nervous system. I'm fully present. This is home.

The intense deregulation of the environment isn't really left outside, it is part of my life, the ground I operate from. However, for few hours, there is a steadier rhythm in my own nervous system and body. By deregulation I mean the intensity of people bumping into one another on the roads; driving too close, bypassing each other no matter what. It is as if the 'other' is always an enemy. There is an atmosphere of nervousness – between cars, between human beings, between bodies and minds. This is also present in the way we treat our streets and public spaces. There is little care given to creating healthy conditions, whether in people's own physical bodies or the collective body – homes, the land, or nature. Being in survival mode excludes such care. A society on high adrenalin, high reactivity, does not quieten enough to take care of its resources, the environment and ground of well being. This continues even in times between wars.

I take time to restore my own balance and regulation through breath and bringing awareness to what is present in my own body, attending to the stress present in me. This quietening enables a shift. I let tension go into the ground, yield into the space, going moment by moment; this in itself is a support. It is a return to internal somatic-mindfulness; a 'being with'; 'being' with self. I enter a 'being' mode, on which my somatic practice is based.

It has been an ongoing question – how to rebalance one's own system in such charged and unregulated environments where a reactive survival energy is present in many daily encounters. Many tourists experience this as 'vitality'. However, we are a society with high levels of strain and psychophysical exhaustion. I live with the question: how can I personally remain connected, embodied, attuned in an environment at war? This is my ongoing personal practice. I gain it and lose it and I gain it again.

My body is aching. My dance is hurting. Mind and body in pain.
Living in this reality every day I must find ways to reclaim myself.

My work as a somatic movement therapist is to facilitate healing in the body-mind. I work with babies and adults with many aspects of discomfort. I work particularly with healing trauma. Every day I must first reclaim myself; regain the process and practice of letting in and letting out – like the breath.

Breathing in, breathing out. Breathing in I'm nourished, breathing out I release. Breathing in I'm sad, breathing out I agree to live in this saddening reality of ongoing conflict, violence and war.

Years of movement and dance is for me a practice of being deeply present in each moment. Sensing, feeling, being moved. Sensing, feeling, being still. Movement and stillness with no hierarchy. Aching and hurting; expanding and widening; disconnection and connectedness are all calling for exploration and presence.

Becoming present in a body-mindful way allows a deep sensing that there is always a question: if, and how, to touch – how to approach – how 'to be with' another. As dancers we know ourselves through sensation and movement.

As I move, I become more of myself, as I move, I feel more of me. And 'me' isn't just the outside senses but all of me: my history, my body, my mind, my feelings ... as I embody all of that, I am ready to be with another person. Fully being with another person is being aware of their tone, rhythm, state of being and so forth. I seek to find ways to mirror, match, meet and respond to it with no plans, no agenda, no greed. Just meeting and attuning.

It was my beloved teacher of twenty-five years, Bonnie Bainbridge Cohen, who presented and embodied a quality that we now call Cellular Presence. My understanding of Cellular Presence is of a state of 'being', a state of receptivity and presence of non striving; a state of 'being' and 'being with', where there is slow pacing and receptivity that isn't guided by the intellect. Bonnie also gave me an understanding of what it means to 'go under' that at times saved my life in the toxic environment I live in. To me 'going under' means going under the presenting conditions to see what else might be there that is eliciting a reaction or a response or an emotion or a *physiological strain*. On a physical level it means going under the superficial tone and tissues of the body in touch, and movement to gain awareness of deeper levels of organisation in the body tissues or organs; a dropping into cellular levels of being and consciousness. (I'd like to thank my colleague Teri Anderson in articulating this complex, subtle term.)

I enter the studio.
This small room is my haven, my container.
Soon, a client with symptoms of post trauma will arrive, seeking help to alleviate the multi-layered nature and suffering of trauma.

I sit with the breath. I remind myself that in the pressing challenge to alleviate trauma in another, I first have to find my own way to be fully present with whatever arrives. To be fully present means to be fully and empathically accepting things as they are, the clients as they are, the disturbing symptoms as they are. Without this deep cellular acceptance, very little can change.

Trauma magnetises; a force field drawing everything to itself.

To meet this charge, I need a full bodily presence and anchorage, to hold and to contain. The symptoms and suffering of trauma are in the body. It is through full body-mind resonance and a deep sense of being-met that an organic inner reorganisation can evolve.

This being in resonance with another person is the ground on which I base my work. It is not always easy to access and cultivate. It's an ongoing daily practice, of being in the body, sensing movement within, allowing body-mind to express. It's a demanding and rewarding practice. It requires trust and it acquires trust. Trust grows in the bodily self and supports our innate ability to heal.

As practitioners we need to generate a healing field that equals the magnetising pull of trauma. One of the hardest challenges is that in a post-traumatised state we lose our innate capacity for homeostasis, the multitude of ways in which we regulate ourselves. It is as if the pendulum is stuck and we lose capacity to move between different states e.g. *between* expansion and contraction. Returning to homeostasis, to restore motion of the pendulum, this is a body-mind healing practice.

Somatic approaches offer a person a handle, a key, an entrance to their own experience, to their own body, including illness. In opening up communication with one's inner world, a sense of presence in one's own process – ownership and ability – is cultivated to engage in the process, however difficult. I feel privileged to be in this practice and to offer it to others in the turmoil.

Michal Shahak is a dance artist living and working in Israel

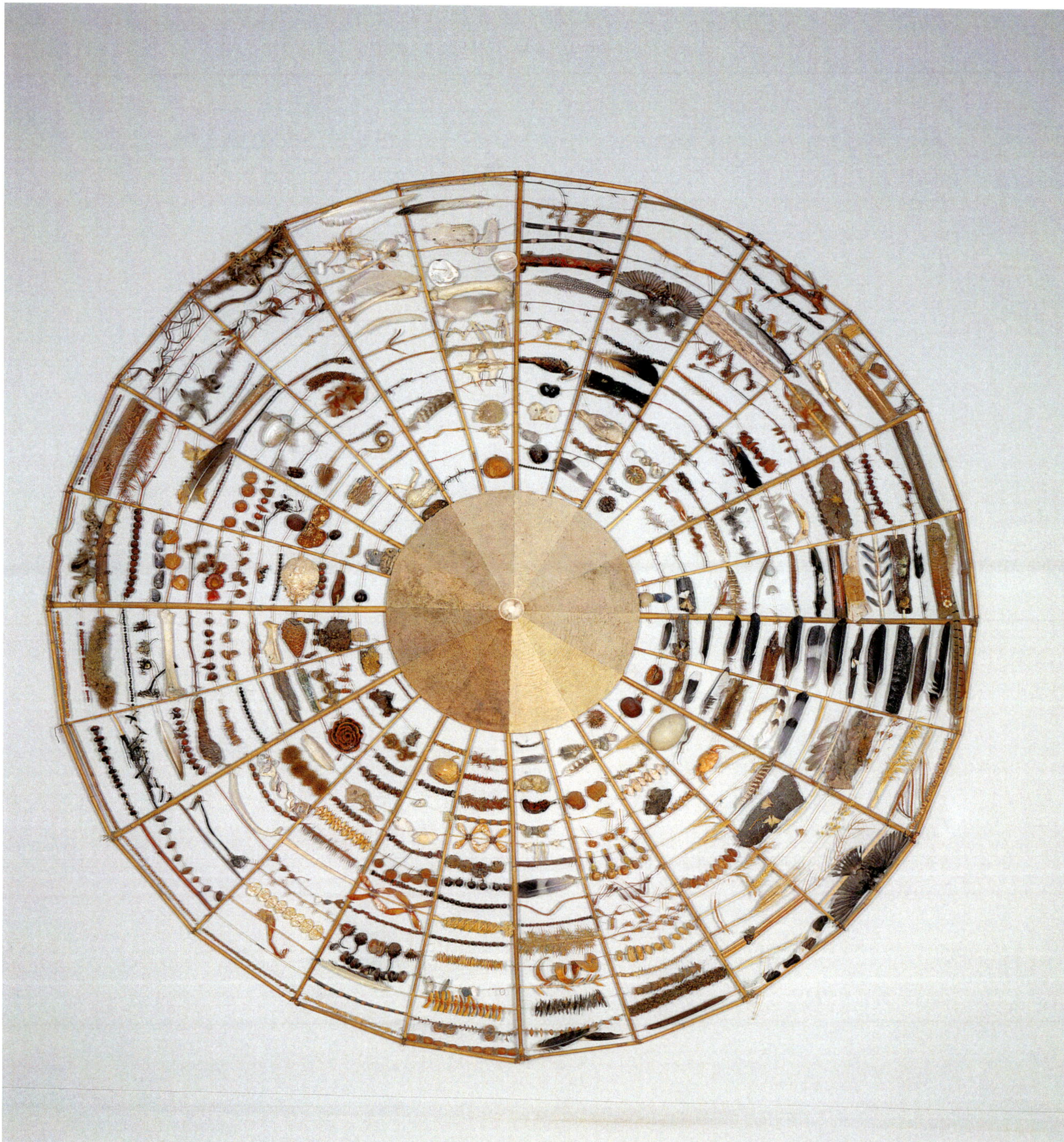

Getting your bearings: movement and sensing

For a new beginning

In out of the way places of the heart,
Where your thoughts never think to wander,
This beginning has been quietly forming,
Waiting until you were ready to emerge.

For a long time it has watched your desire,
Feeling the emptiness growing inside you,
Noticing how you willed yourself on,
Still unable to leave what you had outgrown.

It watched you play with the seduction of safety
And the grey promises that sameness whispered,
Heard the waves of turmoil rise and relent,
Wondered would you always live like this.

Then the delight, when your courage kindled,
And out you stepped onto new ground,
Your eyes young again with energy and dream,
A path of plenitude opening before you.

Though your destination is not yet clear
You can trust the promise of this opening;
Unfurl yourself into the grace of beginning
That is at one with your life's desire.

Awaken your sprit to adventure;
Hold nothing back, learn to find ease in risk;
Soon you will be home in a new rhythm
For your soul senses the world that awaits you.

John O'Donohue, *Benedictus: A Book of Blessings*, p. 32

The accounts and approaches throughout this book have been concerned with seeking health and wellbeing through widening the field of our attention. In getting more in touch with this mystery we call our 'body' – not the mechanical, anatomised, medicalised body, but our sensing and imagining body – we strengthen an innate bodily intelligence, awaken imagination, and ground perception in the world around us.

The chapter that follows goes more deeply into movement and sensing. Taking time to notice and savour what we feel is a vital step in how we look after ourselves. We can repair our worlds only to the extent that we are awake to them.

When working with others, sensing what is appropriate or needed is key. The activities in this chapter can be interpreted in different ways and need to be adapted for particular participants who are more fragile.

To move out of our heads into the sensing world of the body opens us to a slower, deeper world, flowing beneath the surface of everyday consciousness – a numinous landscape of feeling, instinct, image, memory, dream – the infinitely complex terrain of being human and alive. Everything we have ever experienced, even things that have escaped consciousness, nonetheless are remembered in the body. To listen to the body, to listen to the world through the body, profoundly affects how we feel – details come into focus, we notice more of what delights, strengthens, or weakens the rhythms of our breath and heart.

> To acknowledge that 'I am this body' is not to reduce the mystery of my yearnings and fluid thoughts to a set of mechanisms, or my 'self' to a determinate robot. Rather it is to affirm the uncanniness of this physical form. It is not to lock up awareness within the density of a closed and bounded object, for as we shall see, the boundaries of a living body are open and indeterminate; more like membranes than barriers, they define a surface of metamorphosis and exchange
> Far from restricting my access to things and to the world, the body is my means of entering into relation with all things.
>
> David Abram, *The Spell of the Sensuous*

Each day... here and now

Close your eyes

Take time to settle and find stillness... notice... how do you feel?
Acknowledge... sensations... feelings... dreams... grief... hope... concerns

Notice... sensations ***inside your own body****... scan through from head to toes, from front to back... notice movements of breath... details of sensation... sense the beat and pace of your heart... acknowledge comfort or discomfort in any part of your body*

Notice sensations and impressions ***coming from outside you****... from contact with ground or chair from light... weather... time of day*

Acknowledge ***each sense****: sight... hearing... smell... touch... sense of movement... of balance*
Notice ***thoughts****: what's on your mind?... fears... concerns*
What ***emotions*** *are present?... where do you feel them in your body?*
Imagine... their movements... gestures

Breathe... let your shoulders soften and open
Let your spine lengthen... let your back widen
Let your neck be free to carry your head high
Sense space... inside... and outside you

Notice small internal movements... messages... signs... of what is carried in the body
Follow sensation into movement*... sense how movement wakes up other sensations*
Sense breath... as movement... watch how it moves through the body
Notice... changes... how you feel NOW

When you are ready... open your eyes
Notice what you see... what draws your attention?
Take a pen. Moment by moment, ***write****... list what you notice*
Then begin to add other impressions... qualities... associations
Let the writing find its own direction

Coming to our senses

My belief is in the blood and flesh as being wiser than the intellect.
The body unconscious is where life bubbles up in us.
It is how we know we are alive, alive to the depths of our souls
and in touch somewhere with the vivid reaches of the cosmos.

D. H. Lawrence

'How are you? How do you feel?' these are such everyday questions, yet ones that can evoke a curious blank. We mostly respond with bland generalities or a quick 'cover story'. Yet what we actually feel can seem strangely out of sight – a submerged and wordless continent of emotions and concerns. Often what we think we feel – fatigued, depressed or the opposite, cheerful, going strong – overlays deeper strands of feeling which only emerge as we settle and become more imaginatively present. Even when we seem to know what we feel, there are often other currents nudging into our awareness, nuanced, often contradictory feelings and thoughts. Discovering what is at play within us takes time. If we let our attention drop into the body – into weight, breath and sensation – we may begin to perceive a host of details, qualities and associations hidden beneath the surface of everyday awareness, which like pieces of a jigsaw, gradually begin to emerge and reveal a more complex pattern of connections.

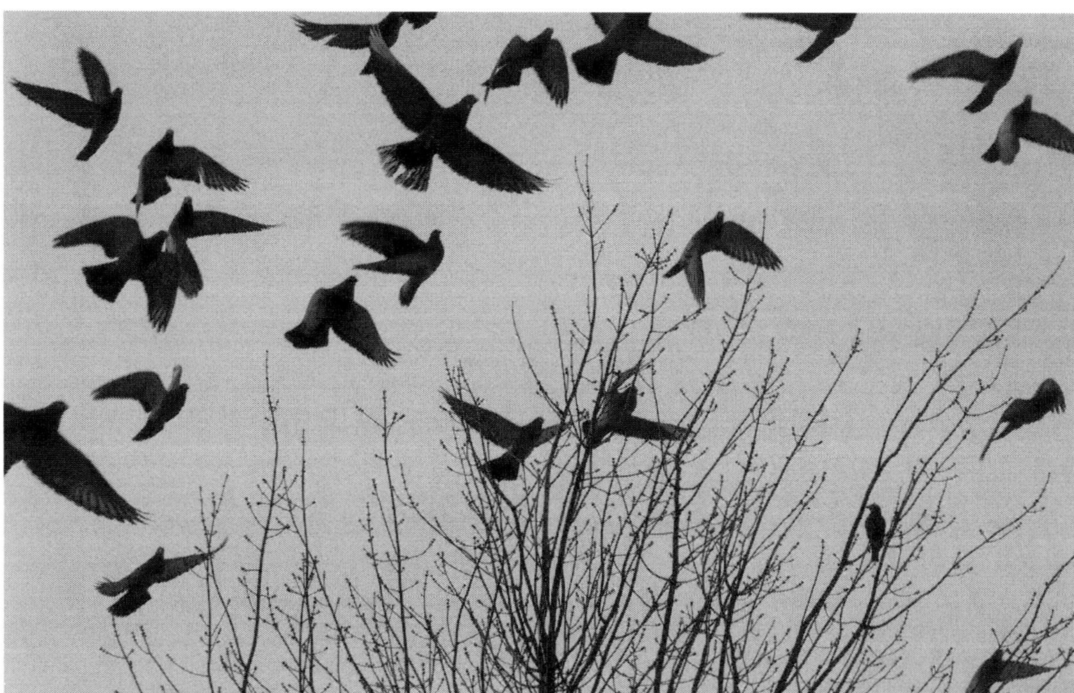

Information from our senses underpins how we establish a coherent sense of self and connection to the world about us. Feeling my feet on the ground, the air on my skin, hearing the sounds immediately around me, quietens the chatter of thoughts and brings awareness to the present moment. Sensing, feeling, intuition, instinct, emotion, proprioception and kinaesthesia all interweave to give us a sense of how and where we are. Recognising these messages in and from the body is a crucial part of how we manage our day-to-day lives, from injury prevention to relating with another and understanding the nuances of non-verbal communication. Despite all that science tells us about our amazing bodies, language traps us in a Cartesian duality of mind as distinct from body.[1] Yet there is no thought in our mind that is not also in our body; thought and feeling pattern our muscle, blood and bone. We sense a person's state of mind immediately in their body language. Connecting to our bodies alters our state of mind as much as our thinking mind influences body chemistries, posture and function. It is this that makes creative work sourced in the body so potent a tool in healthcare.

'The feeling of identity arises from a feeling of contact with the body. To know who one is the person must be aware of what he feels' Alexander Lowen [2]

Getting in tune from Penny Collinson

'The majority of my clients come for sessions to support them towards feeling more connection within their body and to their lives, and to make dedicated time for this 'listening process' to be explored, with me alongside. Fundamentally they know that if they take time to slow down and listen to their bodily 'voices' – sensations, imagination, movements, affects – they may feel more energised and able to participate in all they do more fully. Sensations are always present in the body. I help a person attune to these – to take notice of them – and also to notice their response. Are sensations attended to, ignored, rejected, blamed? Sometimes there are emotional, psychological or physical aspects to integrate, accept and work through. Simply attending to the body, inviting it to reveal how it is, can bring back a sense of flow and more capacity to meet what's going on.'

Sense: of touch... of position... of warmth... of cold... of pressure... of pain... of taste... of gravity... of hunger... of thirst... of time... of sound... of tension... of stretch... of ease...of play... of movement... of balance... of thinking... of space... of cycles and rhythms..

[1] Since the Enlightenment, medical science has tended to regard the human body as an object that can be dissected and analysed scientifically, and its "defects" treated accordingly. The subjective experience of our human mind has been marginalised and the interdependence of body and mind within a unique individual has been largely ignored. Yet psychoneuro-immunology is revealing just how much our body responds to the feelings, and emotions of our mind.

[2] quoted in Deane Juhan, *Job's Body: A handbook for bodywork*

Each day, take time to slow down and acknowledge sensations and perceptions. Take time to listen and inquire into our physical state, noticing small internal movements, buried gestures, qualities of breath – these are messages from the body, fragments of what is present within us. As we wake up to sensation, letting it amplify, move and unfold as weather patterns through our tissues, breath begins to change and we find ourselves gradually feeling more present and in tune with who and how we are.

Choose a spot... *close your eyes... stand still... listen... feel.*
What do you notice?... what does your body see?
What touches your body? speaks to you
sense light... shadow... air

Imagine *your body as soft wax... let what you see touch... leave an imprint*
How does your body respond... move... change shape?
Move to find... a dance for the time of day... for the season... weather

Move... *from sound... from smell... from taste... from touch*

Move... to explore a dream... to tell a story... to make a deliberate mistake[3]

Go outside... *notice what is moving... sense details... qualities*
Let your body join... echo... mirror... a particular movement you see...
let it inspire other movement

[3] Playing with the idea of a mistake can free up any tendency in us towards weighty worthiness.

Stillness

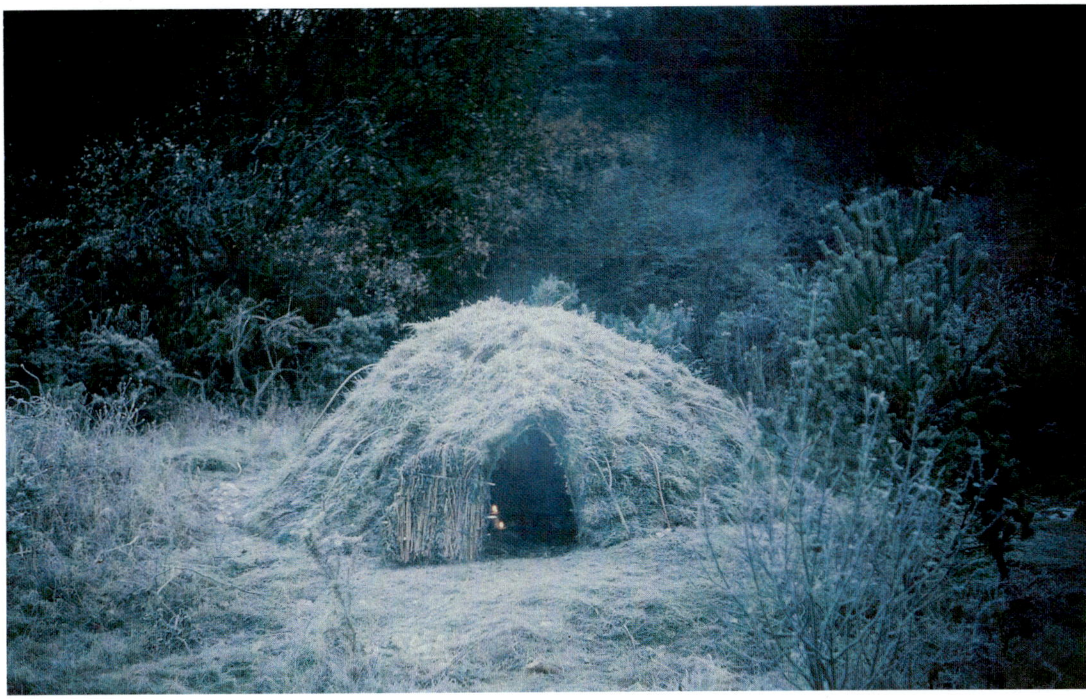

Stillness... of a bird on a nest... of night sky... of a lake... of snow falling... when the wind drops

Giving time for stillness and rest is a vital aspect of learning to care for oneself (and for others). Each day quietening the mind and getting in tune with the rhythms and pace of breath and body is key to restoring balance and wholeness.

fallow – farmland ploughed and harrowed
but left for a period without being sown to restore its fertility

There are many layers within stillness. If we yield and give way into its depths, dropping downwards through eddies, pools, to the ocean floor – a sense of inner spaciousness, of going beyond time begins to open up. Through stillness and slowed time, letting go immediate preoccupations, we discover ever deeper, subtler rhythms of movement and qualities of stillness within the body. Through stillness unforeseen possibilities and directions begin to emerge. This dedicated time of stillness and non-doing swiftly refines awareness of what is going on in mind and body.[4]

[4] F.M. Alexander's insight into the corrosive impact of compression, misalignment and poor posture on health emphasises this need for stillness. His technique recommends lying down for twenty minutes each day for the body to recover its length, width and depth.

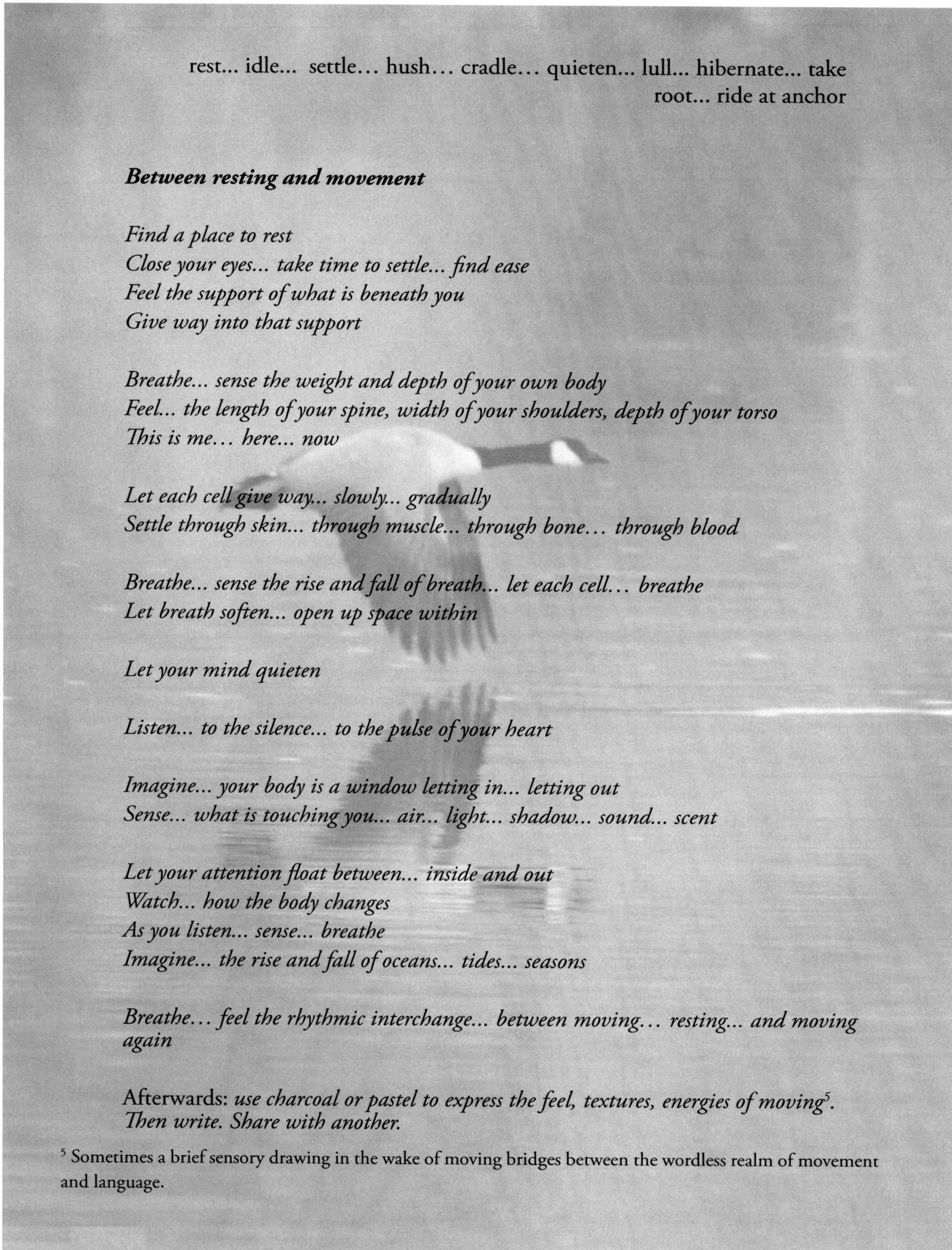

rest... idle... settle... hush... cradle... quieten... lull... hibernate... take root... ride at anchor

Between resting and movement

Find a place to rest
Close your eyes... take time to settle... find ease
Feel the support of what is beneath you
Give way into that support

Breathe... sense the weight and depth of your own body
Feel... the length of your spine, width of your shoulders, depth of your torso
This is me... here... now

Let each cell give way... slowly... gradually
Settle through skin... through muscle... through bone... through blood

Breathe... sense the rise and fall of breath... let each cell... breathe
Let breath soften... open up space within

Let your mind quieten

Listen... to the silence... to the pulse of your heart

Imagine... your body is a window letting in... letting out
Sense... what is touching you... air... light... shadow... sound... scent

Let your attention float between... inside and out
Watch... how the body changes
As you listen... sense... breathe
Imagine... the rise and fall of oceans... tides... seasons

Breathe... feel the rhythmic interchange... between moving... resting... and moving again

Afterwards: *use charcoal or pastel to express the feel, textures, energies of moving*[5]*. Then write. Share with another.*

[5] Sometimes a brief sensory drawing in the wake of moving bridges between the wordless realm of movement and language.

Taking a walk

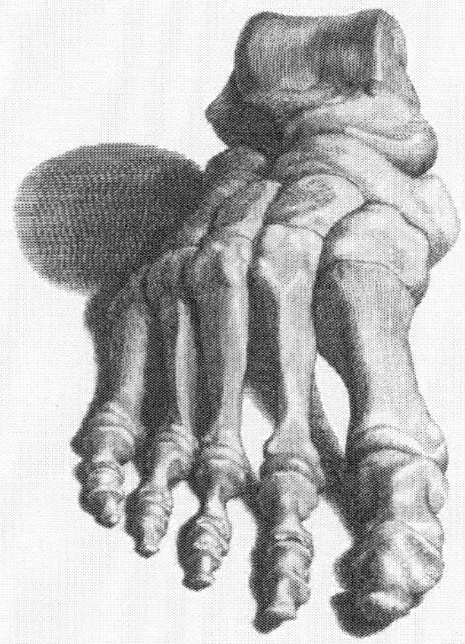

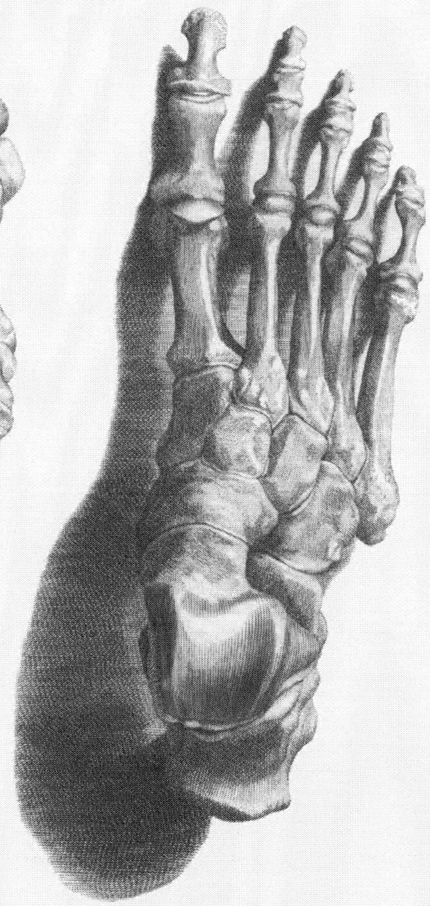

The human foot
is a masterpiece
of engineering
and a work of art.
Leonardo da Vinci

When we feel tired or stuck, simply moving with a focus on our feet loosens and wakes up the rest of the body, speeding the return of blood to the heart and calling up a surprising range of movement as we play with pace, length of stride, distribution of weight on different surfaces of the foot. In our own work, in groups where people were mobile, we often began sessions with walking, an everyday familiar activity which can be played with through games and qualities, both with partners or solo.

Many people go for a walk when they feel stuck and find the action of walking begins to loosen thinking and to free attention. Einstein reckoned his insight and best ideas came not from sitting and trying to work something out, but through getting on the move. New ideas and insights come in, we breathe more deeply, and blood (nutrients, waste removal and information) begins to flow through tissues that have become fixed.[6] Inertia and sensory numbing dissolve as we move and regain a sense of our own pace and rhythm. In the play of dance and movement we find new possibilities and energies. Charlie Chaplin famously found his character of The Tramp through a large pair of shoes and an unforgettable walk.

Each foot is made up of twenty-six uniquely shaped small bones that allow an extraordinary range of movement. The heel is highly sensitive to pressure. Fat pads in the heel (and fat packets throughout the foot) act like bubble wrap, as shock absorbers, and dissipate the impact of the ground. For over three million years we walked barefoot on the ground, the soles of our feet highly sensitive to the surface of the terrain, and informing spine and pelvis to respond appropriately. The feet are sense organs guiding the flexibility and stability of the body in every moment.

> The soles of our own feet are usually out of sight. Making them visible was inspired by the play *Footfalls* by Samuel Beckett. During the course of the play the performer walks 9 paces, backwards and forwards, repeatedly, across the stage. This work is about that touch: of the feet, of stepping and of being in physical contact with the earth. The repetition of walking, of travelling through landscapes and traversing the world is a deep human impulse. It is how our distant ancestors first moved across the continents.
>
> David Ward, artist

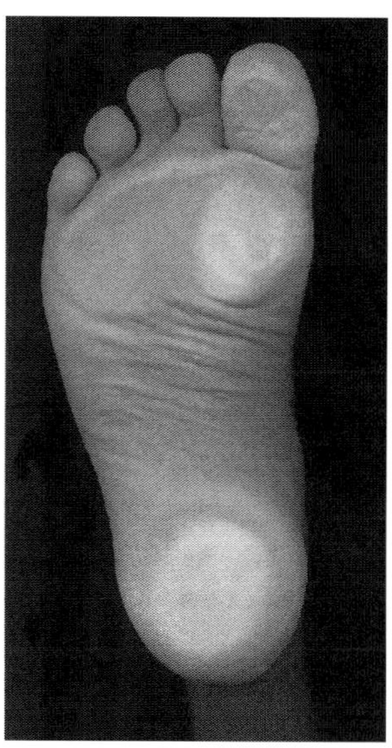

Light on the Feet
(Footfalls for Samuel Beckett)
David Ward

Nine images projected onto fabric.
Dimensions variable
(Originally commissioned by King's College, Cambridge for *Somewhere there where: Samuel Beckett in dialogue with King's College Chapel* in 2015.)

[6] Darwin had his 'Sandwalk' – a gravel track near Down House, his home in Kent. He called it his 'thinking path'. Every day, once in the morning and again in the afternoon, Darwin strolled and reflected amongst the privet and hazel, often alongside his fox terrier. Darwin had a little pile of stones on the path, and he kicked one with each turn; some ideas were four-pebble problems. Filipa Pereira-Stubbs

The most fundamental orientation in the body is to gravity, weight and balance. We stand up from the ground and stride out through a balancing that begins in our feet. Over 200,000 tactile sensory nerve endings in our toes and soles of our feet inform our brain and body of the ground's vital support. Our heads balance, like a crow's nest, high on the tip of the spine, a balancing dependent on the responsiveness and flexibility of our feet. Two condyles, little 'feet' on the base of the skull, rest into two facet joints in the atlas. The **cerebellum**, behind the condyles at the base of the brain, controls fine motor movement, coordination, balance, equilibrium and muscle tone. Chinese medicine aptly names these points 'Heavenly Pillars'. Getting our bearings in relation to gravity is an essential aspect of being present and grounded. Balance is to movement what light is to vision. It is our feet to a large extent that guide these subtle processes of movement and balancing.

Our evolution, and the shape of our bodies, has been driven by rising to the challenge of changing climate. We came out of the trees onto the savannah, walked and ran on our two feet. The unique structure of the human foot gives a spring to our step and the necessary speed for us to survive as hunters. Learning to balance on our two feet and walk upright freed our hands for tool-making and extended the field of our senses to the horizon, all of which helped develop our amazing brain.

Endurance was vital to our ancestors and our bodies evolved for endurance running. Three ligamentous arches extend through the foot which stretch as the foot articulates with the ground. The ligaments and tendons of the foot store energy as we run. Waking up the feet stimulates balance receptors and moves all parts of our body above.

A story: finding balance

'About four years ago I began to have problems with my balance and muscular fatigue (among other symptoms) and lost confidence in my body. I could no longer unconsciously or effortlessly enjoy using my body.

'I took up T'ai Chi. When I practise T'ai Chi I am continuously giving my attention to dropping my weight into the support of the ground, relaxing my shoulders and moving my weight from one foot to the other.

'Before I started T'ai Chi, my experience of using my legs had become such that after some minutes my muscles tired and my balance deteriorated – I got 'wobbly'. It is with wonder that I notice that, contrary to expectation, as I continue my practice my stability gradually improves and therefore my balance. I can move my weight to one side, allow one foot to rise and stay for some moments. Walking and feeling the ground under my feet as I slowly roll from heel to toes can be exquisite. Standing, my balance comes from feeling the contact of the soles of my feet with the ground, noticing the many points where they connect and the constant tiny changes in that contact. Letting go tension in my shoulders and dropping into my core and into my feet, I feel both heavier and lighter and my balance improves.' Lis Heath

Footsteps

Let the feet... take you into walking
Notice what energy... quality... character... feels present today
Walk of clown... bear... wind... judge... bird... giraffe... river... lion tamer

Open the small bones of feet into ground... let the feet play against the ground

walk... stride... jostle... hop... glide
wake up... shake up
move from... heel... toes... sides of foot
skip... gallop... stamp... tumble... trip

Let in... let out... each breath of air
Sense weight... momentum... march... tip toe... spring... meander
Sense space... near... far... to the horizon

Open gateways of joints... knees... elbows... shoulders... ankles... wrists

Sense how the feet guide the body... changing gait... changing shape
Let the feet wake up... stir up... 650 muscles... 208 bones

Notice... what feels stuck... unmoving

Let the movement of the feet... move the body... from head to heel
As you move... notice how needs change... vary... transform

Open the body... let it go... here and there
Falling upwards from the feet
1000 ways of travelling on

Finding the kinetic melody

Following a climbing accident and surgery to repair torn tendons and quadriceps, Dr Oliver Sacks, a Professor of Neurology, found he could not move his left leg. Despite physical therapy he could not find how to re-engage with it and move. Then, out of the blue, he remembered a piece of music by Mendelssohn and suddenly, 'without thinking, without intending whatever, I found myself walking, easily, joyfully, with the music... and in that very moment my "motor" music, my kinetic melody, my walking came back – my leg came back.' Drawn from Oliver Sacks, *A Leg to Stand On*.

The many walks of life from Chris Crickmay

take to your feet – step off – lollop – float – fly along – sail – hare about – trudge – skidaddle – slip past – swagger – nip out – stroll – slide – stamp – limp – lurch – trek – skulk – press on – creep – crawl – wander – amble – scramble – drift – sail along – mill about – trot – back out – slope off – bustle – glide – idle – walk on all fours – blunder in – dawdle – toddle – bounce along – stride out – scatter – flee – meander – hop – sway – stumble – limp – flounder – totter – stomp – breeze in – roll along – loaf – linger – blow in – saunter – burst in – march – shuffle – waltz in – stagger – stride – mince – weave – clamber over – ramble – slip out – crash in – walk in on – skip along – trip over – wade – splash through – catch up – hop – jog – canter – gallop – jump in – a spring in your step – oozle your way in – tear in – hang back – drag your feet – press forward – push in – elbow your way – surge forward – shrink back – sidle up to – wiggle – waddle – tiptoe – hike – frog march – route march – walk tall – step outside – best foot forward – take a step back – one step at a time – dig in your heels – flat footed – walk away – step up to the plate – walk on – pace up and down – walk round – walk along – walk home – scurry – a walkout – trample all over – put your foot in it – out for a walk – stand firm – tread lightly – walk right up to – quicken your step – out of step – walk the plank – get into your stride – pace yourself – a step in the right direction – turn on your heel – a walking disaster – faltering step – with one bound – step aside – trail after – tread softly – in the steps of your ancestors – fall into step

Finding the dance: moving from sensing

Whenever I quieten the persistent chatter of words within my head, I ind this silent wordless dance always already going on.

David Abram, *The Spell of the Sensuous*

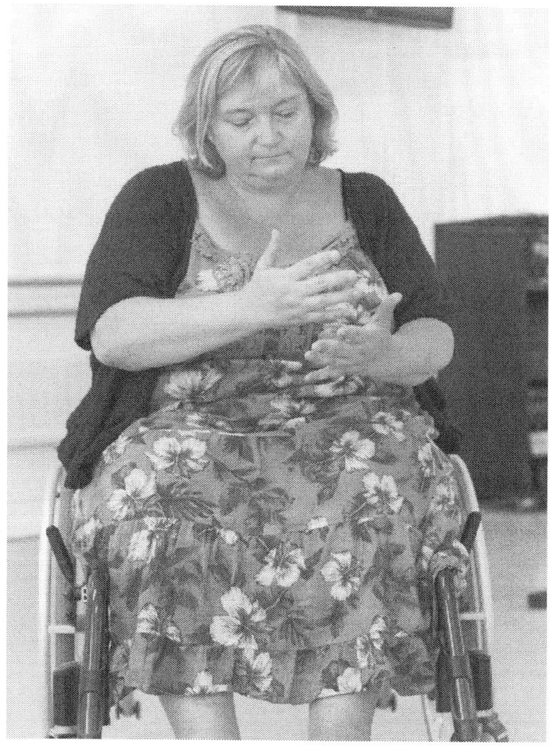

We can begin anywhere, anyhow – listening for a sense of rhythm, or movement.[7] Following the most tentative impulse towards movement, without blocking or forcing, begins to wake up sensation and free our awareness. Listening to the body reveals a vitality that, like living water, twists and turns in so many directions. The living body rarely expresses itself in simple 'linear' or mechanical movement. Linear movement imposed on the body, as in repeating exercises, can dull the senses – there is little room for personal feeling or creativity. A listening, spontaneous approach to the body and movement awakens imagination, opening the door into the unique landscapes of a person's life. Movement becomes a way of bodying forth the unseen within us. Our gestures, however clumsy or small, become a way of entering into what we sense, yet cannot yet give words to. And as we follow moment by moment, allowing a silent inner melody to carry us along, we discover energies, characters, qualities that bring us more fully into connection both with ourselves and with what is around us.

[7] Getting moving can be stimulated in any medium – clay, paint, drawing, making sound, etc.

Life is movement. We tend to forget that our body is a living process in time, not a fixed structure. Moment by moment we are creating and shaping the unique signature of who we are. Though the science of anatomy separates the body into independent parts, in our essence we are the confluence of many spiralling streams of movement. Blood, bone, heart, muscle, dermatomes, nerve pathways all express these spiral forces. In the embryo fluid movement precedes form; blood flows before we have a heart; the spiralling fibres of the heart forming in response to the primordial movement of our lifeblood. The movement, or gesture of our midline at 15 days sets a direction and axis between tail and head, which will later become spinal cord and spine. The living body shimmers with pulsations, micro-movements, our tissues changing, adapting, shedding, re-forming. Nothing is fixed. Through movement we become explorers, actively voyaging into the mysteries of being a body, of being alive.

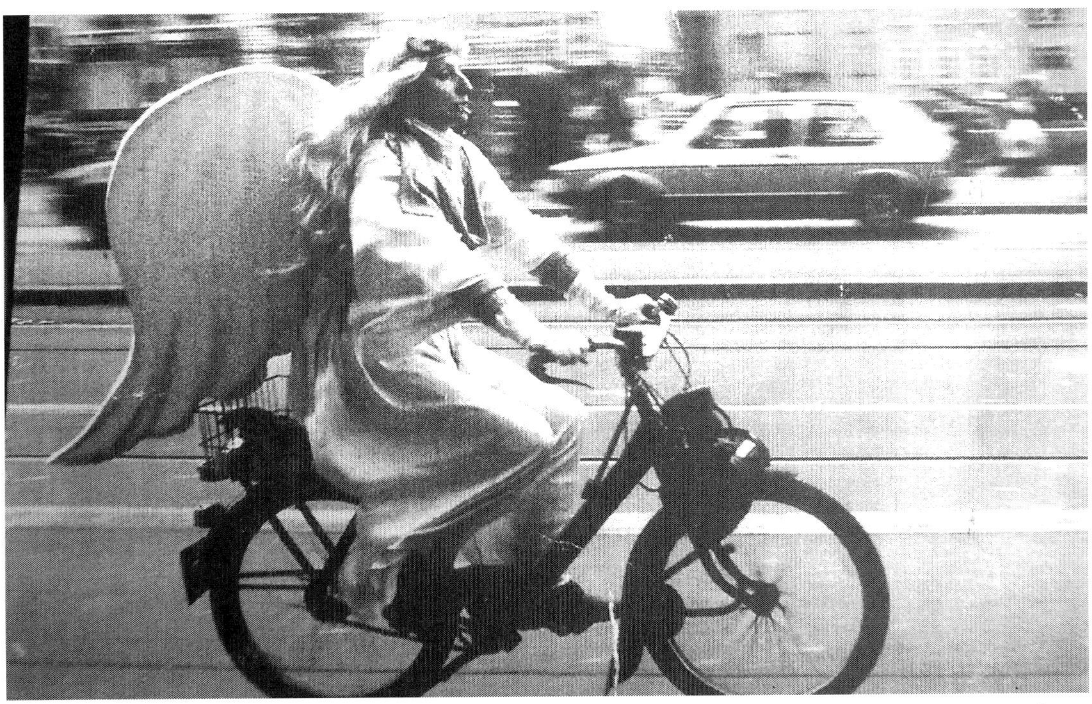

moving

A conversation of parts

Make a simple gesture... repeat it several times,
Slow it down... feel the movement for itself
Feel its weight... quality... pace... tone

Notice sensation... and what happens elsewhere in the body... answering impulses
Sense in your body... as one part awakens another

What else... begins to move... echo… respond… agree... disagree

Follow and notice... let the conversation spread throughout the whole body... and beyond

***Explore... between opposites**... polarities*
between in breath… and out breath
between inside and outside… dark and light... visible and invisible
appear… disappear… be full… empty

***Explore a palette of qualities**... energies*
*Explore... **slowing down**... creep... amble… dawdle… trickle… melt... go slower than slow*
***Speeding up**… stir… whisk... hurry... dash… pelt… flash... whizz…gallop… fast as lightening*
Feel in your body what pace feels comfortable... appeals... now
Watch... as a flowing river... sense different currents... streams... eddies
Surge as a wave... spill... plunge... sink... swirl... drip... ripple... move against the current
Be awake to the need for change

*Let your **field of attention** shift... come close… around the body*
Spread out… sense space beyond the body… outside… to the horizon

Stay awake… follow as energy fluctuates… changes
Expand the time… between one state and another
Between one movement… and another

Creating new pathways: movement, play and improvisation

We live in times when we are increasingly sedentary. What movement we do is compartmentalised into gym or exercise regimes, done routinely and by rote, whilst our mind goes elsewhere, rarely in attendance, or listening to the body itself.

But in our early years, movement is our primary language. Every feeling is expressed through the body – response *is* movement. Yet so quickly this natural physicality is suppressed, can become an embarrassment; the child that sits still is praised, whilst wriggling is frowned on. But research increasingly reveals how fundamental movement is to the growth and maturing of our nervous system. Norman Doidge in his work with Parkinsonian patients writes of how, even in later life, creative, as opposed to functional movement, stimulates the growth of new connections between neurons.

Feldenkrais discovered that monumental gains are made not by mechanical movements done by rote but its opposite – 'random movements'. Children learn to roll over, crawl, sit and walk through experimenting and unencumbered curiosity. Most babies learn to roll over when they follow something with their eyes that interests them, then they follow it so far that, to their surprise, they roll over. They learn to roll over by accident, by 'random' movement. For an artist, or dancer, this is the practice of improvisation. There is no goal, simply a moment-by-moment responsiveness to whatever is occurring.

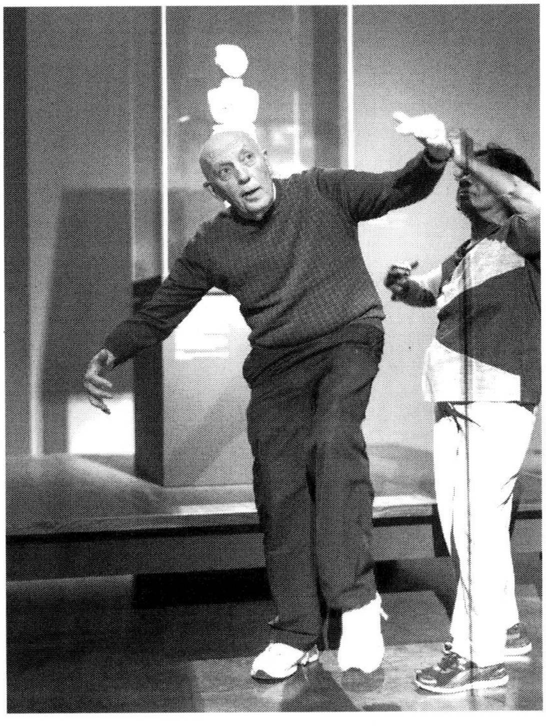

Movement is a medicine that swiftly refreshes, surprising us with unexpected energies, memories and sensations.[8] The ripple effect of any one movement wakes up connection with other parts. As we follow the inner kinetic melodies of dance, body, mind and perception all loosen up. Freeing the body frees the mind so that we see and feel differently, however stuck our conditions may seem.

As we wake up to sensation, letting it amplify, move and unfold as weather patterns through our tissues, breath begins to change and we find ourselves gradually feeling more present and in tune with who and how we are. There are rhythms within rhythms at play in the body – waking up to the shifting needs of pace and time within us refreshes and enlivens our sensory palette. It is all to easy to get stuck in a familiar pace – moving through a range of qualities allows whatever needs to make itself felt to come to the surface.

kinaesthesia from Greek *kinein* – to move
and *aisthesis* – sensation, information we receive from our sensory organs

The fluid body

Our bodies are threaded by a vast and intricate network of sensory receptors in the connective tissues and joints that register the subtlest of internal movements and feeling-states as well as informing us about our environment. Our senses are the prime means by which we make sense of both our internal and external worlds – physical injury, congestion, tension and disassociation all disrupt this vital flow of information.

We are formed out of movement – there is no part of the body that is static or fixed unless we make it so. Every part of the body, including bone, is inherently and subtly mobile in relation to every other part. Our bodies are an ever-shifting, changing constellation of tissues. Blood, bone, organ, muscle and connective tissue form a continuous streaming unified field that is each one of us. We are made up of 206 bones and 360 joints. Bones connect through joints and each joint is a place of meeting, of movement, and of change. Arteries, nerves, veins and lymph vessels are all affected by their transition through a joint. Lack of movement through a joint can cause inflammation.

[8] Our bodies are designed to be on the move, and movement helps keep blood pressure down, generates good cholesterol, stimulates more oxygen to the heart and muscles and keeps our joints healthy and free of pain. Thirty minutes of exercise, or movement, will boost our immune system for a whole day, keeping away infections and mopping up stray cancer cells. However 70% of us don't manage this. Lack of physical activity has the same effect on heart disease as smoking twenty cigarettes a day; it increases the risk of diabetes, colon and breast cancer, osteoporosis, arthritis and, of course, obesity that will affect 60% by 2040. (Drawn from Dr William Bird, strategic health advisor to Natural England, *Resurgence,* Jan/Feb 2010).

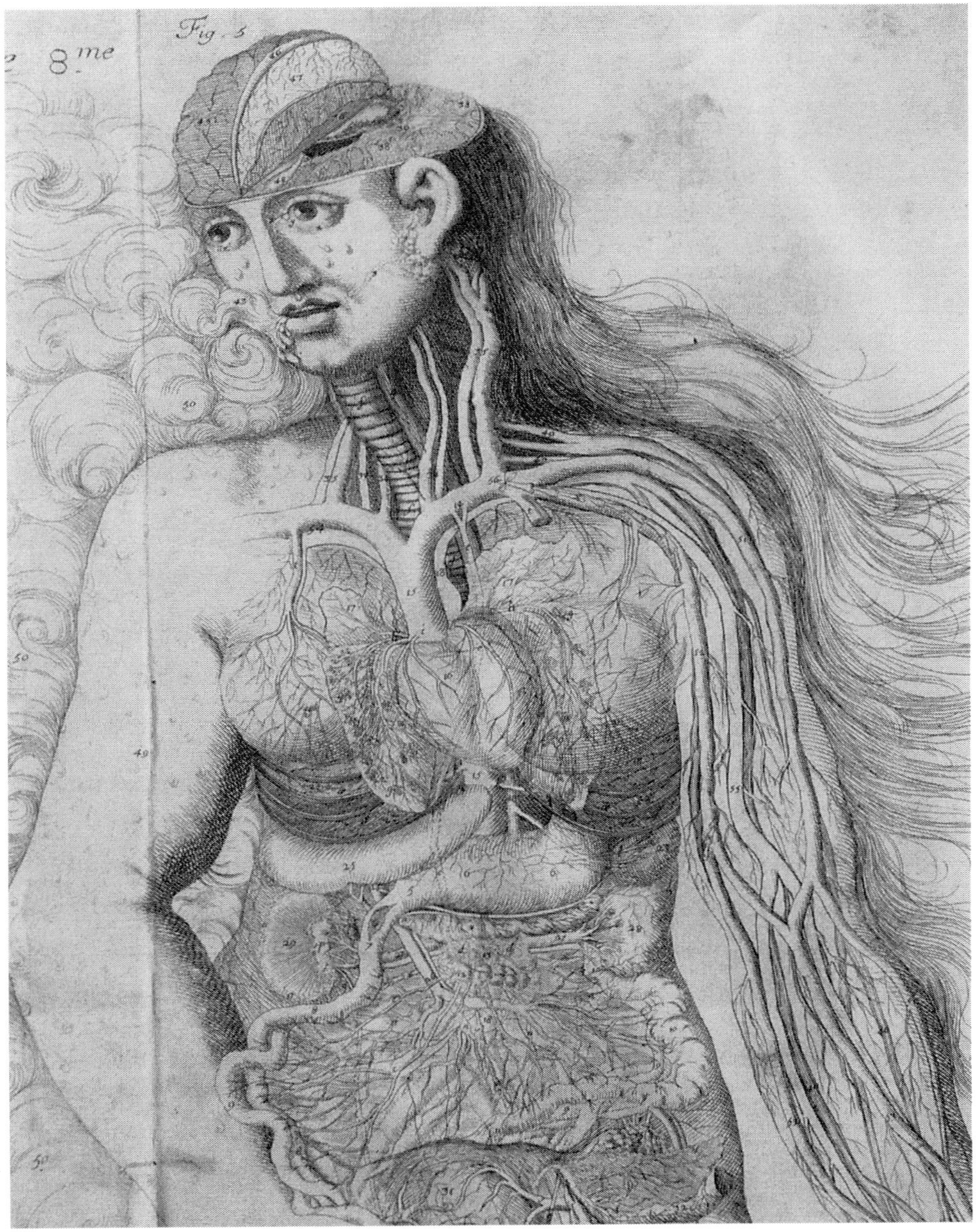

The richest and largest sensory system in the body is not our eyes, ears, skin, or vestibular system, but is in fact our muscles with their related fascia. The nervous system receives its greatest amount of sensory input from 'myofascial' tissues. Yet the majority of these sensory neurones are so small that until recently little has been known about them.[9]

Wherever blood flow is poor, health and healing are compromised. Tension, stress and lack of movement wreak havoc in our bodies. The discs of the spine dry and atrophy

[9] Drawn from Schleip (2003) quoted in Michael Kern, *The Living Matrix* Article published in *The Fulcrum*

when the spine lacks movement. Muscle and connective tissue lose their flexibility, and bones become brittle when they lack movement and fluid exchange.

Our bodies have an incredible capacity for change, renewal and growth. Every day we create 15 million new cells nourished by the vast irrigation system of capillary and blood vessels, (65,000 miles) that if laid end to end would encircle the earth twice. Every one of our 75 trillion cells depends on the movement and exchange of nutrients and waste through the liquid mediums of blood, lymph, cerebrospinal fluid, cellular, intercellular and synovial fluid. These all play their part in nourishing, cleansing, defending and communicating throughout our bodies. This movement of fluids through our tissue field creates a streaming of connection between every part of the body. When we feel lost, confused or fragmented, tuning in to the subtle movements of our fluid body restores a sense of connection and coherence.

Many people want to actively engage with their own recovery and turn to movement to access a more intuitive and instinctual part of themselves. Dr Andrew Still, the founder of Osteopathy, realised that fixity and misalignment of any joint or part of the body, through restricting blood flow and nerve impulse, brought on illness. He understood that a mobile and nuanced relationship of each part to the whole was vital to health and well being. Still's capacity to see into the body and locate the pivot of malfunction was legendary. Visualisation was a vital aspect in how he engaged with a person and their illness, an X-ray inner seeing into a body, knowing intimately the needs of normal function, he spoke of 'living in the liver' or 'being a bone'. He was remarkable for his deep understanding and empathy with each body he treated.[10] Few people are trained in the detailed, clinical anatomy of an osteopath, but dancers particularly are tuned to perceiving movement – and inertia, or lack of movement.

> The 70 to 80% of water that makes up living organisms turns the entire body into a liquid crystalline continuum that permeates throughout the connective tissues into the interior of every single cell. And ALL of the molecules in the body, including the water, are dancing coherently together.
>
> Mae-Wan Ho from *To Science with Love*[11]

[10] Drawn from John Lewis's biography, *A.T. Still: From the Dry Bone to the Living Man* (2012)

[11] Dr Mae-Wan Ho is a scientist and geneticist whose work is concerned with the vital living qualities of cells.

Ariadne's thread: a sense of connection

> Yesterday from my office window I saw a crippled girl negotiating her way across the street, her shoulders squarely braced. At each jerky movement I saw her hair blow back like an annunciatory angel, and I saw that she was the only dancer in the street.
>
> Elisabeth Smart, *The Assumption of the Rogues & Rascals*

Marion Milner – artist, psychoanalyst and author – kept journals throughout her life in which she recorded small, private events, or things that touched her, 'the most important thing that happened each day', transitory events that somehow warmed and resonated for her. Through a process of writing and reflecting on what she called these 'bead memories' – a flower in a garden, a conversation, a painting – she sought to uncover what gave her a sense of happiness, and of living her own life.[12] In this search she writes of the need to 'look with my whole body', which revealed another essential attitude: 'Moments when I had by some chance stood aside and looked at my experience, looked with a wide focus, wanting nothing and prepared for anything. Happiness came when I was most widely aware... and to be more and more aware I had to become more and more still.' Through dwelling on these 'beads', Marion Milner noted 'an answering activity' in herself, an imaginative responsiveness that brought with it a sense of joy and connectedness.

How we feel depends on a sensitivity and responsiveness to the world about us. How we make sense of our lives involves an interweaving of senses, thoughts, feelings, intuitions and imagination. Perception is founded on the way each of us notices, interprets and absorbs these streams of information coming from within our sensing bodies and from what is outside. When we lose touch with what is around us, with the natural environment and a *feeling* kind of attention, we lose inner coherence and a sense of belonging.

What makes you feel alive?

Each day take time to notice what is around you... be curious...
catch sight of the beautiful.
Notice what inspires... lifts your spirits: activities... places... people
Gather materials that evoke qualities you cherish
Find something else... that is awkward... grates... challenges
Explore ways of bringing these opposites together... explore their relationship
What emerges?[13]

12 Marion Milner, *A Life of One's Own*, Routledge (2011 reprint)

13 (including dissonance in both body and in making or writing allows surprising and often vitalising new insights and energies)

Keep a journal to reflect, explore, follow the movements of thought, dreams, ideas, feelings, intuitions – and so become more aware of your responses and what is happening in you. For practitioners, this grounds and strengthens the moment-by-moment awareness vital in working with others. Writing when our mind is scattered can help focus attention and allows whatever needs to be expressed to come to the surface of awareness.

Bring curiosity and imagination to what you see
Choose something that appeals... and let your eye dwell on it for a full minute,
Rest in your breath... let your mind quieten... settle silently into what you see
Then let words come into your mind... write down everything you notice
Colour... tone... position... location... energy
Then allow associations to surface... a cup evokes a listening ear...
An apple calls up a memory of a friend's smile
Imagine what you are looking at as active... what is happening?
Let your imagination... as your breath... fill into whatever you are looking at.
Let in... words... images... voices.. characters... stories
Then move... what energies surface?

Collage things you find, make sketches, take photographs, gather up images that speak to you. C.G. Jung made a mandala each day through which he reflected on what was going on within him. Like preparing a meal, notice what kind of expression draws you – movement, writing, song, percussion, painting. Use your imagination to find ways that satisfy and extend your expression, creating in whatever medium calls to you. Even a small window of time enlivens and strengthens the circulation of creative energy. Sustaining a regular creative process is often easier done with others. Having a companion to create alongside, witness, and share insights or thoughts always deepens and extends our own creative practice.

'I was a young man with uninformed ideas. I threw out queries, suggestions, wondering all the time over everything; and to my astonishment the ideas took like wildfire....'

Charles Darwin

What are you drawn to? *An experiment in looking*
(developed with Chris Crickmay)

To begin... quieten... breathe... settle... close your eyes
Then... slowly... open your eyes... let your attention spread...
open to what is around you...
Be present... receiving what is there

Look freshly... as with the eyes of a child... notice what comes to your eye
Patches of light... scratches on wall... knot of wood in floor... colour of light switch.

Let some particular detail draw your eye
Go closer... let your attention dwell quietly on what you see
Begin to see more... shape... feel... quality... of what is there... what surrounds it?
Details of colour... form... texture

Let associations flow in to what you see...
a small crack may become... a crevasse... a frown line... a border crossing...
edge of a cliff.
Let these associations amplify the qualities of what is there... see it more vividly

Imagine what you are seeing... as active... a verb
What might be happening in this spot?

Walk about... what else draws your eye?

Then, with a partner, take them around to share what you have noticed
Speaking... impressions... qualities... associations[14]
Notice... how each spot resonates in your body

Afterwards... write, or move as response... what does this 'place' speak of?... what emerges?
(An option: as you write, invite a memory to rise from whatever you are looking at.)

aesthetic from Greek *aestheticos* – things perceptible by the senses
anaesthetic from Greek *anaisthaetos* – numb, without feeling

[14] Joining with another and sharing what you see deepens this process, always enhances our own sense of what is there, drawing in a richer field of associations, connections.

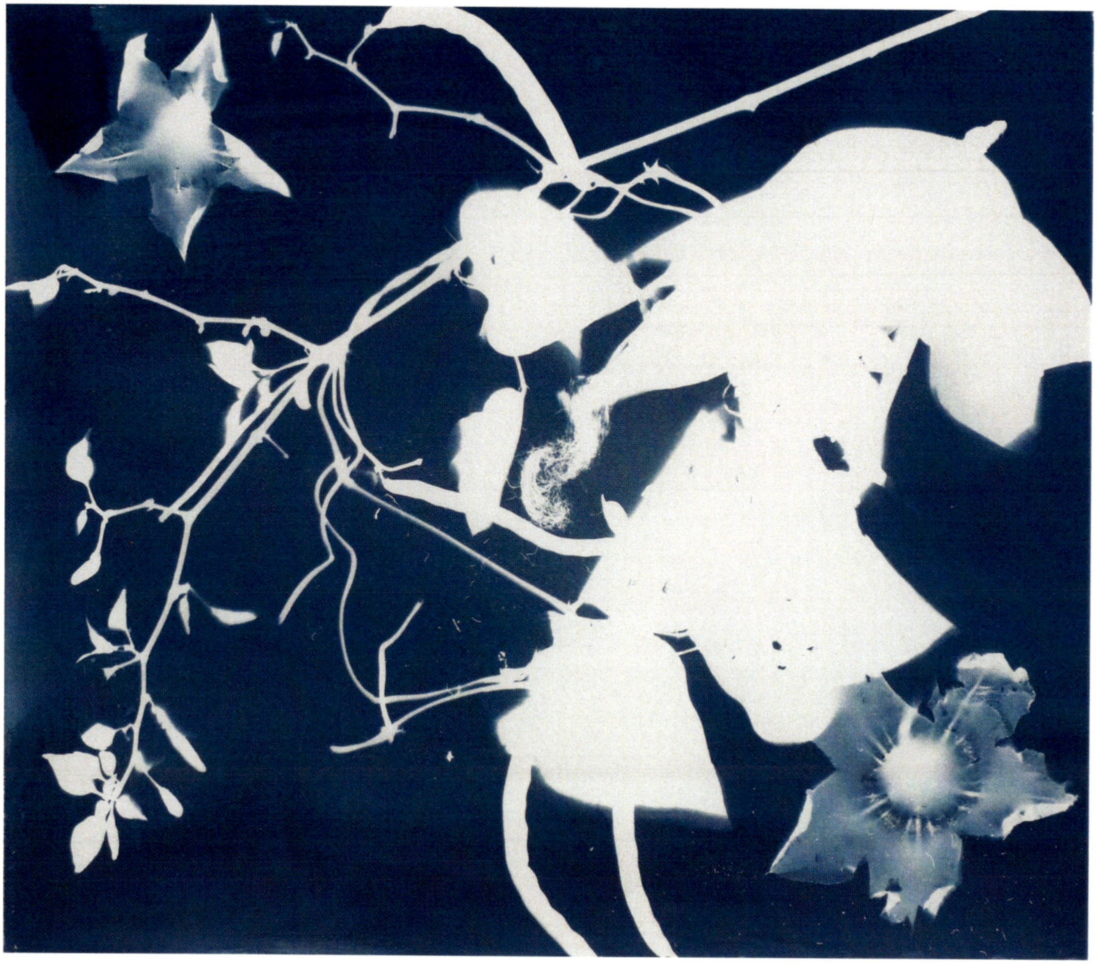

M came to the Breath of Fresh Air project for several months. Her life story seemed locked into ruminations and painful memories of the past. We worked slowly with her body – with breath, her spine, her arms – developing her sense of weight, to bring awareness of herself in present time. One day after wandering around the room in which we were working, she was drawn to a knot of wood in the floor, and spoke about it as evoking a butterfly. After moving in response to it, she began to write, and discovered a memory of herself as a child in a garden at dusk, enchanted by hundreds of tiny moths fluttering in and amongst the seeded grass heads. She said later how much it surprised and warmed her to find a memory of such peace and happiness. 'I am growing stronger', she said, 'and as I get stronger I feel lighter, clearer'.

Finding what matters

To know more of what is going on within us is not a matter of rearranging the all too familiar furniture of our thoughts, but about entering the world differently, opening our eyes and ears and tuning ourselves to different frequencies, textures and details. It involves listening, exploring, and getting to know the many selves and voices at play within us. Through movement, gesture, poem or paint we discover more of who we are and resources that lie hidden within us.

Much of the time our eyes and mind tend to glance and skim over the surface of things, as if passing in a train, as if life were a film. Yet to let our attention settle and dwell on something reveals a wealth of qualities and textures – things that are outside us, and which seem initially to have nothing to do with us, come to feel personally relevant.

Seeking what really matters for us is like approaching a shy wild creature that hides from direct gaze. If we take time to respond creatively to what we notice – a sensation in the body, a spot in the room, a phrase in the mind – layers of connection gradually come to the surface. Creating (moving, drawing, writing) moment by moment, in response to what we notice or feel, allows whatever needs to be expressed to find its way into form. If we then take time to savour and look back at what we have done, we discover connections to many aspects of our lives, much as a poem captures a host of resonant meanings and feelings that everyday linear prose cannot convey. In this open, indirect way of working, we discover what we think and feel *through* what we make or create. Self-understanding is not fuelled simply by a dive inward to our inner worlds, but is formed and re-formed by continual engagement with what is around us.

'And so by indirection find direction out.' *Hamlet*

Any one perception can awaken a host of feelings, memories and associations. Our well being is profoundly affected by how we are able to be in relationship to these ongoing flows of sensation and thoughts as they manifest in our bodies. Being able to observe, feel, sense and move between different states of mind, from the practical, common-sense mind to more sensory, intuitive and imaginative awareness, awakens a more grounded and connected sense of self.

In engaging our senses and imagination – through story, music, poetry, dance, painting – we shift from our familiar thoughts and anxieties into a receptive and creative participation with what is around us. The free play of creativity throws up gestures, rhythms, movements, and energies that open out and refresh how we feel in ourselves. Meaning arises from discovering relationships and connections; imagination a vital force that brings a sense of life and coherence.

> The inner world separated from the outer world is a place of demons. The outer world separated from the inner world is a place of meaningless objects and machines.
>
> Ted Hughes, 'Myth and Education' in *Winter Pollen: Occasional Prose*

A note on looking after ourselves

Artists working in these contexts need to take care of themselves. Periods of stress often precede illness and many people working in health settings become unwell through a tendency to over commit and overextend in caring for others. These areas of work make huge personal demands on artists. The work can be joyous and exhilarating. The changes that occur among people are often profound and moving to witness. Yet at times during the Breath of Fresh Air project Tim Rubidge and I felt very depleted and drained. This was partly due to the pressure of expectations both from patients and from health professionals (who themselves have to meet a target-driven health agenda). At times we found ourselves demoralised by the day-to-day problems of meeting the widely differing needs within our groups. The intimacy of the work, its intensely personal nature, is both beautiful and life affirming, yet at times can also be deeply challenging of one's own personal and professional resources. It takes resilience and strength to accompany others who themselves may be overwhelmed by a sense of futility or hopelessness, facing death or the loss of all that is familiar and treasured. It is essential to find time for one's own creative process and to cultivate a range of other interests. Time with peers, supervision, and bodywork all help replenish.

We all have concerns, stresses and anxieties in our daily lives and need to be aware of how these are held in our bodies, giving dedicated time to easing these. Being touch with our own feeling world means we are less likely project it onto another. There are many challenges in this work; no two contexts, or sessions, are the same when working with people whose health needs fluctuate daily. We can assume nothing. Being creatively resourced and in touch body and soul, underlies any capacity for getting in tune with another. It is easy to override the need for self-care, particularly when there is a pressure of others to be cared for. But each of us needs dedicated time and space to nourish the wellsprings of our lives. Giving time for stillness and rest is a vital aspect of learning to care for and pace oneself, particularly when working with others who are fragile. Taking time each day to quieten the mind and get in tune with the rhythm and pace of breath and body is key to maintaining our own balance and wholeness.

A story of music and movement from Filipa Pereira-Stubbs

M was curled up in a chair next to the nurse. They were in front of a computer screen, watching the rolling words of a Frank Sinatra song, singing along. I asked if M might be interested in joining the music and movement group. She turned a keen bright face to me. 'Really! Here! Dancing?' Yes, downstairs, here at the hospital. The nurse reassured M that this was indeed so, and I was the dancing lady, and reassured me that M could easily and comfortably walk the distance with me. So, after rearranging M's dressing gown just so – 'but I'm not dressed,' was her only protest – we sailed off.

M's steps are light and she glides more than she steps. Her posture is upright and her eyes are searching and curious, even in a face that sometimes drains away into absence. Her smile is luminous, and sparks responding huge smiles. She is charming, like a wise and powerful hostess in an P.G. Wodehouse novel. Decorum and grace seep through her bones. She has presence. And yet her face holds a tightness, an anxious wariness.

As we walk through the hospital, M communicates to me aspects of her relationship with dance, which then becomes a tale about a sister whom she protected. I gather the threads of these stories; M's sentences trail off as her words slip off their shape and identity and become word-like sounds, so the gist of the sentence loosens and floats away. The melody of the sentence is there, but the words dissipate. Even so, the beginnings build a picture about a father who was a musician, and a big sister, herself, who taught a younger sister to dance, and a sense of sad unkindnesses done to a younger sister, who maybe had a cleft lip? M's face is animated, and her eyes fill alternately with tears, and then with laughter and love as she imparts her stories to me.

We reach our dancing space where Debbie, my colleague, is waiting. We settle and arrange ourselves comfortably in chairs, and I tell Debbie of M's great love of dance. I find a first song – a piano piece by Phamie Gow. As the first notes ring out – clear, soft and sweet – M's eyes widen, and her hand flies to her heart. She leans forward and stares into our eyes, hers filled with wonderment – as if to say, 'Really! This? Music? Here? Now!' Debbie and I are both startled by the passion and intensity in her eyes – we are moved by her reaction, and have to laugh to express our delight – we too both love music and dance, and understand her excitement.

Usually we begin movement sessions with a calm warm up, carefully leading people into awareness of their body, but M is lit up, and beseeches us, 'May I,' and springs from her chair. She catches the melody with her hands, and steps into a current of sound and movement, dancing as if at a ball, nimbly and elegantly moving across the floor. Debbie swoops and joins in, as I quickly and quietly push back the small circle of chairs to give M the space she needs.

M holds out a hand to each of us, and knowingly takes us along the floor, swaying one way, then another, her feet stepping out a quick foxtrot rhythm, her hands tracing beautiful lines. But it is the look on her face that is wonderful. Her face is composed and delighted, smiling with the comfort of one who has arrived and finds themselves thankfully and finally in the right place. She smiles to us encouragingly and affirming that, yes, isn't this marvellous, isn't it wonderful to be dancing together.

When we sit back down again, M tells us with thanks how good that was. And yet across her obvious delight she also expresses her confusion that this is in fact what we are doing, dancing, and how could this marvellous thing be true? Her anxiety arrives as she conveys to us that others would disapprove, oh yes, they wouldn't understand. They are stupid. Thick. Then she carefully laughs her unkind words away. We reassure her that it is okay to be doing just this, that we are there to move with her, maybe more gently this time? and her eyes fill with gratitude and calm again.

It is in itself a dance, witnessing M become peacefully at one with her dancing self, and then clouding with a sense of wrongness, that she might be misunderstood, that something isn't quite right. As her words do not deliver entirely, her eyes convey this dance of emotions and feelings. Repeatedly she stops and looks at us as if to read in our eyes that this really is happening. She cries out in recognition when I play songs she loves – Glenn Miller, Nat King Cole – ah yes, yes, yes! And she tells us this is lovely, so lovely, so very lovely, and thank you so very much.

On the ward, the staff know that M loves to dance, and in fact she spins off into dancing at all times. But dancing alone, as I witness her once, standing outside the ward doors, she looks like a restless ghost, her attention is inwards, her smile is a polite statement of protection. When she danced with us, together we were able to acknowledge a vital part of her, she felt our recognition and could be herself, could express niggling fears. Safe, and comforted by familiarity, she could loosen her carefulness and find a connection with herself and others. We are making no demands of her, we are joining in with her, we are listening, we are real.

Where her words fail her, M's movements are clear, expressive, assured and entirely beautiful. As the hospital competently treat the symptoms of her illness, her depression and apathy have lifted. Dancing with companions has given her the further boost of a sense of wellness and a joyous life-affirming experience, that in M's case was an essential part of her personality.

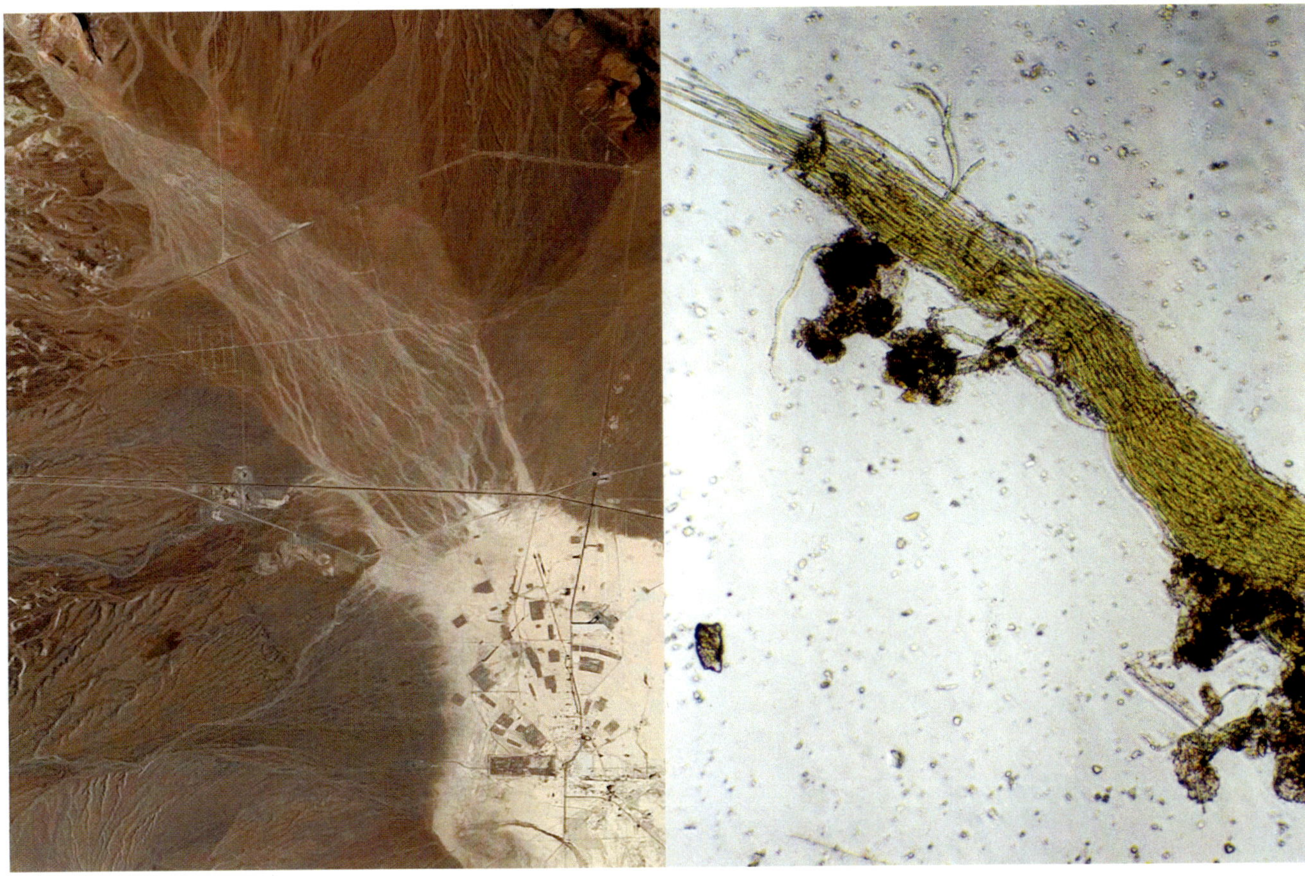

Life in the Field of Death 2012 Chris Drury

Made in collaboration with Dr Lynn Fenstermaker, the work shows a microscope image of Microcoleus Vaginata which is growing in the soils of the Nevada Nuclear Test site where 100 atmospheric bombs were tested. Next to it is an image from space of that same test site. Microcoleus Vaginata is a cyanobacteria, which were the first organisms to convert CO_2 into xygen, paving the way for life on the planet.

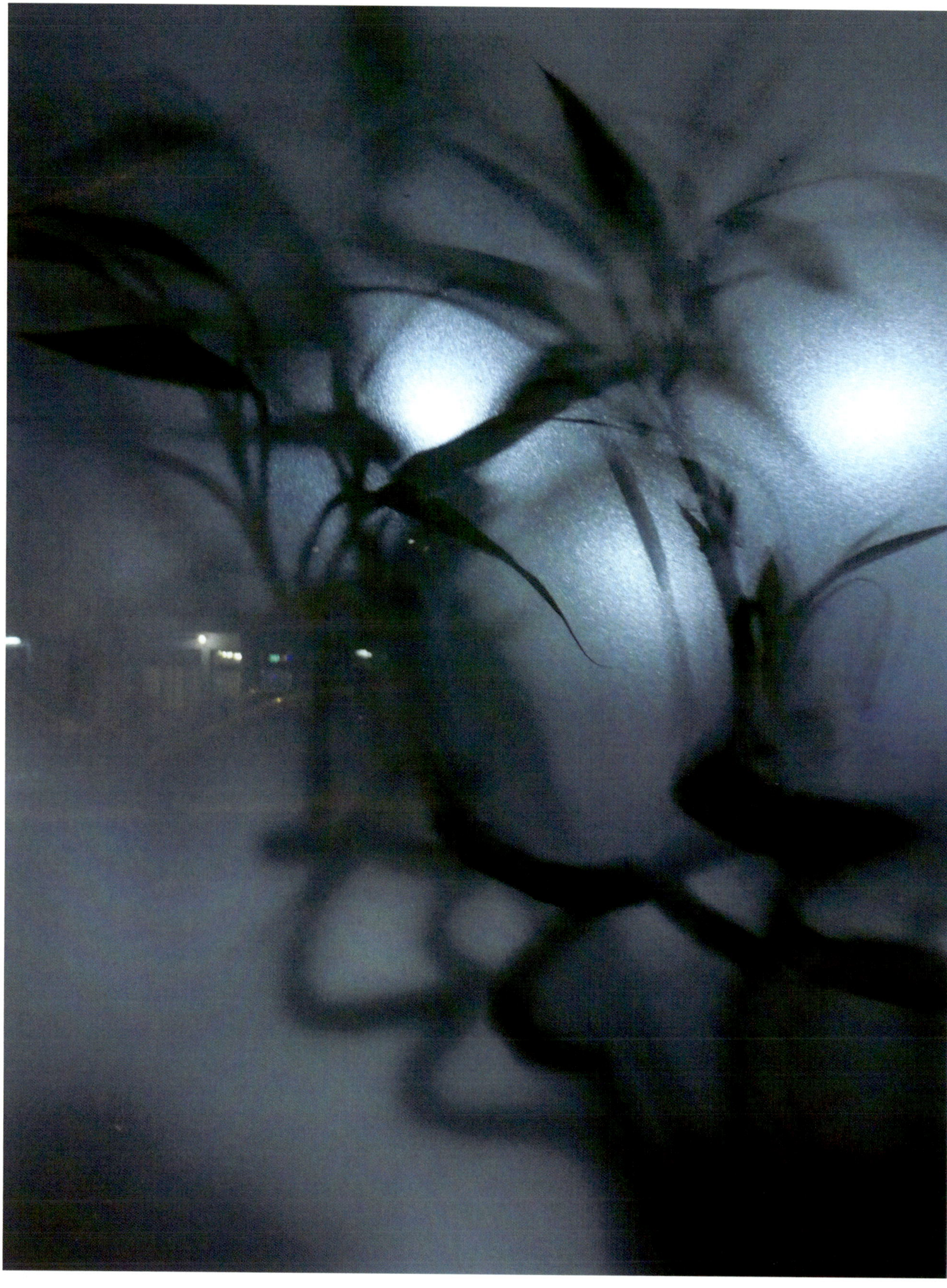

Towards meaning: body, health and imagination

A Short Story of Falling

It is the story of the falling rain
To turn into a leaf and fall again

It is the secret of a summer shower
To steal the light and hide it in a flower

And every flower a tiny tributary
That from the ground flows green and momentary

Is one of water's wishes and this tale
Hangs in a seed head smaller than my thumbnail

If only I a passerby could pass
As clear as water through a plume of grass

To find the sunlight hidden at the tip
Turning to seed a kind of lifting rain drip

Then I might know like water how to balance
The weight of hope against the light of patience

Water which is so raw so earthy-strong
And lurks in cast iron tanks and leaks along

Drawn under gravity towards my tongue
To cool and fill the pipe-work of this song

Which is the story of the falling rain
That rises to the light and falls again

Alice Oswald, from *Falling Awake* (2016)

Finding a language

In every aspect and at any stage of our lives, articulating what we feel is challenging. We all need some means of expression. Our words are often clichés or arbitrary labels and obscure or misrepresent. This can leave us with an even deeper sense of helplessness and isolation. The inarticulacy of feelings that are not expressed or spoken is a recurrent feature of loneliness, and a source of stress and unhappiness. We have continually to refresh our sensing and means of expression – and to find ways of giving form to what is sensed yet invisible and coming towards us from the darkness of ourselves.

When life throws us into crisis we may reach out for the arts – to poetry, music, song and dance – to help make sense of otherwise unbearable circumstances. Only the world of imagery can convey a feeling sense of what we are experiencing. The physicality of movement, of poetic language, of music, or pictorial sensuousness can reveal and extend our perception, helping us both express and contain feelings. The words and images that arise in the wake of moving or making surprise and sharpen our perception, connecting vividly to our feeling world.

Weaving through this book are many accounts where an image speaks for a person and opens out how they feel in themselves. A sailing boat, a queen bee, a clown toy, a pod, are all images that emerged through the free play of creating. A piece of wood placed on a windowsill with feathers and sheep's wool becomes 'a place to rest' embodying a need for the maker. Every image carries a meaning that communicates to body and soul and speaks to what matters to a person, in this they are potent and life affirming.

To know and not to speak
In that way one forgets
What is pronounced strengthens itself
What is not pronounced tends to non-existence

Czesław Miłosz, *New and Collected Poems 1931–2001*

'This being human'[1]

> Our stories, myths and fairy tales are a kind of poetic code similar to our genetic code – and the body a spirit beacon as much as a chemical formula.
>
> Drawn from Seamus Heaney speaking at Ted Hughes' memorial service in 1999.

In 1887, just before he attempted suicide, Gauguin painted a large, colourful painting, one of his rich and glorious works from the South Sea Islands. He gave it the title: *Where do we come from? What are we? Where are we going?* His words express a deep human need to find purpose and meaning in our experience. Dr Mehl-Madrona writes about his Cherokee ancestry and the elders' use of personal narrative in healing processes: 'A traditional elder told me that health and disease evolved from the way we answered four simple questions: Who are you? Where did you come from? Why are you here? Where are you going?'[2] Edward Adamson, the first visual artist to be employed in the NHS, worked with William Kurelek, an artist being treated for schizophrenia, whose now famous painting entitled *Where Am I? Who Am I? Why Am I?* hangs in the American Visionary Arts Museum.

For as long as we humans have existed, we've turned to the arts in order to find meaning, to respond to the world around us, and to articulate what is invisible and buried within us. Art, dance, poetry and music all communicate experiences that are beyond our everyday words. When the circumstances of our lives become unbearable and our prose fails, then we may reach out for new poetic means of expression.

And whatever we make or create brings solace – something expressed and shared. We all have a need to communicate and to be known, recognised for who we are – indeed without some means of expression we become strangers to our deeper selves.

Art making emerged thousands of years ago along with language. The brain's capacity for symbolic thought developing alongside our human need to communicate and give form to the beliefs, prayers and wordless feelings that give meaning to our life experience. Over 35,000 years ago, our hunter-gatherer ancestors went into the quiet and dark of caves and with exquisite sensitivity painted the walls with animals and figures, depicting the creatures, rituals and forces on which their lives depended.

From our earliest beginnings and in every region of the world, the arts have been involved

[1] Drawn from 'The Guest House', a poem by Rumi

[2] Dr Mehl-Madrona, *Coyote Medicine: Lessons from Native American Healing 1998, see also Narrative Medicine the use of history and story in the healing process,* 2007

with healing, with engaging our creativity in a search for connection and meaning. And whatever we create illuminates, opens doors between the hidden inner worlds of our feelings and the outer realities we inhabit. The arts in health do not seek to 'cure', but to bring a greater sense of wholeness to a person; in this they strengthen our capacity to meet and adapt to change.

Dance is often used as a metaphor for life. It is the earliest and the most ephemeral of the arts, rarely leaving a trace. Yet on cave and rock walls there are dancing figures – dances that are invocations, prayers, speaking to the numinous forces of life and to the entwined relationship of human and non-human worlds – the dancing body a portal through which elemental life forces are sensed and communicated with.

Finding ways to engage creatively, opening eyes, ears and other senses, reconnects us to essential aspects of who we are, strengthening how we live with illness and how we look after ourselves. In whatever way art making engages and absorbs us – music, movement, paint, poems – anxiety quietens as we delve creatively, a moving out of clock time into a deeper realm of feelings, dreams and intuitions. And whatever emerges infuses new content into our lives.

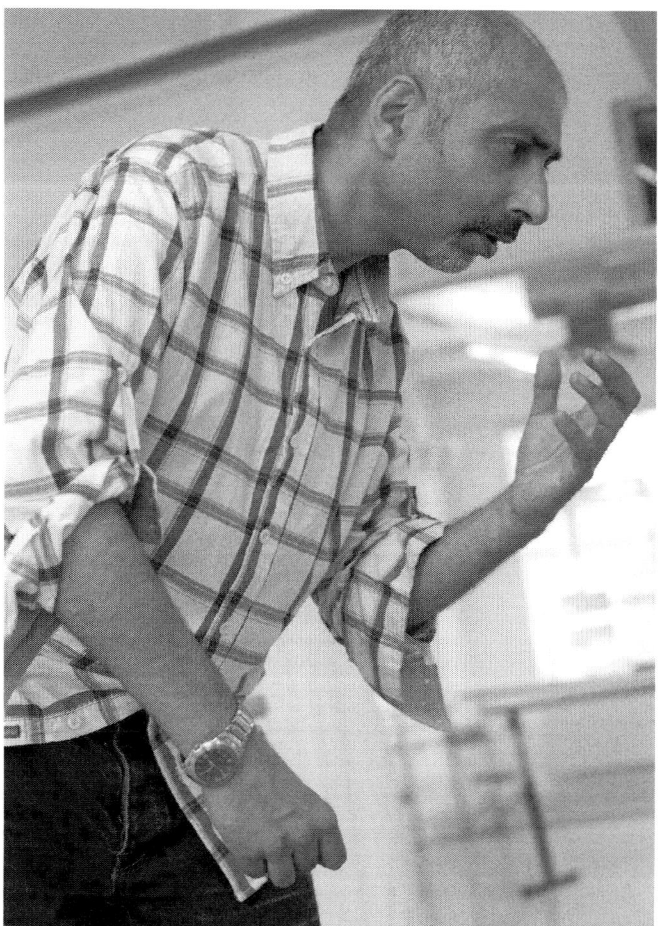

Gerhard Dorn,
a sixteenth century
alchemist, writes:
'In order to heal,
one must learn from
what one depends
and to whom
one belongs and to
what end one
has been created.'

Being well

Hippocrates, whose oath underlies the principles of modern medicine, taught that health lies in balance, in harmony between the different aspects of our lives. In any one moment our body is a confluence of many streams of information communicating between body and brain, between what is inside us and our surrounding world. Research increasingly reveals the impact of emotions on every aspect of our physiology, from heart and circulation to digestion and gastrointestinal activity, respiration and immune functioning – all respond swiftly to how we think and feel (and vice versa).

Many of the problems and concerns people bring to their doctor do not conform to simple diagnostic labels. Unhappiness, depression, insoluble life predicaments and social problems, all significantly impact on a person's health.

> My twenty-four years as a family doctor have convinced me that many 'medical' complaints reported by patients are in fact physical manifestations of social, psychological and emotional problems. To create a healthier nation we must start by encouraging inclusive, harmonious relationships in a society where so many find themselves socially excluded. The principal killers are not cancer and heart disease but lack of social support, poor education and stagnant economies.
>
> Dr Malcolm Rigler, General Practitioner

Despite the miraculous advances of modern medicine, it is rarely concerned with the individual and with what makes life significant. Standards of healthcare are dictated more and more by evidence-based protocols, which by their nature regard patients as standardised units of disease. Such protocols have no way of accommodating the unique story of the individual. Yet our well being is intricately bound up with the personal and particular, with what gives each of our lives meaning and value.

> There is nothing alive which is not individual; our health is ours; our diseases are ours; our reactions are ours – no less than our minds or our faces.
>
> Oliver Sacks, *Awakenings*

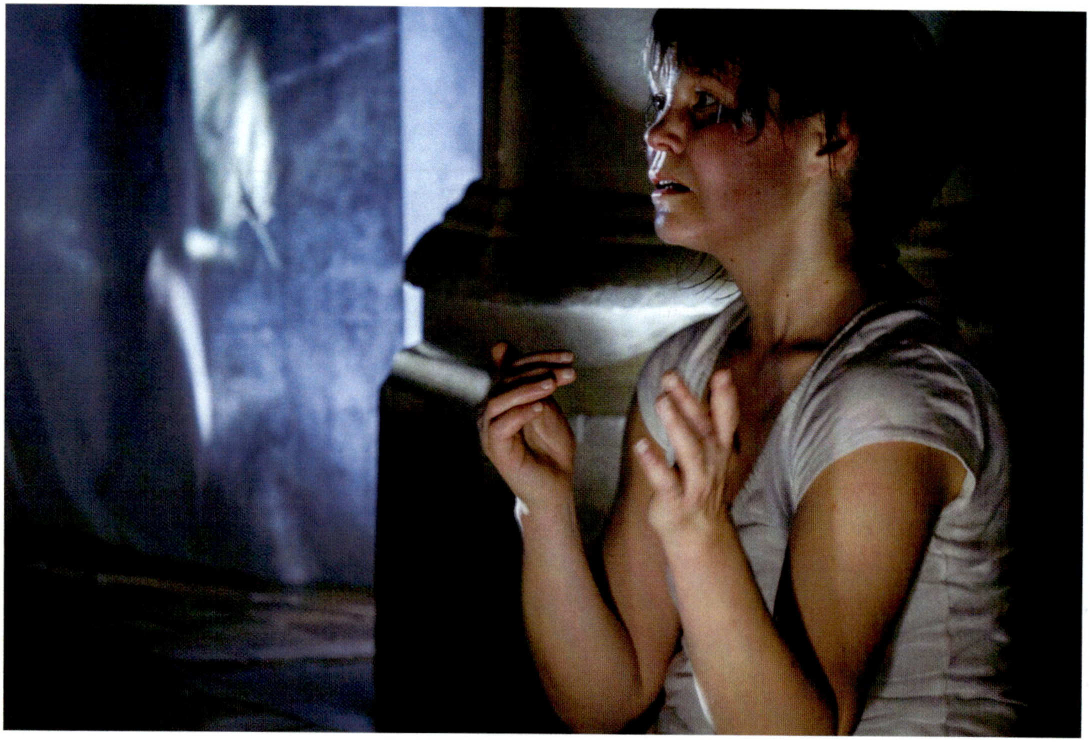

The healing image – towards an embodied imagination

> Healing through the arts is one of the oldest cultural practices in every region of the world.... The arts heal by activating the powers of the imagination... If we can liberate the creative process in our lives it will always find the way to whatever needs attention and transformation.
>
> Drawn from Shaun McNiff, *How Art Heals*

Imagination and imagery have always played a role in both illness and healing. There are stories from around the globe and across the ages, of the power of imagination, of story and image in easing pain, nausea, reducing ulcers, tumours and other ills. In traditional societies illness and disease are perceived as a rift in relationship between the human and non-human worlds. Shamans journey into the imagination to discover the source of illness and restore balance and relationship – both within the individual body and within the community.

In ancient Greece, the healing centre of the *Asclepium*[3] received patients to dream until

[3] From Asclepius, the Greek god of healing.

their dreaming revealed some metaphor or image that made visible the source of their disease. They dreamed to find what they could not see with their everyday eyes. The arts are a form of reverie. All forms of art making give rise to imagery that makes tangible the inner world of our feelings.

We all tend to ruminate and worry, our mind trapped in concerns about past or future-a sadly familiar way we engage our imagination. Yet if we can come back to the body and the sensuous detail of what is at hand, imagination begins to open out our seeing and reveal the multi layered nature of our feelings. As we create forms – through dance, writing, sculpting, painting – we take possession of our experiences rather than letting our responses get stuck within us as symptoms. As we detach from what seem the insistent imperatives of our lives and allow ourselves to wander and wonder, play, upset and reverse our familiar world orders, we begin to find voice, give shape, colour, pattern and coherence to more of what we feel. The stories and images we find as we sense and create are a means of feeling our way towards new understanding.

> For an animal its natural environment and habitat are a given – despite the faith of the empiricists reality is not a given; it has to be continually sought out and held – I am tempted to say salvaged. One is taught to oppose the real to the imaginary, as though the first were always at hand and the second distant, far away. This opposition is false. Events are always to hand. But the coherence of these events – which is what one means by reality – is an imaginative construction. Reality always lies beyond – and this is true for materialists as for idealists. For Plato, or Marx. Reality, however one interprets it, lies beyond a screen of clichés.
>
> John Berger, *And our Faces, My Heart, Brief as Photos,* p. 72

The making of personal and potent images is itself therapeutic and life enhancing moving us from the passivity of being a patient into artist and maker, actively responding to and shaping our world. Edward Adamson, the first visual artist to be employed in the NHS, witnessed patients recovering and healing from illness, simply through the opportunity to create and express. He wrote of the therapeutic potency of art making, and stressed that patients drew on his knowledge and skill as artist and painter rather than on any psychological framework.[4]

The story of our lives, like a river, is always changing, retold in the light of new events, a circling and re-circling as we attempt to give form and meaning to events. And it is within our bodies, in our instinctual and sensory responses, that the metaphors and images that underlie our seeing and sense of meaning are revealed. To listen and move as the impulse

[4] Many of the practices in this book may seem to overlap with arts therapy but the intention differs and lies in engaging the artist in each person.

takes us allows what lies within us to swim up to the surface of awareness. And the images and metaphors that emerge are as bridges by which we connect what we feel within us, outwards to the objects and people of the everyday world of which we are part. An image becomes a window through which I 'see', which lets in, lets through meaning – through image we touch our feeling world.

Creating in any medium shifts the focus from self as centre, to a 'self among',[5] a belonging with and in relation to others and the world about us. The arts engage our senses and imagination in story, colour, music, and gesture. In the free play of creativity we discover other and often surprising voices, movements and stories that open out how we feel in ourselves, profoundly altering the feeling tone of our bodies.

Dance is ephemeral, and leaves no visible trace of itself; like a message on water, it rises, plays through the body and vanishes. In our own projects, we encouraged people to move between different media, engaging creatively in whatever way seemed possible or accessible for a person; a story, a memory, a song or piece of music, could each open a door into movement and bring to the fore what mattered to a person. To sift and evoke the experience of moving through other media – stories, poems, paint, or sculpting materials – amplifies this wordless realm, offering a tangible means of reflection which extends the resonances of whatever is created.

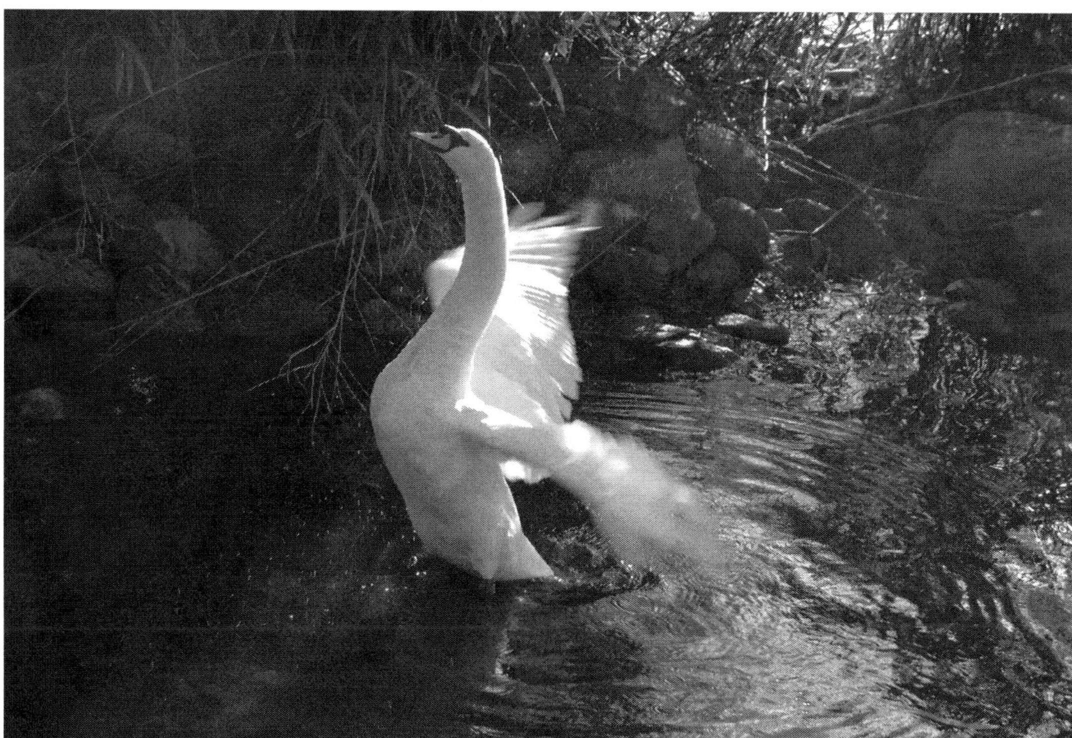

5 An insight from James Hillman, psychologist. See *The Soul's Code:In search of character and calling.*

On the movement of painting and words

> My words join the edges of pages, inside them other words, around them winds, beneath them streams, and every word has a root and a leaf and a becoming. I know it now, can feel still the wide circular strokes, finding the years, knowing through all the strokes the binding of all things, the interlacing, interacting, need of each thing for the other. Paints and hands and heart moved into the moving on the page, a past, a present and future within the breath on the page and a moving transcribing itself into unimagined ways of new logic. No words can say this and make it true, only the breath, becoming dance, becoming yes, becoming movement, translating a new language and shifting it to this page of emerging life.
>
> Sr Bridget Folkard working with breath in a hospital

When we become ill our familiar life narratives fall apart. It is here that the creative space of art making offers a context where we can begin to find a new coherence. In the stress of managing illness it is often difficult to remember that movement and change (as in Alice Oswald's poem above) are fundamental to being alive. Listening to the body as movement and creating with what we find can re-awaken us to the richness and diversity of life. As we gain trust and articulateness in our bodies, in our senses, our feelings and imagination, we discover the multi layered nature of experience. Through this we discover new stories through we which we may recover a sense of meaning and purpose in our lives.

Each day the poet Mary Oliver records something seen in the natural world. In her introduction to the collection *Wild Geese* she writes of this life-saving practice:

> I stood willingly and gladly in the characters of everything – other people, trees, clouds – and this is what I learned, that the world's otherness is antidote to confusion... that standing within this otherness... the beauty and the mystery of the world, out in the fields or deep inside books, can re-dignify the worst-stung heart.
>
> Mary Oliver[6]

[6] *Wild Geese: Selected Poems.*

Chance of fair ...

writing with people with mental and physical health issues

Kay Syrad

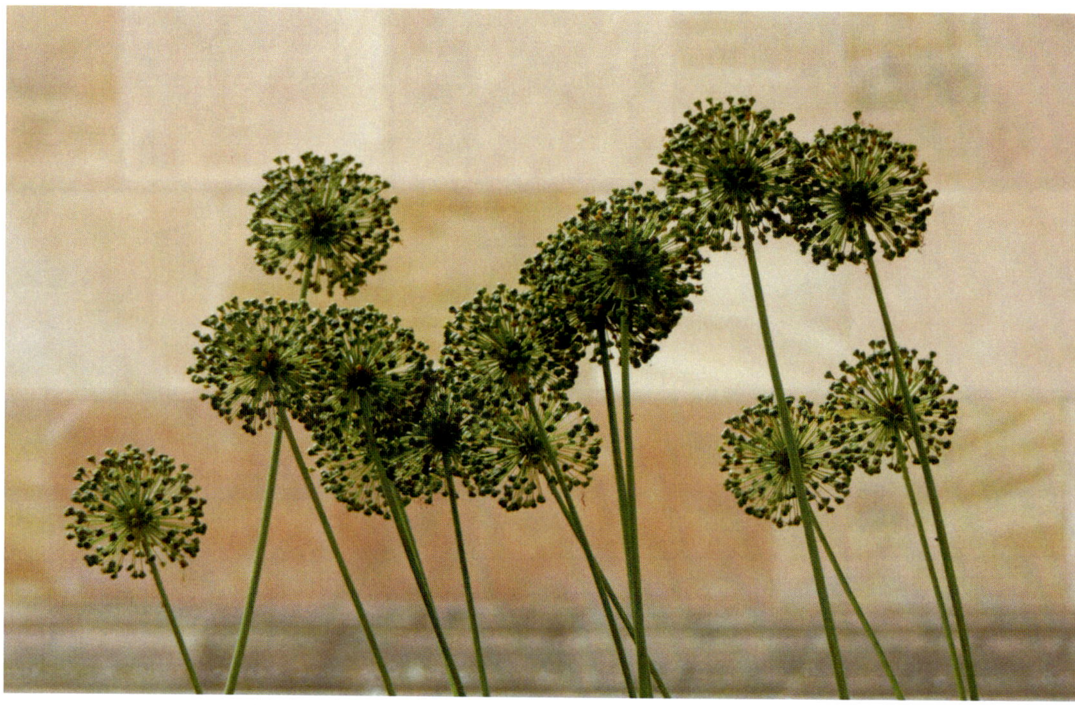

I am a poet and novelist who runs creative writing classes at a drop-in centre for people with experience of mental illness and/or emotional distress, and also for people with acquired brain injury (ABI) at a Headway day centre in East Sussex. I am outside these people's lives, in that I am not given specific information about my students' situations or conditions; I haven't been trained to work with people with ABI, and have only a little training (plus family experience) in mental health. What I discover about each person, therefore, is by chance and through their creative work. The groups have some long-standing members but there is also a changing constituency and, in the case of the ABI group, a number of different carers or support workers each week as well. Consequently, the writing activities I devise have an almost theatrical or performance quality, and require from me a great deal of energy and nerve to 'hold' the situation.

Working with a group at the mental health drop-in centre, I set a writing task entitled 'Imagining Cuckmere Haven', in which participants were invited to write about that beautiful coastal area near Eastbourne, incorporating or inspired by one of the following words or phrases:

a grey heron ... the wreck of the Polynesia ... a lime-green pool ... an excess of light
the seventh sister (Went Hill) ... an ox-bow lake ... whiteness ... unexplained laughter
dusk ... the first sister (Haven Brow) ... 'the sea has fallen on us' [1]

Offering such phrases or words gives students confidence and helps to frame their thoughts and ideas:

> Chance of fair, going on first light.
> We can see the ox-bow lake at first light,
> time to set sail through the twists and turns
> and at the ox-bow lake, an excess of light...'
>
> Stephen, from his poem 'An Excess of Light and an Ox-bow Lake'

Another confidence-enhancing activity is the creation of group poems, where students are asked to contribute their best or favourite line from the poetry or prose they have written during the class that day. We then collectively agree on the best order for the disparate lines to create a coherent (if surreal) poem. In the example below, each line is exactly the line that each student gave me, including the title:

> ***Don't swing on the bars***
>
> I prayed I'd be back in this place -
> the expectation was to blossom out of the sickroom
> looking elegant.
> The tranquillity allowed the imagination to run freely and relax -
> (serenity is a safe place
> and Christ, not Man, is King).
> Fickle, reflective glass ushering in one image after another.

At Headway, my students, whose ages range from 20 to 75, and who have suffered life-changing strokes, accidents or illnesses, have, with varying degrees of help, been able to attempt the writing of sonnets, ballads, clerihews, limericks and haiku:

[1] A line from Janet Sutherland's poem 'Sea Level' in her collection *Hangman's Acre*.

The light makes a flame
On a sad face
Shows which way to go

Nathan Milham

And also love letters, prison letters and flash fiction. They have deployed classic plots (rags to riches; quest; overcoming the monster; journey). We have worked with the conventions of myth, fairy tales and legends and with the genres of mystery and romantic comedy; students have also contributed to a group detective story, and to the storylines for a 3-episode soap opera based on the Wimbledon Tennis Championships.

Unlike some of my colleagues, I don't encourage directly personal writing although of course the students' prose and poetry is imbued with their feelings, thoughts and world views. I find what works well is giving students a clear structure and form (particularly, in poetry, where it is musical, with a distinct rhythm); it is within a strong framework that everyone's rich imaginations can be activated.

Barometer

From Clear to Dry, From Close to Fair
It weighs the sky and it weighs the air
It measures the pressures, which warn of the storm –
Warning of the hurricane, from cold onto warm –
I watched the barometer, as I sat on the stair,
Silently rotating and measuring the air
And measuring the pressure, with its needle of gold –
From Rain to Moisture, from Warm to Cold –
I wondered at its needles as it spun against the sky –
From Warm to Cold, from Rain to Dry –
When I was so young, when I was a boy
I watched the barometer, I made it my toy
As it hung by the picture, firmly fixed to the wall –
I watched the slow needle, its rise and its fall –
The barometer was my father's, it was mine in my eyes,
I watched the slow pressure, its fall and its rise –
I watched dad's barometer, so calm and so old:
As it warned of the storm, as it warned of the cold.

Poem by Ben Gribbin at Headway Centre for ABI

The students with ABI all have memory loss, particularly short-term memory, so what we accomplish during each class is made special by its temporality. Sometimes earlier memories are activated: one student, working with the ballad form, remembered in detail the Arthur Scargill/Margaret Thatcher conflict of the 1980s. Without this formal cue, we may never have known that this student was interested in politics in this way.

I often give students a prompt such as an image (we've used a drawing by Leonardo da Vinci for his Ornithopter Flying Machine, the first ice cream parlour in New York, the book covers of famous novels), or an unusual juxtaposition of characters, which always produces great hilarity. I suggest contemporary figures such as politicians, celebrities, and characters from literature, history, films or TV. The following story was written about the invented character of the second Mrs Leonardo da Vinci:

Leonardo's Wish

> 'Signora da Vinci – the new incarnation – stepped out into the hot Italian sun. Leonardo traced her shadow. She daintily collected the whirling washing from the line and he stole a shadowed glance. His calculating mind and artistic vision pictured her on canvas. The sun beat down on the pair as they whirled indoors. The chore was over for the day. Leonardo asked his wife if she'd like him to invent a new-fangled automatic clothes drier. "Yes, Leonardo, sounds good to me," she gasped, and fields of vision collided.'
>
> Saeed Mesbah

Sometimes I give an ending perhaps taken from a famous novel ('There was the hum of bees, and the musky odour of pinks filled the air' from Kate Chopin's *The Awakening*), or an opening line such as '*He thought he heard a flock of geese overhead, but...*' which works well for short stories and flash fiction.

The carers and support staff contribute to the writing exercises, helping the student to say what they want to say, however slowly, and they often write their own creative piece too – and as the carers get to know their clients through the imaginative writing they do, so we get to know the carers, the writing exercises supporting everyone in quiet and unpredictable ways. As one of my students said, 'Betterment Occurred'.[2]

[2] 'Betterment Occurred' became the title of the student Saeed Mesbah's poem.

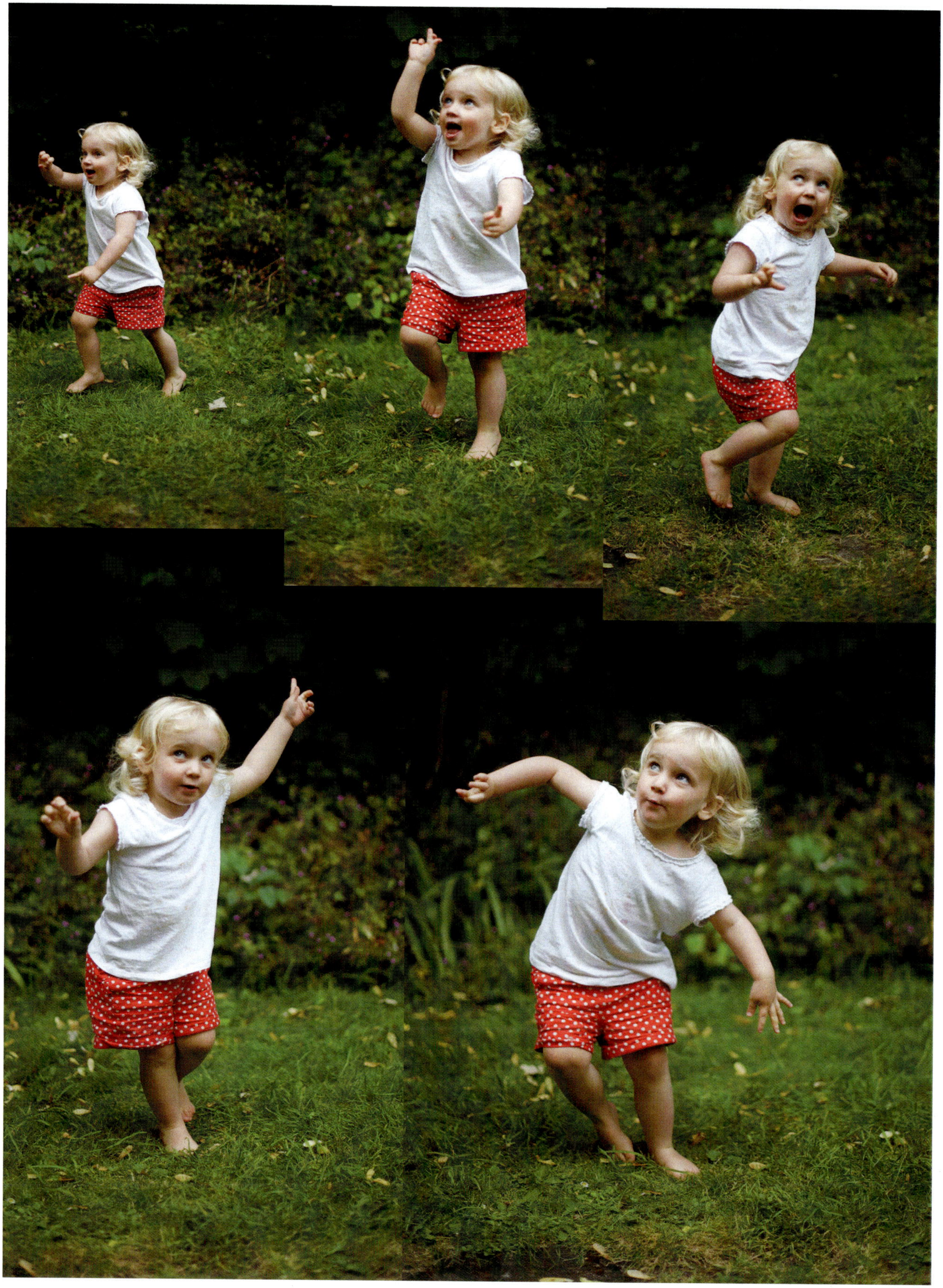

Laying the Foundations
Karen Adcock Doyle and Jasmine Pasch

Jasmine Pasch trained as a professional dancer, teacher and counselor. She has worked across the arts, health and education sectors for over thirty years. She currently works in the London boroughs of Brent and Tower Hamlets with babies, toddlers, young children and their families, and supports early years educators and parents develop their understanding of the particular developmental, learning and play needs of this age group.

Karen Adcock Doyle is a family and pupil support manager in a North Yorkshire school, working with early years and primary age children and their families. Karen trained as a learning disability nurse, and worked in Barnardo's for many years as a therapeutic worker. Karen supports children with social, emotional and mental health needs and is interested in how movement can support children to develop sensate language and have greater agency over their bodies.

A young boy whose difficulties with movement, balance and coordination affected his confidence and ability to join in with his school friends, chose to come along to movement sessions. He said at the end that being able to do things now made him HAPPY!!

Such a simple statement from a five-year-old tells a story.

Making relationships and feeling good about oneself, having a sense of agency and competence, being able to think, learn creatively and make connections are at the heart of well being and happiness. Body movement underpins these essential capacities throughout life, with the early years being particularly significant.

> Trust the body, to have the solutions
> Trust the child, to show you the way

In early development, some children may not have had the opportunity to move and play on the floor, and so have missed out on building significant foundations. This affects sensory and movement integration, later behaviour, self-esteem and confidence, and basic skills such as holding a pen to write.

Through movement, play and dance, we help children get the experiences they need to grow to their full potential.

The magic of trust – Karen

> By taking on an animal nature we are better able to express feelings. It can give us permission to express and experience certain qualities of movement not readily available to us in everyday life.
>
> Anna Halprin

I met C while offering somatic movement sessions in a Lancashire primary school. In class, he was unable to sit on his bottom with feet on the ground, preferring to squat. He found it difficult to pick up a pencil and place recognisable letters on the paper. I worked with him one to one.

The first time we met I offered him a deck of animal cards. We placed all the cards out on the floor in a circle, then slowly walked all the way around, looking at the cards and speaking about some of them.

He chose the aardvark, although he didn't know its name. We discussed the animal, its armour, qualities. We spent the session moving as aardvarks. I followed him and tried to embody his patterns! His crawling was side to side, on knees, calf and foot pointing to the sky – which was very painful. At times, I witnessed[1] whilst inviting him through story to rest, sleep, hunt, eat as the aardvark.

C made marks on paper of his journey as an aardvark. I was witness, watching and listening as C's breath settled into his moving and drawing. Names were given to important places on the paper. These became a dance score, choreographed by C with me as audience. He asked me to use the camera to film him as he shared his dance. I called out the words he had asked me to write on his picture: claw, wave, bone; and he would find a movement in response. He loved watching this back. It was his dance, and he chose not to share with anyone else.

> I am constantly amazed by the magic of trust. Going with an older child back to a place where they can start to revisit early childhood patterns – like creeping and crawling. These patterns make changes to their emotional and physical well being. These are joyous, playful, self-esteem-building ways to help children.

Week 7, his teacher asked me with interest: 'What did you two do today?' I explained

[1] Linda Hartley, *Somatic Psychology*, 2004, describes the witness as someone who: 'pays attention to the feelings, images, sensations, memories, and movement impulses that arise in her, evoked by the presence of the person moving. She owns these as her own experience ... she does not attempt to interpret or analyse the mover's experience ... but owns these for what they are – her own direct experience, evoked by the presence and activity of the mover.'

that we did exactly the same as we had done for the last six weeks: crawled, ate, slept as an aardvark; from his painting score, C had then developed his dance. She told me that C came back to class, sat at his table, picked up his pen, and wrote on paper. His writing was readable, better than anything she'd ever seen him produce, and this was the first time he'd actually sat properly on a chair, feet on the ground.

Become your animal

Choose an animal
Close your eyes
Imagine you are this animal
Do you have fur, skin, feathers, a shell?
Scales, spikes, hooves, horns, wings?
Do you stand on the earth, live underground or in the sky?
When do you move – in the dark, daylight?
Can I see you, hear you, smell you?

Imagine being this animal
How do you meet the ground – heavy, light, solid, fragile?
Where are you resting?
In a cave, hole, nest, shell, log pile, tree, field?
Can anyone see you?

It's time to wake up
How do you wake? slowwwwwww, stretching, taking time? or alert – ready for action!
Become your animal
Take flight, poke your snout out of your hole, roll onto your paws
Are you slow, inquisitive, timid, fierce, fast, unpredictable?

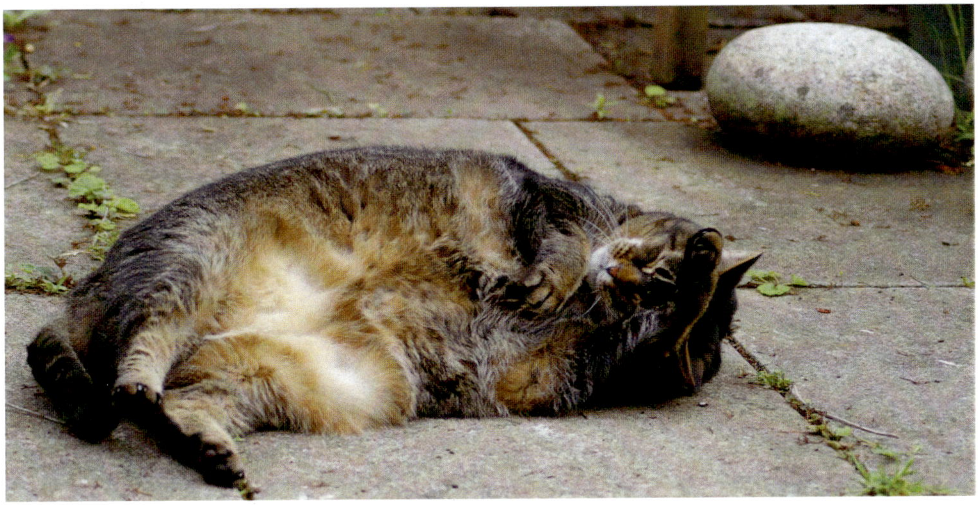

Getting connected in the early years – Jasmine

Babies, toddlers and young children need movement and play experiences in the loving arms of their parents and caregivers, with that shared rhythm of the heartbeat and breath, the familiar voice, song and dance, reassuring touch and warmth. This is a vital part of the bonding process, and helps them to feel safe and secure, and good about themselves. The parent or carer's body is the best piece of play equipment, and far more interesting than any toy or baby gym.

> Enjoying one another's company, having fun and laughing together produces dopamine: 'the big, buzz reward hormone that actively stimulates brain growth.'
>
> R Bowlby, *Attachment Videos*

From the beginning of life, body movement stimulates the growth of brain circuitry, the 'wiring'. This is then insulated by myelin which is a white, fatty substance which forms a protective sheath around nerve fibres and allows for more efficient transmission of impulses. Through movement and play we grow our neural networks, and thus our potential functioning. So babies need plenty of opportunity for unrestricted movement to make those vital connections, and enough space to move around in so that they can practice over and over again, strengthening the connections as they move, play and actively explore the world around them.[2]

The belly crawl is a top-to-toe workout, and very hard work. It may be a brief phase, but is a critical and distinct phase that puts many specific and necessary pieces into place. According to Bette Lamont: 'Many people allow or encourage children to skip it because when they put them down they hear grunting and fussing that sounds like distress. In many cases this is simply the infant trying to sort out breathing from moving, so the grunts are understandable ... and necessary.'[3] Babies put onto their backs will wriggle and roll over, finding the prone position by themselves if we give them the freedom to move and get comfortable. Gaining head control is the baby's first and most important task as many other movement abilities are built on this foundation skill. Towards the second half of the first year, the baby may push up onto hands and knees and, after a bit of rocking back and forth, pushing off and going backwards instead of forwards, the infant begins to creep on all fours. Two significant early patterns are the belly crawl, and creeping on hands and knees, described by Bette Lamont as 'double clicks on the brain'.[4]

[2] A montage of the movements a baby does in the first year of life can be found at www.thenext25years.com 'Baby Liv' and is a useful resource for parents as they can identify and track the moves their baby is making.

[3] Bette Lamont, personal communication with Jasmine Pasch (2006)

[4] *Ibid.*

Ten good reasons to get your baby Crawling on its Belly ... a 'double click' on the brain[5]

Stimulates **horizontal eye tracking**, *and helps the eyes to work together in correct alignment.*

Early head movement helps the neck to grow strong and the skull to round out, **preventing flat head syndrome**[6]

Strengthens the arches in the feet, helps with heel to coccyx alignment, and **stabilises the hip sockets.**

Promotes cervical and lumbar spine stability, and neck strength, so helps the **development of the mature S curve** *from the infant C curve.*

Makes the child aware of the genital area through ventral stimulation, and helps with **on time toilet training.**

Helps with the supination and pronation of the lower arm, and helps the hands to open out from the grasp reflex to eventual **cortical control**[7]

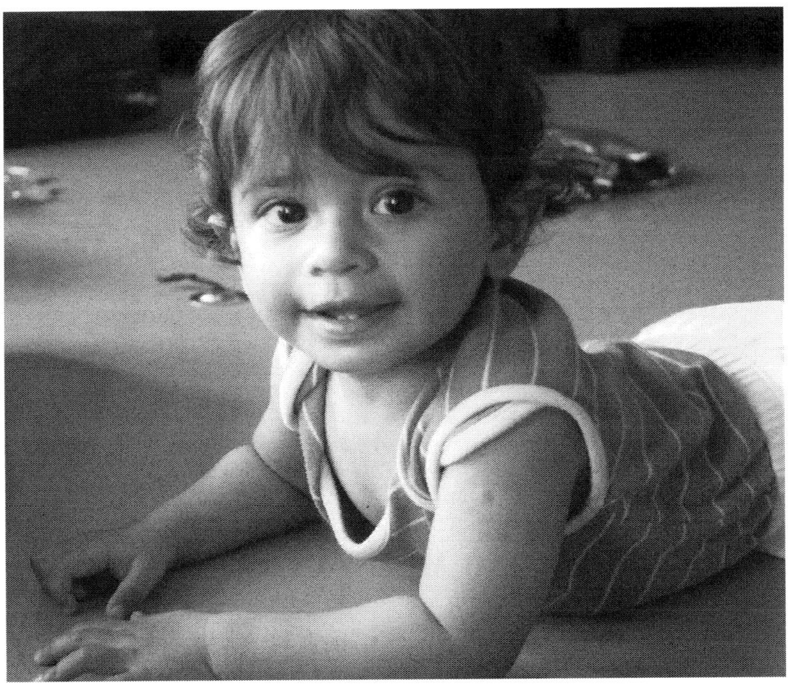

[5] Taken from the work of Bette Lamont, Seattle USA (Jasmine Pasch 2010)

[6] Positional plagiocephaly

[7] Fine motor skills

Creates a feeling of vertical throughness[8] *which helps the child to feel* **grounded**.
is the first **self-determined** *movement.*

Seems to be connected with **brain stem development**, *and functions that ensure survival: accurate perception of pain, heat, cold and hunger.*

Builds a sense of self, and is the basis for development of **empathy and compassion.**

Ten good reasons to get your baby Creeping on its Hands and Knees ... a 'double click' on the brain[9]

Stimulates **vertical eye tracking**, *visual convergence, teaches the eyes to cross the midline and practice near and far point vision.*

Promotes **hand to eye** *coordination.*

Shoulders and hips *are further rotated into alignment.*

The **hands** *are more fully opened out as they support the weight.*

Balance away from the floor *is explored through much trial and error, and mastered gradually. This forms the basis of balance throughout life.*

Goes through a number of stages which the child must practice and play with before arriving at the **cross pattern crawl**.

Supports the development of the **corpus callosum**[10]

Fires connections between the two hemispheres of the brain supporting retrieval, filtering, sorting and sifting, and sequencing, and without the connections we may see difficulties with **learning and memory**[11]

Seems to be connected to development of the **mid brain**, *building a bridge between oneself and the world and* **making relationships.**

Enables the vestibular, proprioceptive and visual systems to connect and operate together for the first time. Without this **integration** *there can be a poorly developed sense of balance and poor space and depth perception.*

[8] 'Throughness' is a sense of connection right through the body

[9] Taken from the work of Bette Lamont, Seattle USA, and Jane Field, Jasmine Pasch, 2010.

[10] The corpus callosum is the major inter-hemispheric communicator and as such it mediates between the hemispheres to synchronise their particular specialisations, Field, 1995.

[11] Such as difficulties in knowing right from left, letter, word and number reversals, e.g. b/d, p/q, on/no, patterns of learning and forgetting the same thing several times.

What are we seeing in the early years setting – Karen

Children in early years come to school: in cars, buggies, prams, on buggy boards, wearing safety harness, backpack, wrist links, reins, enabling carers to restrict how far away the child can move from the adult. Mobile phones and iPads are placed in the buggy to entertain on the move. In the home, carers are encouraged to use Bumbos[12], door jumpers, bouncers and baby walkers.

All these restrictive devices and the lack of creeping and crawling hinder development and can store up a wide range of problems for later. These include poor depth perception, poor balance, poor ability to walk and see at the same time. When children start school, some are: unable to hold a spoon or pencil (but able to swipe a phone or tablet); unable to sense danger, climbing onto high walls, leaning out of tall buildings, and walking downstairs 45 degrees forwards; not able to balance, coordinate their movements, with lack of proprioception and kinaesthetic awareness; struggling to transition from sitting to standing, bumping into objects and others, can't stop and start when asked, unable to walk backwards. Often there is poor concentration or focus, impulsive behaviour (including hitting and hurting), poor speech and language (12-24 months below age-related expectations), not toilet trained, suffering constipation, poor vision, lack of empathy, high sensitivity to all or to some senses.

Children walk around the school in herds, charging down four flights of stairs and leaping off the last four steps. They race in to cloakrooms, knocking over smaller, more timid children, stimulating already over-stimulated children, leaving some fearful and feeling they have been pushed and knocked over.

Children are outraged when their experiments with their bodies are classed as 'purposeful violence'! Teachers and parents are confused, not wanting to make communal spaces like an army camp, but at the same time, needing to consider child and adult safety, a need to feel safe and secure, a need to help children who become overwhelmed through sensory overload to stay calm. Such a confusing world! These same children spend far too many hours on electronic games and computers.

Not... moving...

Missing early foundations

I'm in a clothes shop when a family from school comes to say hello. Their three year old runs up to me: 'I'm a ballerina', and spins and spins and spins. I watch, fascinated, transported back, a memory of climbing my dad's legs and tipple-tailing over, of spinning on ice as a skater, faster and faster. She

[12] A baby-sitting seat that helps infants to prematurely prop themselves up, impeding their natural movement development.

> starts nursery this autumn. How wonderful! Other children will be inspired by her mastery and enthusiasm.

So many children so early on are stuck, hesitant, and fearful of their bodies. Scared of spiders and worms; unable to balance on a log, pile of twigs; can't judge the edges of surfaces.

> I watch another child, two years old, just learning to walk. He cannot hold his weight, his muscles aren't strong enough. His parents are desperate to show he can walk. They pull him up by the hands to standing – he hasn't learn to do this himself. He is disorganised, in heavy boots, all the pressure on him reaching age-related expectations by three years, so everyone feels they 'did their job'.

Pulling infants up to encourage early walking misses out on the early foundations put in place by creeping and crawling[13] and stores up problems for later in primary school years.

> I'm on Facebook and see a post, a little baby and a caption: 'can't wait till he's walking' – it's in response to another of a child less than 12 months old, proud dad posting: 'he's walking, so clever'. Such a rush to get children standing. So dangerous.

[13] See 'ten good reasons'.

Movement, play and dance with infants – Jasmine

I was invited to work with babies, toddlers and their families at Rich Mix Cultural Foundation in 2009. I noticed how in many groups the babies were passive or moved around whilst being held by adults, and the more active children were restrained by parents who were uncomfortable or embarrassed with their need to escape and move freely.

In Early Years we talk about the importance of physical development in young children, but for some reason adults feel a need to put a stop to children moving in ways of their choosing. So I set about providing a session where there are no adult-led activities. The movement work is entirely child initiated and supported by the watchful adults, the environment is uncluttered and safe, and the time unhurried. Into this mix I create invitations to move in a variety of ways with minimal open-ended resources to cater for the very young babies through to the more active toddlers. The floor is an important workplace for this age group, the 'athletic field of the child'[14]. We are fortunate to have theatre lighting and sound, so the space has a magical quality and atmosphere.

Movement, play and dance are fundamental. Crucial for development at the beginning of life, and just as vital for health and well being throughout life.

I support parents through one-to-one conversations, and through observing and feeding back or voicing over what I see happening in terms of movement and development with their child. We are all learning together 'in the moment' as each child is different from any other, and yet there are some well-known universal milestones. Bonnie Bainbridge Cohen talks about how in this first year of life: 'The relation of the perceptual process (the way one sees) and the motor process (the way one moves or acts in the world) is established. This is the baseline for how you will be processing activity, either in receiving or expressing, throughout your life.'[15] My understanding of infant development has been deepened by working with Bette Lamont from the USA, who is a Neurological Reorganisation Therapist.

Movement, play and dance with young children... indoors – Jasmine

Following a planning visit to a primary school we had a staff twilight session, two parents' sessions, and two practical sessions with nursery children. The nursery teachers and I exchanged lots of articles on movement, play and physical development and talked of letting the project grow according to what we felt was needed. We spoke of indoor and

[14] Arnold Gesell

[15] *Contact Quarterly* (1984)

outdoor opportunities for children, but parents were worried about their children's safety when outdoors.[16] Their own memories of growing up, however, included a great deal of outdoor play experiences.

For the follow-up visit, R (one of the two nursery teachers) asked me to bring Lycra, as they do not have theirs yet. Chose four different colour squares, including the red one with holes in it, and one long Lycra; set up the hall with two mats and the squares rolled up in the middle of the mats; offering rather than telling them what to do – I know they know all about how to use this approach. We made a rest area with a number of big, colourful soft cushions with the option to take time out as required during the session. Safety rule in place: take care and look where you are going so as not to bump anyone else.

We had three groups over the course of the afternoon, and they tried out a variety of activities with adults in supporting roles, but not telling them what to do. I suggested the big Lycra swings, and demonstrated the safety rules for everyone with volunteers. It ties in nicely with the caterpillar rearing they had been doing in class, the notion of cocoons. I knew nothing about this beforehand. Serendipity.

Soundproofing in the hall ceiling was helpful. I wonder how long it has been there? I can't remember seeing it before. I made a note of things Karen noticed about the sessions and the children at the school. She remarked on how they came into the hall space, how they moved in the space, and how they negotiated tasks with no adult direction.

They collaborated, communicated clearly, worked well together and managed their bodies in a tuned-in way. They were excited and giggling when they walked in anticipation of the activities, and confident in their bodies. There was no need for adults to calm things down as they were regulating themselves well.

They were listening and moving.

Running around was allowed.

Children were encouraged to have a go, but without compulsion. Most wanted to take up what was on offer.

At one point Karen noticed nursery teacher R and a group playing 'like a lioness and her cubs'.

Connections were allowed, bodily communication encouraged.

Children could say 'Stop!' if there was something happening they did not like or wish to continue.

At changeover time, everyone managed to take off or to put on their socks and shoes independently.

[16] I sent a map put together by PATH (self-play access) which was available online and could be sent to parents' phones. PATH had started some Friday afternoon sessions in Mile End Park.

Movement, play and dance with young children... outdoors – Jasmine

There are connections between balance and the eyes, balance and the ears, and balance and body movement; the young child spends much time practising and playing the systems into good working order. The baby is rocked gently, bounced on the knee, twirled around and thrown high in the air. The young child swings, spins, tips, twirls, rocks and rolls over and over, stimulating the vestibular system, then hops, skips, climbs, jumps and runs, improving coordination between the vestibular and motor systems.

The most advanced level of movement is the ability to stay totally still. This requires muscle groups to operate together in perfect synchrony with the balance mechanism, and is dependent on a certain level of maturity in the nervous system. The typically developing child wriggles, 'fidgets' and dashes about as the system is still immature.[17]

> Like a coin spinning on its axis, 'balance is only initially maintained by moving fast, and wobble sets in as the movement slows down, stops or starts. As control over balance improves, the amount of movement required to remain upright can be reduced.'[18]

Some activities that help the vestibular system to develop and which the youngster may engage in spontaneously:

Jumping on the bed
Hanging upside down
Space hopping or bouncing on a ball
Twisting the chains of a swing and untwisting
Cartwheels and somersaults
Piggyback rides
Rolling down hill
Jumping down from a high place (for them)
Swinging around a pole
Sliding down stairs on their bottoms
Rough and tumble play

Each of the three semi-circular canals in the inner ear respond to movement in different planes. Most children love doing the things listed below, for very good reasons:

[17] Rowe in Sally Goddard Blythe, *Reflexes, Learning and Behaviour,* Fern Ridge Press ,2002.

[18] Sally Goddard Blythe, *The Well-Balanced Child,* Hawthorn Press, 2004.

*BOING... **up and down** movement on the vertical axis:*
Being bounced on the knee, being lifted up and down in the air or tossed high in the air, bouncing on the bed, hanging upside down, climbing and jumping off, hopping, skipping and jumping, playing on a see-saw, going on a bouncy castle.

*WHOOOSH... **to and fro** movement:*
Being rocked side to side, rocking forwards and backwards on hands and knees, running, starting and stopping, swinging, going on a zip wire, using bikes, scooters and slides, sliding down stairs on your bottom.

*ROLY POLY... movement where **the body rotates**:*
Being twirled around, rolling over, spinning round on your bottom, spinning around a pole, dancing, rolling down a hill, doing somersaults and cartwheels.

I heard that the school were redesigning their outdoor play space over the summer break. Nursery teacher R explained how the plans have changed since we started working together. The new play space will incorporate thinking and ideas offered in the physical development training, redesigned with boing, whoosh and roly poly in mind.

Developing sensation language – Karen

> Decisions begin with sensation[19]

I'm reading *Bad Sir Brian Botany.*[20] C lay over a yoga ball to listen, and immediately said that 'it hurt'. He then stood up with a big smile: 'I feel hungry'. He chuckled. Why did a soft yoga ball hurt so much? But how wonderful that C had noticed that he was hungry and felt good about having noticed!

> The language of sensation is, to many, a foreign language.
>
> Peter Levine

We have a world of sensation and sensation-based feelings inside our body. A sense of well being is based on our bodies' ability to self-regulate – rather than to escalate out of control. When we don't notice these sensations, our self-awareness and decision-making ability is limited, causing us to react in a predetermined way.

The human body has a triune brain, each part speaking its own 'language'. Together they

[19] Dr Cherionna Menzam-Sills

[20] A. A. Milne

form the body-brain connection. Neocortical speaks the language of words. Mammalian (mid-brain) speaks with the language of feeling. Reptilian brain speaks the language of sensation (primitive response of sensory and motor systems that moves us out of danger; no words, just sensations).

> If your body could speak, what would it say?
>
> Anne-Marie Nissen

Children learn to describe feelings and emotions. Children need to learn the language of sensation. Words for feelings, emotion and sensation can become a jumble. Children will say 'I'm happy' with a gloomy face. I try to go below the language of feelings and emotions, to sensation. We often need to relearn the voice of the body. We may have stopped listening to our bodies as a self-protective strategy, learning to ignore what our bodies are telling us.

'I now realise that when I am angry I clench my fist, my jaw goes tight and I feel hot. I have been able to walk away rather than hitting my sister when she upsets me.' 13-year-old

One way I invite children to learn the language of sensation is by taking objects from a treasure box; holding, exploring and coming up with words to describe it – sharp, heavy, prickly, cold, fuzzy, smooth, floaty.[21] Once a child has a language for sensation, they can begin to notice and locate sensation, describe the sensation first around them, then on them, and then in the body. When I see children start to notice sensation, I am excited. They begin to communicate this: through movement, physically, verbally, in stories and pictures. Things start to change, bed-wetting reduces, hitting out at others lessens, children remove themselves from tricky or anxiety-provoking situations, they verbalise to others when they are struggling – 'my head is hurting', 'it's spikey, 'it's too noisy' – often taking themselves away from the situation.[22]

21 Peter A. Levine and Maggie Kline, *Trauma-Proofing Your Kids*, 2008.

22 Peter Levine talks about somatisation in Levine and Kline, 2008. He introduces parents to a range of activities that they can do with their children to develop a sensate language.

About self-regulation – Karen

Children don't always arrive at school ready to learn. Some children are overstimulated or unable to self-regulate.

> *'How can a child come into school at nine am, say they are "ten plus",[23] and within fifteen minutes the child has lost control of their temper and is hitting out?'* Teacher

Many children I encounter spend most of their time being ALERT! All the body's energy is at the periphery. This puts them in a place where they cannot digest... food, information, emotion. They are in the sympathetic nervous system, where the body needs to be when it's ready for action.

Hyper vigilance is an enhanced state of sensory sensitivity accompanied by an exaggerated intensity of behaviours whose purpose is to detect threat.

The 'river of integration'[24] is when our senses are integrated and our central nervous system has balance between action and digestion; we see harmony in the emotional and physical body.[25]

Within the 'window of tolerance'[26] is where we manage to regulate our emotions and feelings. Once we step out of the window, we have lost control. Most of us can keep within this window most of the time. Maybe stopping an explosive situation by walking away, having a growl at a friend, counting to ten. Our windows are reasonably big, and therefore we have plenty of space to slow things back down. However some of the children I am observing have very tiny windows. Very little (if any) space to de-escalate the situation, to self-soothe, to self-regulate. So they spend most of their time popping out of the window and hitting, hurting, running, sleeping, zoning out, shouting, and collapsing.

Recognising sensation and moving is so important, and in school I have seen some huge changes: children learning about personal space (kinaesthetic awareness) has made so much difference to how they sit, line up, walk around school, greet each other and adults; learning about how everyone needs space, and knowing what you need, how to ask for what you want and negotiate with others – this reduces the falling out, the lashing out

[23] 'Ten plus' is the best that they can be.

[24] Daniel J. Siegel, *Pocket Guide to Interpersonal Neurobiology: An Integrative Handbook of the Mind*, W. W. Norton & Company, New York, 2012.

[25] Siegel discusses how, when we are not fully integrated, we end up on the banks of chaos or rigidity (either living in chaos, with poor focus, concentration, easily overloaded, becoming inflexible in our thoughts and actions). Bessel van der Kolk talks of the importance of children learning about 'feeling into your body, calming your body, befriending your body'.

[26] P. Ogden, K Minton & C Pain, *Trauma and the Body: A Sensorimotor Approach to Psychotherapy*, W. W. Norton & Company, New York, 2006.

and, most of all, I see a huge shift in empathy; children are proud in year 3 to say they are a 'class team', a 'family' – when a child said that he found the cloakroom 'scary', his team worked together to learn how to move in and out of a cramped area more safely; when a child becomes upset, I now see the class going to the child to offer support – an arm on their shoulder, a rub on the back...

Children want to come to school; children feel safer; they start to make friends; they find what it is they enjoy; some go from risk of exclusion to asking for help, taking more self-control.

In school, learning through movement allows children to share what is happening, to move away from uncomfortable, overwhelming situations, and towards something that supports. Going into the den, wrapping in a blanket, putting a weighted pad on their lap – to help ground; running, rolling, spinning; hands in clay... They have greater choices and agency over their body. These children's lives change.

Language, thought and feeling – Jasmine

In addition to working with the senses, body movement as supports for the growing child and his or her awareness of self, language and thought have a role to play too. Here Byron Katie helps us to understand ways to work with cognitive processing, and helping the child and family to think about unmanageable 'big' feelings.

Sometimes the movement patterns in the programme stimulate early memories and emotions, and lead to a regression in behaviour. It helps to know that this might happen, and how to respond with sensitivity when it does.

Strategies for dealing with behavioural issues ... 'turnarounds'

Jack's mother described difficulties she was having with her son:

'Jack started having some challenging behaviour prior to us knowing that he would change school. He is a bit aggressive and verbally abusive especially towards me. When he is upset he often says to me: "I will kill you". You can imagine how distressing those words are to me. He is also very rough in his display of affection, even towards my parents. He is behaving like a toddler. Whenever we tell him to stop, he starts giggling and ignores our requests. He is at times defiant and oppositional. Our boy has also started to complain about doing the walking pattern. There are days when he is so uncooperative.'

Bette Lamont suggested using a technique called 'turnarounds', adapted from the work of Byron Katie.[27]

> '*When a child says something like "I want to kill you", he is really just expressing a huge, undefined, raw emotional state, and there you are standing in front of him, so this stuff lands on you. What I would love to have you do for an exercise for YOU, is to write down any nasty thing he directs at you, and "turn it around". Write it down during the day, then after he goes to bed, do YOUR work on it. So, for instance if he says "I want to KILL YOU!" Change out every word in the sentence in as many ways as possible, for instance:*
>
> "I want to kill myself." (because I don't feel worthy of all of the wonderful things you give me)
>
> "I don't want to kill you." (but I don't know why you don't want to kill me because I am so bad)
>
> "You want to kill me." (I'm afraid)
>
> "I don't want to die."
>
> '*You see what I am doing – just turning it all around so we can look at this wad of nasty feelings like a gem of insights with many facets that can give you insight into Jack. It might be that all of the above are true. He may not know what he feels. It may give you new perspective and insight that guides how you respond when he is in this mood.*'

[27] Byron Katie, *Loving What Is,* 2002.

Story, imagination and sensation – Karen

M was six years old and had just started his class. I was asked to work with M as he was new to the school and had been having difficulty with making friends, controlling his anger, staying in the class circle. He had hurt others, disrupted lessons and seemed very unhappy.

> *I asked M what he would like to do. He told me that he wanted to make a comic. Totally thrown. How do you get a child that wants to write a comic to start moving...?*
>
> *We start with a basket of objects, and M chooses a crystal.*
>
> *Hold the crystal in your hand... close your eyes... imagine all the adventures this crystal has had... feel the edges... is it cold, warm, crunchy...? heavy, smooth...? where has it come from...? who owned it before you...? what's your adventure...?*

M was a great storyteller and had so many ideas about the general who likes to gallop on his horse over sand dunes and kill people. I constantly guided him to landscapes where his imagination could also get in contact with his lived body. He had already brought in sand dunes, men dying and the crystal being propelled into the sea. It was then easy to use sound and to introduce the idea of the waves. This, without me knowing, became a very important part of the sessions.

After a tentative start, M would join me in making the sound and movement of waves crashing, becoming seaweed on the sea bed, swaying side to side in intercellular moves. M's body took him to movements that he needed. In a playful and imaginative way, these moves worked at a silent level, and over the weeks they settled in the body, and new patterns formed:

> *Shhhh shhhh shhhh*
> *This is a crystal from the sword of a general.*
> *The crystal flew from his sword up high into the sky and landed in the sea*
> *Sinking down, down, down to the bottom of the sea*
>
> *We sit on the sand watching the sea as the crystal flies high above us and with a splash... lands in the sea.*
> *We can hear the sea, the sound of waves crashing*
> *Shhhhhh shhhhhhh shhhh*
> *Waves come up to our toes and then out again*
> *Up and down, up and down*

We make the sound of the sea, shhhh shhhh
Moving our arms, tracing the waves' departure
Arms sweeping from floor to sky
Body folded forward, to lifted straight (raised and upright)
Then repeat the pattern until arms by our side

We would then make the comic strip.

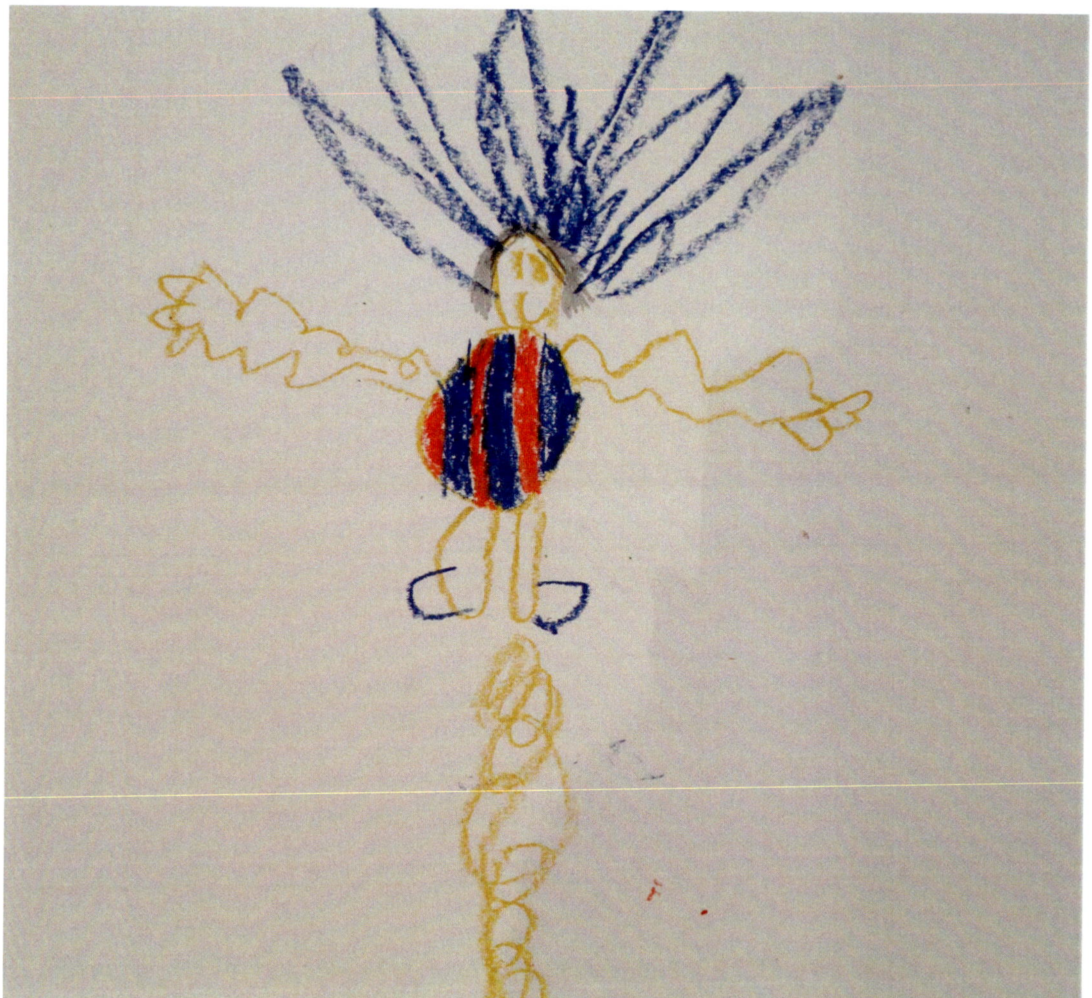

Meeting the teacher after several sessions, she stopped me and said: 'I can tell you've been teaching M breathing techniques, it's really working. Yesterday he had a fight with a child. He was very distressed and came to sit next to me. I noticed how he was practising breathing in and out to calm himself down. Usually he can't calm himself and it takes a long time for him to settle.'

Movement, imagination and creativity – Jasmine

There is a connection between the movement experiences that support physical development, and the imaginative and creative ways that support children to find what they need to do in the more therapeutic interactions, which involve skilled and tuned-in adults who can travel alongside, or be their companion.

We provide the environment to encourage moving in all the ways described, and offer our attentiveness, awareness of what is happening, and support.

In therapeutic interactions, there is more of the understanding of the therapeutic process, and the willingness of the adult to trust the child to find the solutions through imagery, story and exploration – often repeated exploration.

It involves trusting the mind of the child as well as the body. We know that they know exactly what to do.

Play is a common feature of both.

This can be done at any time. You can be a ninety year old, and still revisit, recover and awaken your body – it is always ready. There's never a time when it's too late.

Laying the foundations – Jasmine and Karen

What do babies and toddlers need to build firm foundations for later learning, health and well being? What experiences might the children we have described have missed out on? They need plenty of time to move freely, and to crawl and creep, roll and tumble, pull to stand, cruise along, squat down and reach up, and to master the movement of the body in relation to gravity.

> Trust the body, to have the solutions
> Trust the child, to show you the way

Children instinctively know where their bodies need to go to find the source of difficulties and the solutions. Follow their lead; tune in to their interests; give them time to be creative; open their imagination; invite story, pictures, landscapes... be a companion[28] on the journey. The knowing body does the rest.

[28] When witnessing, Miranda Tufnell describes herself as a 'companion'.

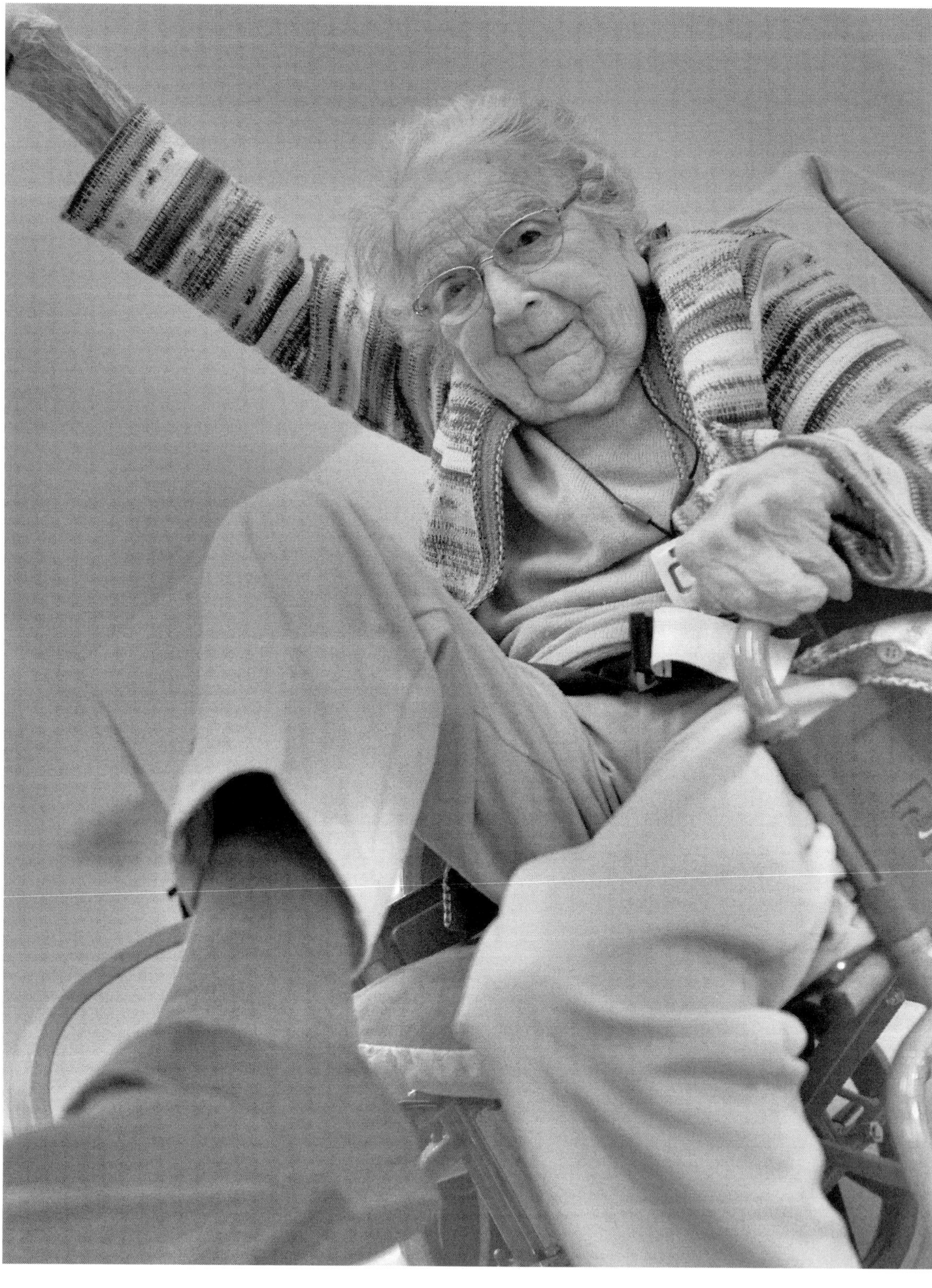

What is this pill called dance?

music and movement in hospital

Filipa Pereira-Stubbs

Working in hospitals upholds my respect for the human capacity, for connection, compassion and endurance, and our human need to source beyond ourselves in our healing journeys, to source through the Arts and Nature. A thread connecting the movement projects and programmes, is the ethos of inviting people to participate in what I am offering. There needs to be a willingness to join in, and an understanding of what is being embarked on. I offer myself as a companion, as someone who will calibrate my expertise to participants' resources. Someone who travels alongside. Regardless of age or experience, there is always something to share, there is always a mutually interesting journey to be found.

Personal interest, confidence, trust and comfort are important for good work to be done. Working in hospital, one is encountering people temporarily or chronically living with high levels of distress and anxiety. Patients and visitors are displaced out of their usual time frames and life structures. Mind, body and spirit are weakened and unsteady, at the very time when integration is most needed. Hospitals are holding stations, where crucial work is being done, delivered by staff working within insecure structures, most of whom are shouldering huge burdens and pressures one way or another. The usual human groundwork systems that successfully bolster communities such as shared open conversation, sharing of skills, and mutual support are fragile and erratic, if not absent.

Patients who come into this skew-whiff world are grappling with developing new relationships with changing constellations of healthcare staff. Making and maintaining good relationships is crucial to getting through the hospital stay and getting 'out'. There is much unhappy and negative focus on the ordeal of hospital, there is the glowing promise of getting better, and getting out. In the meantime the work is to fathom how to make the best use of all that the hospital offers.

Working in the Department of Medicine for the Elderly (DME) wards, many of the people I see have reached an unhappy and unhealthy low point in their personal resources. There is much disorientation through ongoing ill health and resulting tired, pained, medicated and disconnected bodies. For many of the elderly, the hospital stay is a purgatorial space they are parked in, whilst core life changes are arranged around them; life as it was will irrevocably change. Their fears and anxieties are well grounded. The unhurried and patient conversation needed with a health professional to reach clarity and comfort is hard to have. The mental wherewithal to know which questions to ask to lead to useful answers is hard to achieve amidst the confusion, noise, the busyness, and the disorienting periods of empty waiting time that make up ward life.

The elderly are also contending with: life weariness, social isolation, loss of family and social structure and support, grief over the loss of life partners, loss of personal communication skills, cognitive confusion, a loss of appetite and zest for life, and anxiety about prognosis and the future. They can be living within a bleak climate of feeling unimportant, unheard, and misunderstood. The fear the advanced elderly carry of being at the end of the road, of being an unwelcome burden, is tangible. Privacy, familiarity, control, and pleasure are for the most part gone. Regardless, these elderly patients have to muster enough patience, trust, ease of mind, and physical well being to assimilate and integrate the medical treatment offered to them.

So along comes a dancer, into this surreal world. An invitation to come and join in with 'movement and lovely music' is offered. Every time, I am fascinated by the exchange of information and understanding, and the ways in which the invitation is accepted, or rejected. Incomprehension and some outrage – *who* did I say I was? what do I mean by movement? *what kind* of music? and a fresh fear that yet another thing is being asked of one. Tired eyes appraise me, peering timidly from swaddled and oddly muffled bodies – how dare I presume this body could muster enough energy to move when pain is so prevalent? Or I get an instant bright smile, and an approving nod, yes dear – music is so important and oh I did so used to love to dance with ... but *where* exactly are we going, and *will* I miss lunch/relatives/the doctor...?

These first points of contact are so important. Important to make eye contact, to talk clearly – not necessarily loudly – to shake hands, touch a hello, introduce oneself fully, and above all take the time to ensure that what you are offering makes sense. Important to be genuine, to be enthusiastic but not insistent. When possible, having a trusted nurse

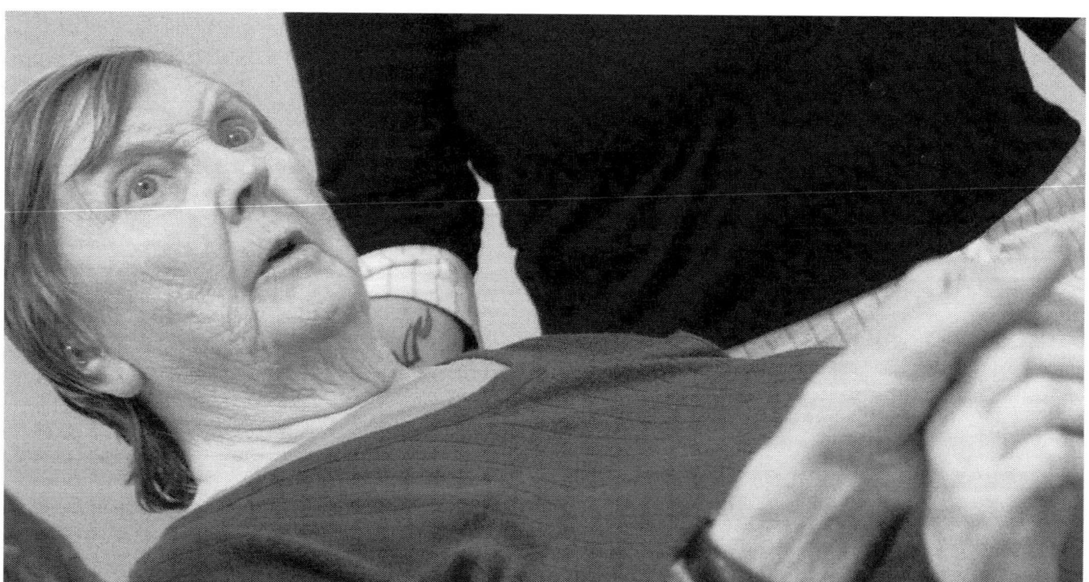

or HCA[1] mediate makes the idea of trying something new more palatable.

Dance usually conjures rhythmical movement, music, a sense of a social occasion and performance. In the world of health, dance is more about expressive movement, somatic movement and dance/movement therapy. There is a belief that the body holds consciousness and kinaesthetic knowledge. Movement can be experienced, sensed, regulated and shaped from within rather than from an external source. Using breath, touch, imagery and sensed movement, individuals and groups can be guided into self-understanding and expression.

When you engage with the body you are engaging directly with the processes of life and, therefore, of ageing. Dance can transform obstacles into potential material, and problems into opportunity. The ability of dance practitioners to attend to physical ability, vitality and engagement (by no means exclusive to ageing) is crucial. In dance with older people, expression and meaning are increasingly important.

So much has been written about the ideal space to deliver movement and dance. A quiet room, with doors that can close against the bustle of the hospital ward. A non-carpeted floor that allows for shuffles and that supports, without the clinical shininess that bewilders the confused mind. Quiet and tasteful decor. Natural light, windows with a view, fresh air, and comfortable flexible seating. Realistically, you just take what you can. If you have a few of the above features you are lucky. Space is a premium, and staff will charge in as and when they need to, not intending disrespect, but too busy to extend that extra sensitivity to the environment of a room.

One of the ward rooms we dance in at Addenbrooke's, is located on the top floors. The windows of the staff room overlook the wide Cambridge skies, and gentle hills. As patients come into the space, sit in their chairs, and patiently wait for all to arrive, we turn our gaze to the windows, remind one another of the world of seasons, of growth and change. The sky is always a point of interest, no matter the weather. It feels good to take attention outwards, and to bring the vastness of the sky into our room, into our group.

I introduce the idea that we can access what is working well through listening to and engaging with our bodies. We invite people to take control in choosing what and how much movement they would like to engage with. A key intention of the movement sessions is to restore a sense of self, and connection to what feels well.

Taking into full consideration and with absolute respect all the ailments and limitations they introduce themselves as having, we are inviting people to move beyond their perceived barriers. It is important to begin with a notion of comfort – as much as possible finding a supported and comfortable position in the chair. Allowing oneself to shift the body in small ways to ease pressure, and awaken sensation. I am often touched by how docile the elderly are, sitting quietly as instructed, disregarding their own comfort levels. Pain creates schisms in the body and mind; our response to pain and discomfort is often to compartmentalise the pain, and the parts of the body the pain is lodged in, and dissociate from that part of the body, that part of ourselves. We withdraw from discomfort, we erect

[1] Healthcare Assistant

barriers and blockades to protect ourselves. There is a sense that our body has let us down, and is behaving badly, and is shamefully beyond our control.

The bodies that sit in the chairs are invariably full of stiffness, of fragmentation, and of fear. Full of 'No's. The first step is to unknot the pain, to create ease and comfort around held and blocked areas. Gentle, flowing, peripheral movement. Gestural, simple, and just a bit at a time. Unhurriedly unravel the tightness and restriction. Each person finds their own way of moving. Coming into awareness of the anatomical connections of hand to wrist to elbow to shoulder – how can they enjoy the journey from hand to neck? What rhythm do they encounter along the way? Is it easier to do with eyes closed? Or is it easier to follow someone else's movement initially?

My voice is quiet and calm as I embark on invitations, as I explain. I reassure people that we have ample time together, but that we will only work for as long as they feel they can. I am establishing the rules of this group – we listen to each other, we work together. We are going to have fun. I smile a lot, listen a lot and take plenty of time to check in with each individual. The HCAs and nurses I work with are astute and compassionate, and between us we create an environment of camaraderie and possibility.

The group begins by everyone saying who they are, telling the group their name (and more if we like). By doing this we establish membership in the activity. If we can't remember our name, someone will say or sing it for us. Being named, heard, validated.

As we begin moving the quality in the room shifts, as we watch and glean from one another. Attention is brought into the present moment. We are focused on what we can do, rather than on symptoms and what we can't do. We're taking respite from the gargantuan task of fixing ourselves, fixing our lives. We focus on breathing, which encourages steadiness and calmness. We are secure within the structure of the group. We move slowly to ensure stability and confidence, and we move to ease flexibility and coordination. We are coming into awareness of ourselves. Through working on releasing tonal tension we begin to relax.

We work with touch. The elderly in particular are condemned to living long days without touch, without contact. Critical then to take time to offer the companionship of supporting hands, the comfort of warm hands on aching bones, tense shoulders. With permission, myself and staff and volunteers use our hands to guide perception of sensation, to awaken minute shifts and changes in proprioception. Our aim is to help people remap their awareness of their body landscapes. I find people love to hear about how their body is constructed in intricate and almost miraculous ways, and that they can directly effect positive change by beginning the smallest of movements. Even sitting in a hospital chair. Where does that breaking spine meet a too-heavy head? How does the paralysed frozen arm hinge on a bony shoulder? Bodies respond to warmth, to touch – sometimes the movement is so small it can barely be seen. But to the mover, concentrating with eyes closed, somewhere inside is coming alive, and is being invited to participate – and unlocking is happening.

When I am in the group, I am fully engaged with the myriad shapes and qualities of the different bodies – the pattern of skin wrinkled across finger knuckles, how a torso fills the entire width and depth of a hospital chair. Some feet dangle daintily, childlike, and others are like large inanimate logs, giant-like. Some movement is ephemeral and barely perceptible, look away and you've missed it, slow tracings of minute circles. Sometimes just a flutter of fingers across green hospital gown. Sometimes majestic wide reaching movements across the space. Sometimes a rhythm or refrain will bring the whole body – nodding, tapping, gesticulating into a coordinated dance. Sometimes there is hip shimmying, or even cancan high kicks. It is such a rich palette of qualities and personalities to draw from, and to dance with. My mind is stimulated, wondering about the experiences these folk carry, that have carved out these body attitudes.

Our intention is to restore a sense of self. We become more fully present and engaged,. through imagination and creativity. Offering a piece of melody, an idea, a colour, a metaphor – these engage the imagination, evoke response and effortlessly unlock ability. Invitation to imagine a spring breeze into one's fingers, or to dance a hand duet with another, facilitates movement. Instruction on what the body *needs* to do to get better or stronger is not the most compatible and encouraging place to begin. Being told one *must* stretch far and wide so as to get better awakens fear of failure, of not being able to do it well, and so brings in resistance, more tightness. Moving through imagination and metaphor allows a person to relate in their own way.

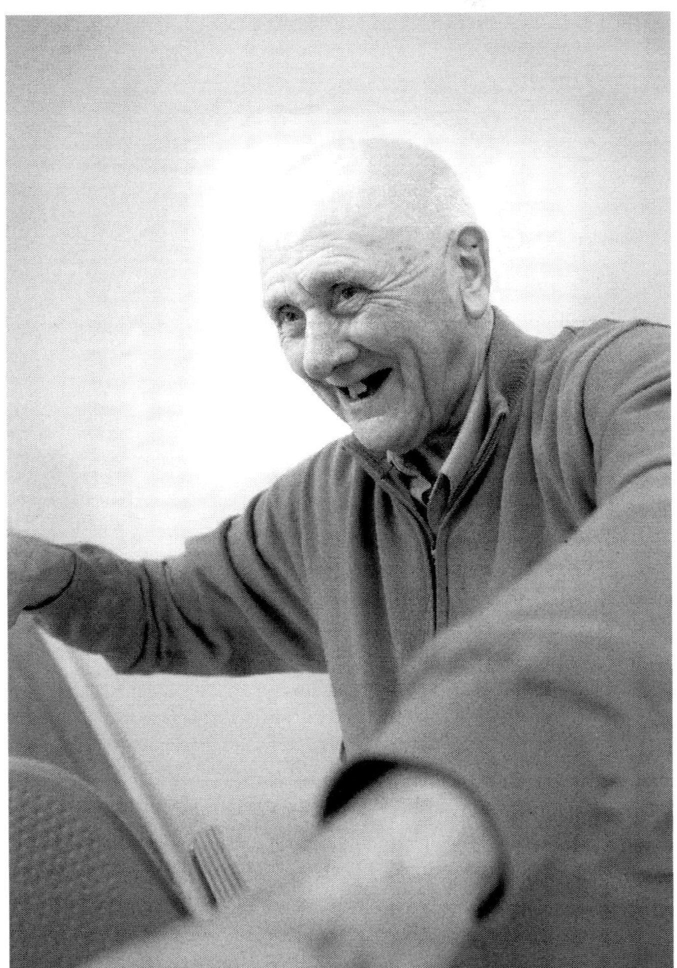

Another intention is to enjoy ourselves, to engage with one another, and to come together as a group. Through moving together in duets, or in a whole group response to a melody or rhythm, we come into non-verbal communication with one another. Establishing a safe, welcoming place where time is given awakens more modes of communication. Memories, stories, feelings arise. What we need to say will find its way, as the body breathes and becomes freer.

Once we have warmed up, and established that movement is possible and enjoyable, the soundscape shifts to include familiar songs, catchy tunes, songs that one can sing along. Releasing voice and sound is a well-established healing process. The breadth of connection with one another widens, opportunities for conversation and reminiscing come into play.

Narratives and stories arise freshly in the context of creating movement; this is different from reminiscence work. Rather than revisiting *a time before*, or allowing nostalgia to creep in, in movement we spark new connections, new conversations. We are all finding out about each other; that our favourite HCA loves to sing; that this young man sings the very songs we loved when young. We recreate some of the energy and vigour enjoyed when younger, and harness it to heal our older, tireder selves.

Improvisation is the art of listening and spontaneously responding to whatever arises in the body. We hold an attitude of openness, curiosity and compassion. Rather than teaching prescribed steps or established routines, I encourage people to find and follow their own movement in the face of the unknown. We work in the moment, focusing on what is immediately present. The old adage of 'there is no right or wrong' firmly and crucially anchors the group ethos. Improvisation supports choice and individual expression. Essentially, improvisation is a tool in this orientation – it helps you know who you are and what is going on.

An intention of the group is to give patients and staff the opportunity to work, move and be together. Because the work is personal, the usual clinical division of roles of carer and cared-for shifts into a more equal and open footing. We move and create together. The responsibility of caring becomes shared. This shared and playful participation improves staff patient communication. Inevitably, your trust in the person you have just enjoyed dancing with increases. Inevitably, you care more emphatically for someone whose story you have just heard. Volunteers and visitors also make up the group – they enrich the group with their personalities, experiences and interest. Essentially, the group is inclusive, and all are encouraged to participate fully. Staff too release tension, relax, breath more fully, and engage their imaginative and playful selves, whilst looking after their patients.

Sometimes the group feels able to choreograph a dance together. Sometimes the need is to enjoy simple meditative, repetitive movements, like a moving mantra. Sometimes the energy and mood is high, and we swing into rock 'n' roll and vigorous dance. Any which way, we need then to find a way of ending the dancing together. Often we take hands, making the circle clear. Bodies and minds are tired, and we slow right down to enjoy the ritual of a final song. We end the session with five minutes of basic massage and relaxation for both staff and patients. People leave slowly and in their own time. One of the greatest pleasures of doing this work, is seeing the difference in how people leave the room – gait is eased, spines are longer, faces are softer, smiling. As patients make their way back to their beds they are greeted cheerfully by staff – how was that? how did you get on? everyone on the ward enjoys that a positive activity has happened.

Dance engages creativity, imagination, and playfulness. It wakes up people's vitality and shifts physiological functioning. It involves moving with others, touch and creating connection. Engaging in dance reconnects a disconnected body, and returns a sense of ability and wholeness in bodies that feel broken or damaged through ill health. Illness affects the person and it is the person who ultimately has to deal with their condition.

Good hospital practice is increasingly about delivering health programmes that encourage patients to find alternative and additional ways to healing and health – through the help of professionals, and through their own initiative. It is well established that the arts go some way in creating the right healing environments and providing the right processes to help people heal. Dance is an arts form that deals directly with the body, and as such is extremely well placed in hospital to provide healing and well being. In bringing together the world of dance and the world of the hospital, the common factors are humans, bodies, health, and well being.

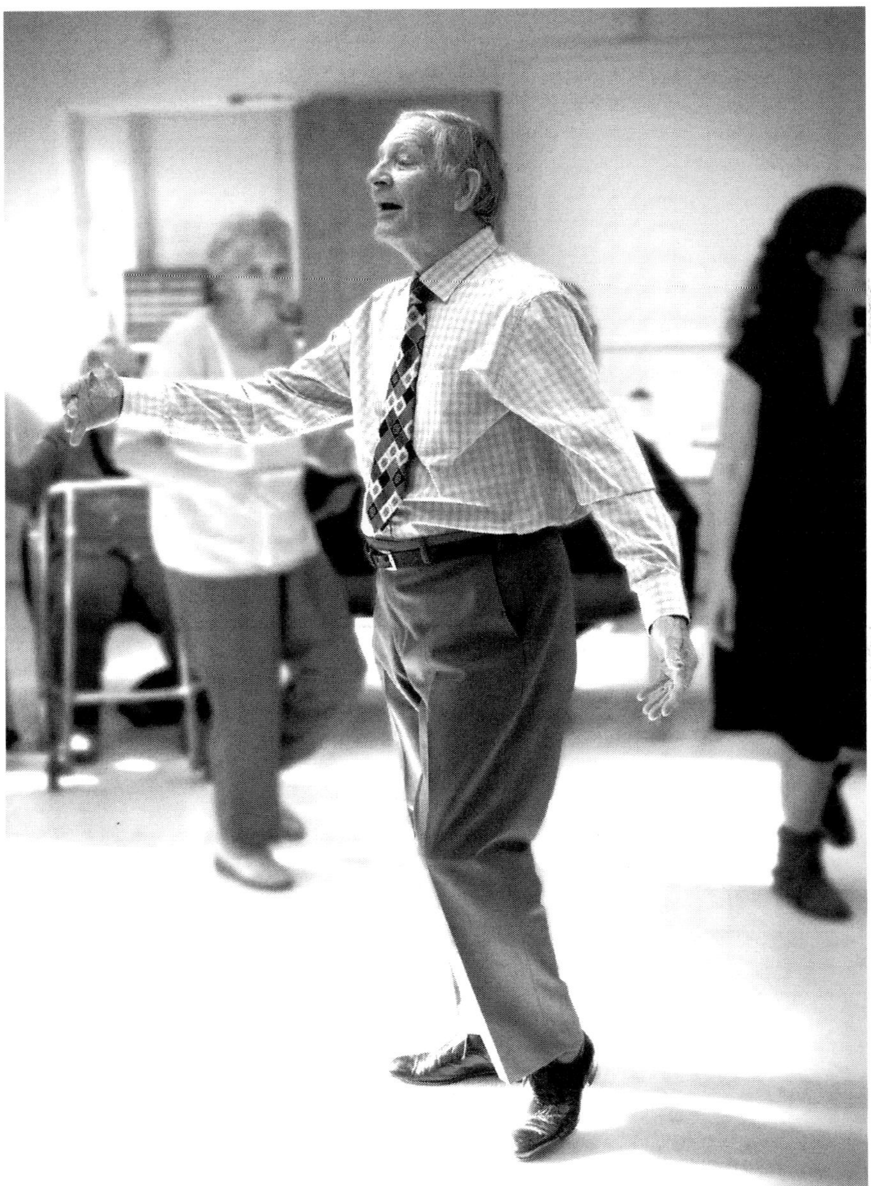

Harry: the story of a child in hospital

Lisa Dowler with Kellie Rixon

Since 2006 I have been a dance artist in residence at Alder Hey Children's Hospital. I have worked across many wards with infants, children, young people and their families including cardiac, orthopaedic, renal, cystic fibrosis and psychiatric units. I have the most experience however, on the neuromedical ward, where I have continued to explore and evolve my practice over these nine years.

The neuromedical ward is essentially a rehabilitation unit and its patients include those with complex and multiple disabilities, including those with chromosomal and genetic disorders and children and young people with acquired brain injury following illness or injury.

My practice is to work one to one with improvisation, movement and touch. As in the duet form of Contact Improvisation, these are shared dances which unfold moment to moment and often over long periods of time with patients who are long term, as we get to know each other through the non-verbal and creative languages of movement and touch.

My experience of working with touch has been influenced significantly by my studies in the somatic practice of Body-Mind Centering over the last ten years. I believe BMC has provided me with more choice in what I can offer a person or how I can respond to them through touch, voice and movement; a myriad of possibilities to make a connection. The shifts in quality may be barely perceptible to someone on the outside, so parents may comment that I have 'magic hands', but it isn't magic, it is one of many somatic approaches that enable the practitioner to tune in to the subtleties of the living body, following, tracking, listening for vitality and making a connection there, bringing this quality of wellness to the fore.

Evolving my practice in this context has been a research project for me, I had no specific training in working with acquired brain injury (ABI), so I gently offered my practice, and the patients I have been privileged to work with have been my teachers. Every ABI is unique, as is every child and their recovery, so it simply is not possible for me to know what each individual person may want or need, I have to listen to what they are communicating through their body. This takes time and space, elements often missing in our busy modern lives and in the clinical environment, so I need to slow down myself, often by becoming aware of my own breath, gravity acting on my body, my feet on the ground. This enables me to open and hold a quiet creative space where it may become possible to sense even the faintest of sounds reverberating through the body of another.

I have been very lucky to work with some wonderful children and their families. Parents, although often a little confused at first as to the benefits of a dance artist working with

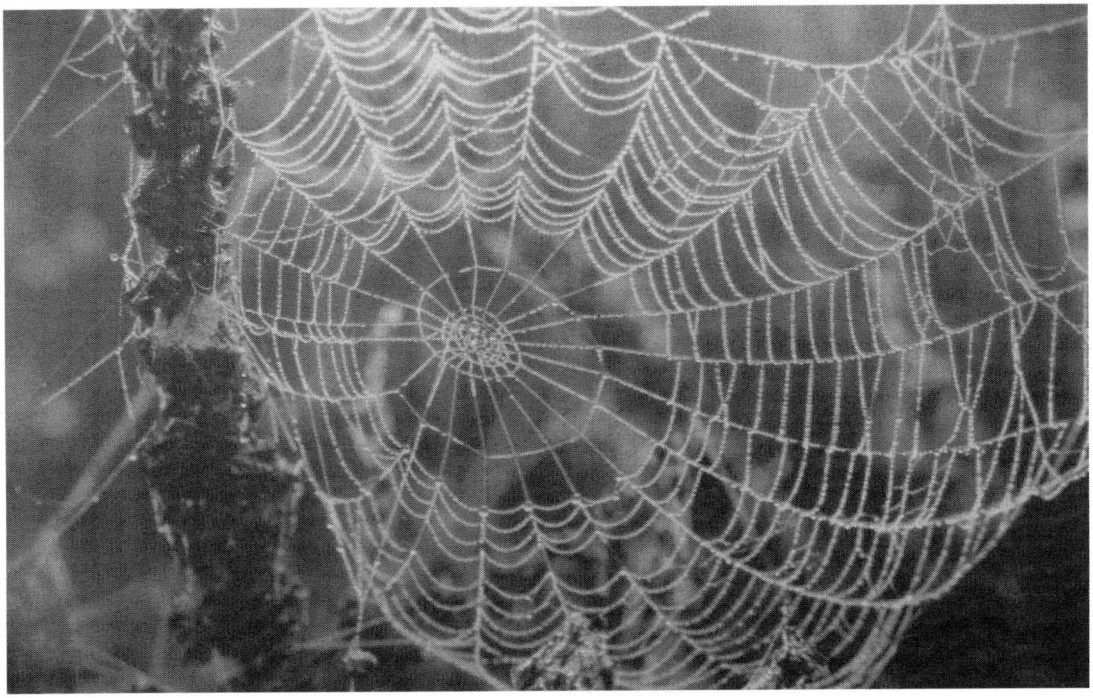

their child, are often open to trying anything at this traumatic time in their lives. One such parent was Kellie Rixon MBE whose son experienced catastrophic head injuries in a car accident and was given hours to live. Kellie was so positive about the benefits of the work of Cath Hawkins and I, of Small Things Dance Collective, that she agreed to present at our symposium 'The Significance of Improvisation in Paediatric Healthcare' in 2013. Her moving account identifies so clearly and passionately the importance of dance in these contexts and it felt important to publish and share her reflections from a parent's perspective. The following are Kellie's words (in italics) alongside my reflective writings written immediately after sessions with Harry.

> *My name's Kellie Rixon, I'm a mum. I'm not here to talk from a clinical perspective, or a medical perspective or a dance artist perspective. I'm here from the parents' perspective.*

> *On December 5th 2012 we were involved in a road traffic accident. We were a normal family who didn't know anything about disability, didn't think we were prejudiced in any way, just a normal hardworking family ... and fate, whatever it is, stepped in and changed our lives that night. I was driving a big Range Rover and Harry was in the back of the car asleep. We were driven off the road by a dangerous driver, we went down an embankment and as our car came to rest we were hit by a train. Amazingly the three of us, Harry, my elder son and I,*

survived the accident, although Harry bore the brunt of the impact.

That leads me to his recovery.... Part one was critical care, or 'saving his life', which took place in Newcastle. A few weeks later he moved to Alder Hey, in Liverpool, and Part two began, which was about 'bringing him back to life'. We had saved him and now we had to get our boy back! So ... doctors do their bit, nurses do their bit and dance artists did their bit (sorry if that sounds random!) to bring our boy back to life.

We had every therapy known to man, physiotherapy, hydrotherapy, speech and language therapy... When Helen the play specialist approached me and said we have dance artists, I could see my husband rolling his eyes ... my son was in a coma and hadn't moved and he was having dance...! I could see people saying, 'I've seen it all now, she's definitely lost it!' ... and I was saying, 'No we'll have it! Who knows, this could be it!'

Our first session with Harry, 9th January. I explored cellular touch with Harry on his arms and shoulders. I noticed when we began, his breathing and heart rate increased, probably due to anxiety as it was our first session. He didn't know us and due to his recent experiences, I imagined he was afraid we were about to do medical procedures. I kept a calm presence through the gentle touch and he began to relax a little and open his fingers. He relaxed into the bed and his range of movement increased. His feet were very stiff but softened and opened, his toes were moving.

Following the same session Cath wrote: 'I offered touch to the arm that had been badly injured in Harry's accident. I felt many clicks in Harry's shoulder joint and then his arm seemed to settle.'

He wasn't awake, he didn't actually wake up for three and a half months. Watching Harry sleep, as beautiful as he is, wasn't enough, we had to push him, we didn't know what the key was. We were offered something that we like to think of in our family as not a therapy but an alternative to therapy. When your boy is lying in bed and all he gets is pummelled, prodded, poked, stabbed, moved and is completely immobile ... as a parent watching your son go through that is heartbreaking and I couldn't see the light and shade, I couldn't see when he was awake, I couldn't see when he was asleep because he was out. We couldn't see when he was relaxed and I couldn't tell what was going on in his head.

And as he started to wake up, I just started imagining what would I be going through if I was in that bed, when all I got was hard work and push, and 'come on Harry, you must do this Harry', and another injection and more medication, and I'm foggy with a headache. So when we were introduced to Lisa and Cath, this was an alternative. It didn't replace the other therapies, but actually it was a moment of peace, it was a moment of Zen-like relaxation and we loved it straight away. So what did they do, these wonderful magical women? Well this kind of dance artistry doesn't come without its challenges, you know, from clinical practitioners. Lisa and Cath would be working with Harry, relaxing him, stroking him, moving his hands for him, but we could see little tiny responses. Then clinical practitioners would come in with their big boots and clipboards, throw the curtain back, march in, start talking to us as parents, start talking to Harry. And this was just the challenge, because you are seen as you are in hospital and so you have got to get fixed, but I'm a great believer that it takes a whole host of things to fix a boy, takes a whole host of things to bring our boy back!

If you knew Harry before the accident he wasn't one of these kids that if you bullied him he'd do it, he was one of these kids that if you praised him he'd do whatever, if you suggested he might do something fantastic. If you told him other kids might do it he would just run for it, but that was never taken into consideration from a clinical perspective. So for us we had some challenges to make it known that for us this was as important as the medication being administered by the nurses. So it's a challenge both as a dance artist and as a parent.

Cath held Harry's hand and rolled a soft ball on his arms. I held his feet, gently listening here. When we first touched him his heart rate went up, showing his anxiety. However, very quickly he relaxed and his heart rate dropped significantly. His face softened, as did the high tone of his legs. His feet became heavy and the tension in his ankles reduced. Cath noticed the same at his wrists. He fell into a deep sleep having been very unsettled.

I'm going to briefly touch on the impact but I think it's too massive, you know he relaxed and as he started to wake up over the period of time Lisa and Cath worked with him, it took time, and you heard it from other parents too, he physically relaxed. He never slept in the day, he'd be restless and his stats monitor would be off the charts, when he was awake he looked really distressed and they'd come in and ... well they had some names, 'tickle therapy' was one of them, because they'd come in and just suggest movement...

27th February. I had planned to go to the sensory room with Harry, but when I got there he was really sleepy and I thought a more restful session might be better. We did some 'hands on' with his arms and he really relaxed, taking big sighs. I used the red overball and he seemed to really like this on his legs. His arms were so much more relaxed and I could help him lift them. He doesn't move his right arm so much, so I gave lots of stimulation, brushing and tickling and was getting subtle jerky responses. I helped him bring his hands together and stroked his hands, he seemed to like that and was really concentrating. He was really interested in the ball and moving it with his left hand. I helped him to grasp it and he was squeezing it in response to being asked and moving it. I brought his left over to rest onto it and when I was supporting his elbow he was able to squeeze his arm in towards his side a bit. He had tight hold of the ball so I left him for a little doze with it. Lovely session.

> *And it's a real challenge not to come off as waffly baffly mumbo jumbo, and people would question me about him having dance as part of his treatment, but I would say, 'look at that boy beforehand and then look at him after! ... he relaxed, his stats came down and then, more importantly, they were working with him one day and one finger moved. They were stroking the back of his hand and it lifted. When as a mother you have watched the light in your life lie still for four months and he moves his finger, it's as if all your Christmases come at once. Then the next week it was an arm slightly raised... Then a leg.*

Harry had some movement in his left leg, he kept extending but this seemed painful. Cath was working mainly with his upper body and I worked mainly with his legs. I placed hands underneath his hamstrings, which felt very high tone, so I gently supported his legs and his weight. He was able to flex his leg a few inches and also after extending it relaxed more quickly. His hip joints softened too and there was a release here. In the same session Cath wrote: 'It was very visible that Harry's upper body relaxed as Lisa worked with his legs. Harry seems a lot more responsive today.'

> *We noticed with every dance intervention that we actually got the same if not more than from physiotherapy. In physio, he fought, he went for it, he had a go. He came into dance and – so unbelievably – he stretched further.*

6th March Harry with Nan. Last call of the day for me ... you were tired. Nan was against me working with you, as she felt you needed to rest, but you said yes (with your eye-blink) you wanted to. We had a lovely duet, you holding my hand, us both listening and responding. You came to midline and sat up really straight, so I engaged your other arm. You were really looking at me and concentrating, it was very moving. I said you had worked very hard and you blinked yes. I said you were a gorgeous boy and you blinked/said yes! I left you to rest.

15th May. With Harry in sensory room. Great session, explored rolling a little. I stimulated the reflexes in the soles of Harry's feet to support him in flexing his legs and hips, then gentle rocking of the pelvis. I followed and supported his initiation to roll to the side. We rested there, he really relaxed, mum noticed this. When he signalled he was ready we explored rolling to prone, again he really enjoyed this. It gave some time to do some 'hands on' on his back, tracing his spine and relaxing the muscles in his back. It was our first opportunity for this and he loved it. An exciting session!

Then it got really exciting, he started sitting up and laughing. We know our boy's coming back, he's coming back faster than anyone could have predicted, we are nine months in, we were told that this kind of brain injury takes years. He's walking, he's eating, he's up and about, he's the boy that we remember and every day he gets stronger and stronger.

You might say it was the drugs, you might say it was the physiotherapy, you might say it was the drive of his family to bring him back, but I'm telling you: everybody played their part and none more so than Lisa and Cath in his rehabilitation. So if you're a dancer and want to do something significant with your life, go out and do something fabulous, really amazing (then, turning to me and Cath) *there must be some gold in there, you are part of team Harry! I'm an advocate and I will speak passionately about the part these women played in Harry's recuperation.*

5th June. Last session with Harry. Can't believe it was our last session! We played a lot with the huge earth balloon. Harry was really happy and excited by it, he was sitting and able to reach out and hit it to Cath and I. We were all giggling and having lots of fun. He did so well and I'm going to miss him!

Dancing recall: making connections

Daphne Cushnie

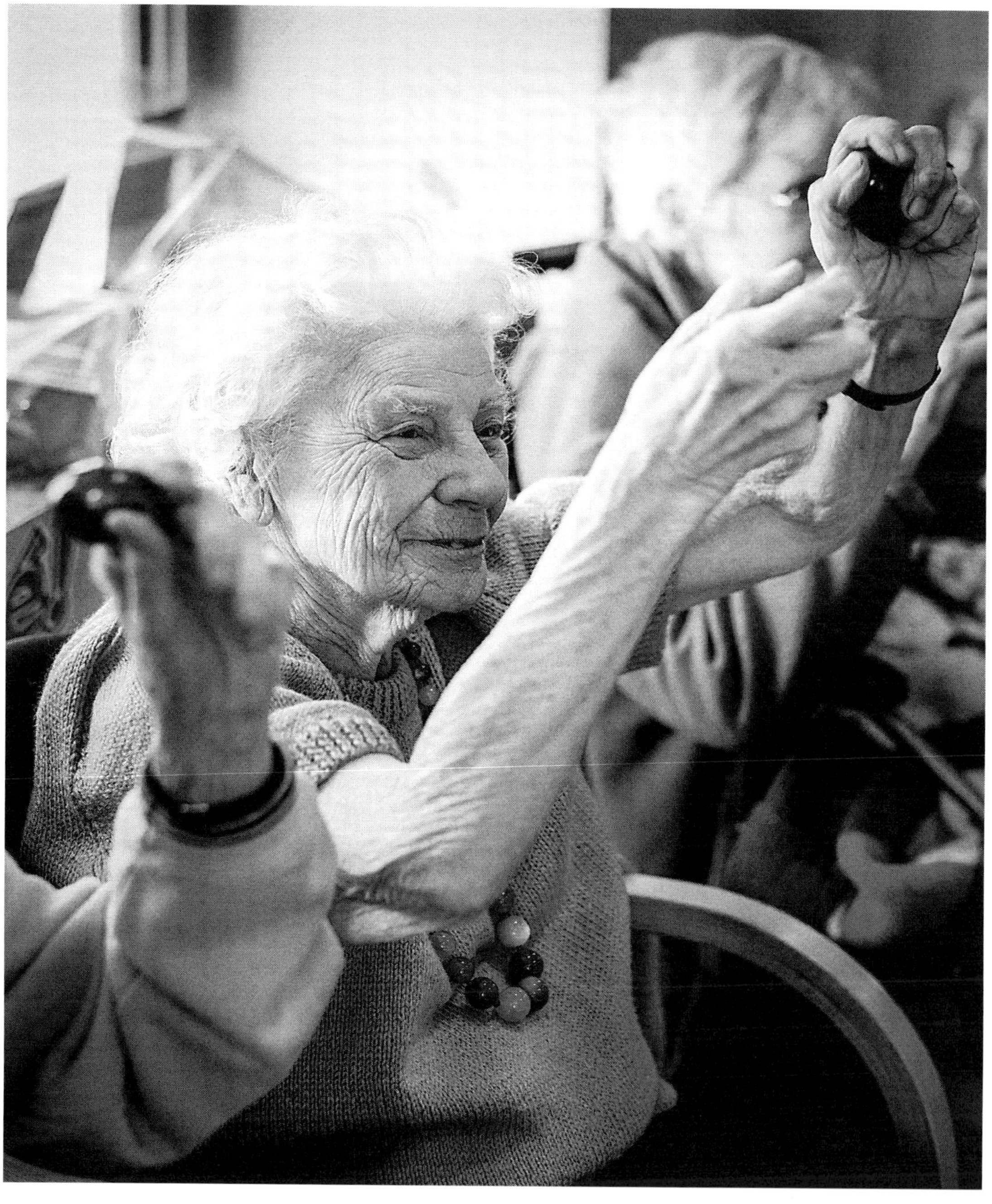

Let's all sit down, take a collective deep breath and look carefully at these recent figures from the Alzheimer's Society:

> 800,000 people in the UK are currently living with dementia.
> 670,000 people in the UK are caring for those with dementia.

And what about this figure:

> By 2021, *over a million people in the UK will be diagnosed with dementia.*

Just imagine the implications of this on a personal and collective level. Dementia is a progressive, remorseless decline in cognition, function and behaviour. The collateral impact is also vast. Carer burden in terms of physical work, psychological distress and financial obligations is huge. The cost to the state is vast too. We don't need to imagine the financial implications because another statistic tells us that the estimated healthcare cost to the UK in 2021 tops £23 billion!

My work, though I should add that it is also my passion, straddles two worlds: neurophysiotherapy and community dance. For many years I have argued the case for the effectiveness of dance and movement in the treatment of neurodegenerative disorders. In comparison to pharmaceutical or surgical treatments it's cheap, it's non-invasive, has only positive side effects and tackles many of the problems of social isolation as well as the clinical symptoms. It's a message which has been slowly gaining ground.

There have been huge strides in the field of dance for Parkinson's, especially since the founding of Dance for Parkinson's Network UK. But dance for dementia has lagged behind despite beacons of light from people like Dr Richard Coaten working with the South West Yorkshire NHS Trust.

In an article in *The Guardian* (11 April 2013) Halima Khan, Director of People Powered Health said that 'the NHS is ... is still finding its way towards a model that effectively manages long-term conditions.' She argues for a person-centred approach that includes exercise and that, by her estimate, could save the NHS up to £4.4 billion a year. She also highlights the challenge of nurturing compassion in large, formal institutions where staff are under considerable financial pressure.

There are many misunderstandings about what dance is, and what its potential may be to make a positive, *measurable* difference to the lives of those living daily with lifelong conditions that will almost certainly get worse. So I was delighted to be invited by Active Cumbria to help develop 'Dancing Recall: Making Connections', a dance for dementia pilot project aiming to bring a clinical perspective to the practice of community dance.

The programme is delivered as a series of training days for dance practitioners followed up by mentoring sessions, observing and supporting them in action as they team-teach. The model is founded on the values of community dance where relationship, creativity and community building are key, but bringing in a logical structure based on clinical understanding. We aim to address, simultaneously, the physical, cognitive, social and emotional effects of dementia in its various forms, in one place and at one time through community dance.

The focus of the training is about developing what could be called 'the clinical eye'. That is: the ability to recognise the clinical condition through posture, gesture and every other aspect of physical movement; to know what is happening beneath the surface of the body and beyond the muscularity. We look at the ways we sit, look up, or out, glance, wave, stand, reach out, grasp another's hand and drop it again. We take into account what is involved when we turn, clap high, stamp a foot and hold our balance.

All of these seemingly simple movements are in fact highly complex. The interactions of the network of nerves and muscles is highly nuanced and, when all works smoothly in a well-orchestrated nervous system, we can take this facility for granted. But when the signals become muddled and muted, as they do in the various forms of dementia, the effects on mind and body are profound and widespread. Our inbuilt ability to process information and respond verbally and through movement can be incrementally compromised. It is hard to think of an area of life which is left untouched by dementia as it progresses.

However, research has shown over and over again that dance, the lyrical, non-didactic flow of movement, can still engage the latent muscle memory that survives the onset of the disorder. According to leading neurologist Doctor Oliver Sacks, part of the mind does remain responsive:

> Some form of memory and response always survives, above all the sort of motor memory and response which goes with dancing.
>
> Oliver Sacks, *Musicophilia: Tales of Music and the Brain* (2007)

This has most positive implications for community dance artists and musicians. The surviving ability to respond to music and dance offers us a clear way to directly engage with our participants. And using a structured, well-considered approach with a reason for everything we do means we have a vocabulary and a rationale to engage with health professionals at every level. It by no means detracts from the level of enjoyment, creative expression and full-hearted response we see at each and every session.

So, here in the workshop, dancing, singing, music and laughter are filling the room and animating faces every week as the first phase of Dancing Recall takes place. The participants arrive as 'people with dementia' but soon become simply people again as the dance begins.

> Peter has no knowledge of the model we are using, the clinical effect we are seeking or even the circumstances which have brought him to this dance studio in Kendal. He just lights up when he hears the music and is moved, from whatever 'within' means, to respond in his own way to its invitation.

> Flora can't remember that she used to win competitions for her beautiful embroidery, or how she met Mike, her husband of many years who accompanies her each week to dance. But she is full of grace and gentle gesture and her smile warms the assembled group. Flora has a natural flow and harmony of movement which makes her so expressive. Neurologists sometimes use the term 'kinetic melody' to describe the fluidity of human movement. Flora oozes her own special kind of kinetic melody. Mike wishes Flora was her old self, but can see her blossoming before his eyes as she tilts her head and smiles, or lifts a graceful hand, or waltzes across the floor with him.

Our groups have been attended by people with various different manifestations and stages of dementia. Some have the stiffening, fixing and flexing of the body which makes movement so impoverished and unreliable; but even they soften in the dance.

So here I am with both my hats on: neurophysiotherapist; and the dancer. What works in practice? What doesn't? What do we need to do more of and what do we need to stop doing? I believe we should do what the latest National Institute for Clinical Excellence (NICE) guidelines suggest. We should converge social and medical streams of healthcare, listen to what real people have to say about what types of healthcare they find most useful, and offer community dance for neurodegenerative conditions as one option. The government's National Dementia Strategy identified key needs for the population which support my own view. It is wonderful to see funding finally being diverted to support initiatives that improve the quality of life for the many thousands of people living with dementia.

We are only part way through the Dancing Recall project. The next groups of participants are in Keswick, Carlisle, Whitehaven and Penrith. By the time the pilot ends we'll have danced our way around all six regions of Cumbria and created a network of trained dance and dementia practitioners. What about the future? So many people have been and will be involved in the running of this project. This network continues to evolve and will serve us well as we move ahead into the evaluation phase. Our evaluation processes are inevitably complex, looking at both the training and the delivery. We have a considerable body of information to look at and use, to help shape the future of this work.

I have had a vision for many years that community dance for people living with neurodegenerative conditions would be made available within the NHS. Dancing Recall, coming at a time when there is national recognition of the scale of the problem, brings us closer to that vision. And the only way that vision will become reality is if it is shared. If together we act positively, decisively and collectively.

Moving forward with Parkinson's

Amanda Fogg

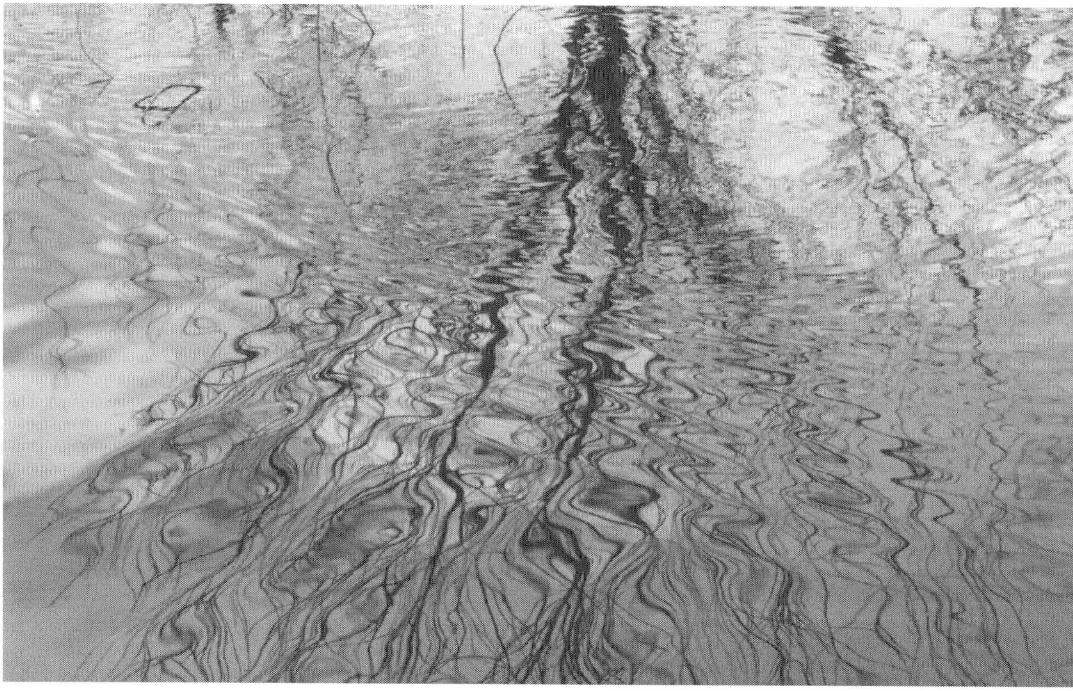

After running movement/dance sessions for people with Parkinson's for many years I now guest teach and co-teach and advocate for this area of work, espousing the aim of our national network[1], to provide opportunities for people with Parkinson's to have access to high-quality dance classes in their area, wherever they are in the UK.

In the dance class the goal is to have fun, to express ourselves creatively, to maintain fitness and find ways of coping with the particular motor challenges of the disease through dance. Over the years my groups and their partners have taught me at least as much as I have taught them. They are truly in the front line and often come up with solutions of their own which help them with their individual problems – solutions which are then tried and adopted or adapted by other group members where appropriate. Sessions combine precepts of general keep fit, Tai Chi, Yoga, Pilates, Conductive Education and exercises recommended by physiotherapists specific to Parkinson's, all via the medium of dance. We also sing and include vocal and facial exercises (since the facial muscles and the vocal folds may be affected by Parkinson's) combining gesture, movement, imagery and dance.

Many elements in the session are pertinent for any dance or fitness class, but they become even more critical in promoting well being and functionality with reference to Parkinson's. We work on posture throughout the session, aiming to correct the pitched-forward stance

1 Amanda Fogg is a founding member of Dance for Parkinson's Network UK.

characteristic of the condition, and where such posture has already become habitual we work to restore mobility in the upper spine and to realign focus. There is a lot of work with the breath, using Pilates breathing as a model, aiming to increase lung capacity and mobility of the inter-costal muscles. This leads to seated Tai Chi inspired warm-up exercises and ports de bras, again using the breath and including gentle but powerful arm movements to open the chest, improve posture and allow full tidal breathing, without strain. Some of the participants may choose to stand during the Tai Chi/ports de bras section of movements, but they may choose to sit at any time, and are encouraged to adapt their practice to how they are feeling.

We do general exercise, seated and standing in rhythmically-driven or flowing movement sequences (music is the transformative factor here), taking all the joints through as comprehensive a range of movement as is individually possible, using the large, then small muscle groups, offering variations to suit each person's needs on that particular day. We work particularly to strengthen the quadriceps, to maintain flexibility in the hamstrings, calves, ankles and feet, whilst aiming for freedom of movement in the upper body, with (for example) oppositional arm swing and an erect, well-supported head. We build movement sequences in various dance styles to encourage cognitive engagement and muscle memory and explore opportunities for creativity and sharing movement ideas.

In standing, initially we work between chairs, holding onto the backs of heavy chairs, so that there is support on both sides. Many specific problems of Parkinson's are addressed in this section as we warm up, practising heel strike, changes of weight from one foot to the other, shifts of centre of gravity towards different sides of the foot, gentle knee bends, hip circles, and low leg swings to keep hip joints free and loose. This work also has the benefit of strengthening both the supporting and working legs, and of course, the importance of good posture and eye focus are also stressed. The use of chairs also assists work on balance, which is monitored so that it is appropriate to the needs of each individual on that particular day. This section of the class equates to the ballet barre, preparing for work in the centre.

A variety of props may be used in the sessions, fulfilling different purposes. Often people with Parkinson's find that their range of movement increases if their focus is outside the body, i.e. taking their awareness away from any movement limitations they may have in ordinary circumstances. In this way they may stretch further than they thought they could to reach a balloon. Focusing on the brightness and movement of a baton may enable greater freedom of arm swing, with easier oppositional movement in the trunk. Other props (small sponge balls, TheraBands) can be used to strengthen or stretch various muscle groups or to aid coordination. Tennis balls may be rolled under foot to both massage the foot and to stimulate nerve endings and enhance sensitivity of small muscles essential to balance. Any variety of objects (feathers, fabric, pebbles, driftwood etc.) may be passed from hand to hand, using different fingers with the thumb, aiding dexterity and encouraging awareness of texture. Quality of movement may also be enhanced by the subtle use of props, and props can also be a vehicle for communication and self-expression as they are passed from person to person.

We try various walking techniques, and for safety, participants with difficulties are accompanied by their partners. Rhythmic music and imagery may override 'freezing' problems and allow people to access a greater freedom of movement. Sometimes we use the Conductive Education approach, counting our steps aloud as we walk round the space, telling ourselves to stop, and then recommencing. The louder and firmer the instruction, the more the body obeys, in most cases producing a larger, more confident stride and improved arm swing. We estimate individually how many paces may be required to cross a certain distance and then see if we are right, encouraging people to weigh up a 'journey', to 'prepare' themselves before they begin to move. Walking in different directions is practised, and sometimes participants work through a Conductive Education sequence which incorporates weight change and changes of direction. (NB: In all parts of the class seated and standing differentiations are given, with the option to sit or stand at will.) This part of the class lends itself to different dance genres, e.g. folk dance or ballroom etc.

Weight transference, incorporating balance work, forms part of this section of the session, as do techniques for turning round (especially in confined spaces) and coping with 'freezing'.

The more (carefully monitored) strenuous movement in the class is interspersed with work, which is less physically tiring, so that overexertion is avoided, since fatigue is a common symptom of the condition. Paying attention to the dynamic arc of the session and making adjustments in response to how people are on any particular day is vital in this work, and the final 'cool down' often revisits elements from different sections of the class which correspond at this point to 'reverence' in the ballet class, followed by a Yoga-based relaxation. Having worked hard for an hour or more, the participants sit back, well supported in armchairs or (if appropriate) lie on the floor and progressively relax each part of the body.

Tea and refreshments and social time provide a popular and essential finale!

Although I have described stages in the class where elements of Tai Chi, Pilates, Yoga, and Conductive Education are drawn upon, dance pervades every part. Music of all styles accompanies our work, and acts like yeast with dough, giving an external rhythm or impulse – an impetus to stimulate the desire to move and to elicit the appropriate movement quality. Also, of course, it makes it much more fun. The use of imagery and metaphor, allied to varied dance styles and/or themes, and teaching according to the precepts of the dance class rather than to symptoms or employing a mechanistic approach, enhances the positive effects of moving, enlivening the body and spirit and encouraging creativity and joy.

As well as having fun, making sessions useful and effective for each individual is an imperative. Safety is the first requirement and everyone has to be aware of the needs of other members of the group. Close monitoring is essential at all times, but especially when someone wishes to attempt movements which might pose significant challenges. Careful judgement is required in the balancing of confidence building/extending someone's ability, against the risks of falling, for example. Where people have difficulties we are always searching for ways of overcoming them. Sometimes the appropriate imagery, or intonation of voice in an instruction or suggestion may unlock the desired effect. Often a piece of music, especially where it has particular relevance for the individual, can help to override difficulties. Where there is great rigidity in muscles and tendons I encourage maintaining as much range of movement as already exists, trying to extend it of course, but also focusing on improving posture and strength, to aid balance. Some people wish to work from an understanding of how the body works, whilst others prefer to explore movement purely as dance.

Much of our effort goes into developing routines and strategies for coping with particular Parkinson's problems before they occur or become insurmountable. Thus we have evolved ways of turning round in small spaces, getting up and down from the floor or out of a chair etc., as discussed earlier. When initiating movement, or resuming it after 'freezing', is posing difficulties, our approach is to take a deep breath, in order to mentally take a step back from the difficulty and calm the system. After a deep breath, the weight may be shifted and the required foot freed in order to step over the threshold – or whatever. Sometimes it may take more than one breath, but the important thing is to slow right down and to think objectively through the mechanics of the movement required. Obviously, there is no magic wand, but there may be alternative ways of dealing with challenges.

There are several precepts which underpin our work. As far as possible people are encouraged to be responsible for themselves and to take account of how they are feeling and what they want to work for or achieve in any particular session. The ethos of the groups is mutually supportive and not competitive. Everyone is unique, despite the Parkinson's umbrella, and people are encouraged to value and respect their own and everyone's effort.

This all sounds like very hard work – as indeed it is – but we think of it as serious fun! We work playfully and we play hard in our sessions, bearing in mind a quote of George Bernard Shaw:

> *Man does not cease to play because he grows old;*
> *He grows old because he ceases to play.*

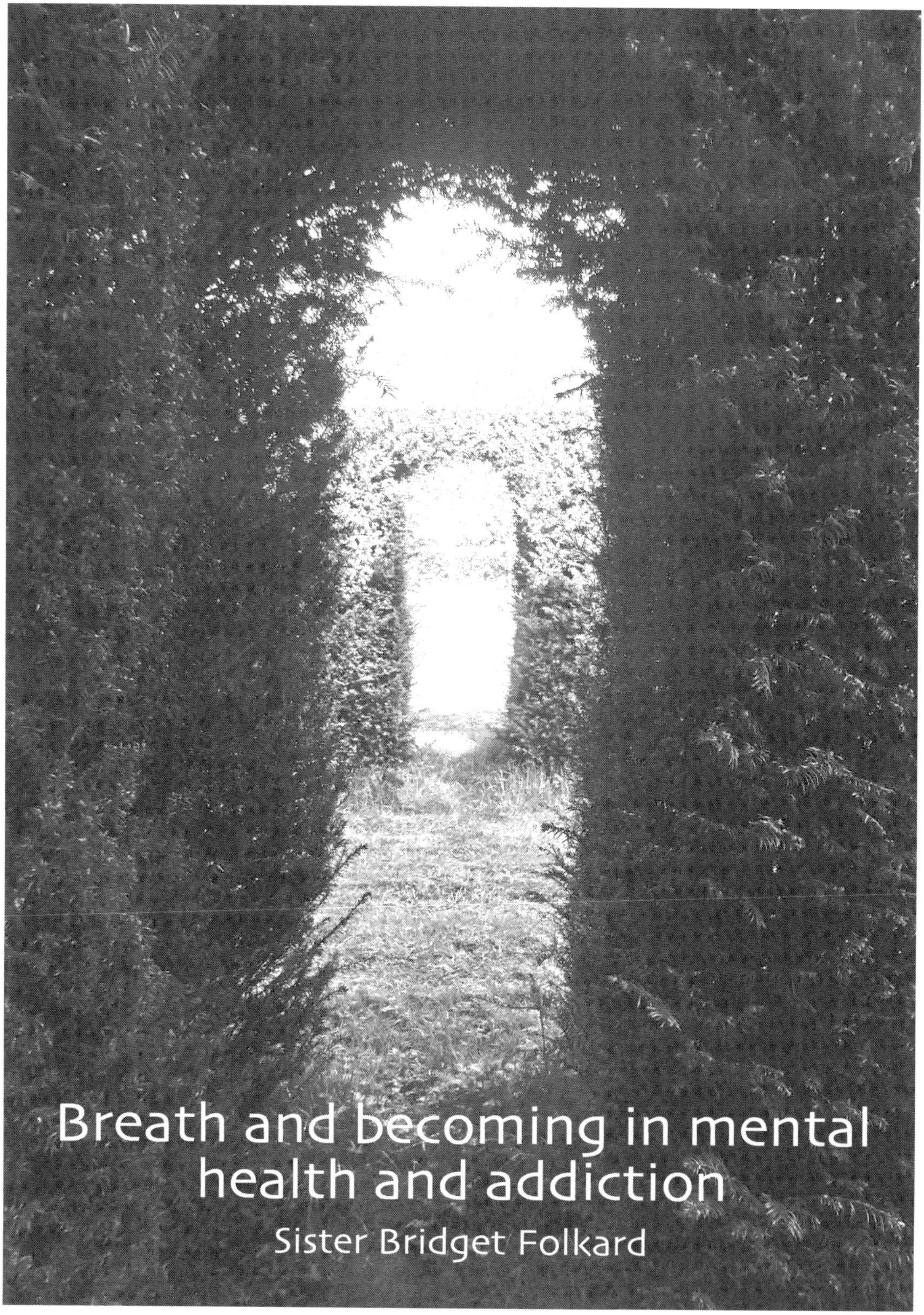

Breath and becoming in mental health and addiction

Sister Bridget Folkard

I was 63 years old when I found that 'gravity' could be inside the body and soul, gravity which was at once true-weighted seriousness, lightness of being, settling, truth and new beginning. It was 2011, a year after I had begun working in a mental hospital where dance, movement and breathing were offered weekly to clients, and to staff wishing to participate.

Years of nursing experience had kept in me sure instincts that 'life is inextricably linked to movement,' that all medicine is a 'dialogue with the process of life.' Moving to new places in life urges us to find new possibilities, sounds, pathways of breath and becoming. Breath and movement are new languages of engaging with what is happening: finding connection, possibility, imagination, understanding and creativity in breath, movement, sound, art and silence. Life too, as I go on learning, emerges from the very place where it lies itself down.

The year 2010 took me into mental healthcare wards and a detox unit for those braving 'life beyond addiction.' Every Monday morning, I share with the patients an hour of movement and dance offered by experienced young artists who reach people where they are, adapting to the group. We have sat, breathed, opened our eyes wider than ever before, laughed, clapped our hands and blown out our breaths, speaking our names, throwing balls to each other, playing with ribbons, flags, balloons and feathers. We have learned Chinese dancing, Tai Chi, become Spanish matadors, Irish dancers, people of South America, Africa and India, learning to stretch, sway, move through water, be blown by the wind, pass between each other in the space of the room, smiling, mirroring movements and creating something between us, in us and around us.

In sickness and health, movement may offer generously new languages of change, perhaps a sudden elasticity, ways through, in and beyond fixed thought patterns. Suddenly we are all swaying, it is not only the music, it is our bodies, and the creation of something within each of us and all of us in the room. In another moment we are all 'Vogue models', posing for ourselves and others, we break the mould of who we are with single poses, suddenly proud, helplessly laughing, unexpectedly glimpsed and allowed to be as 'other'. For this one moment everything is different from 'what it has always been.'

We finish with gentle breathing, calming and distilling what has been in the hour. The hands of all of us float down through the water we imagine, each of us 'doing this for himself, herself.'

Mirroring the actions of each other, following hands, expressions, feelings of each other, one leading and then the other leading without words; this requires and reveals a concentration, a language, incredible strength of soul inside the pain and confusion. Whatever the heaviness/pain, the hour may find us all blowing feathers into the air, tossing balloons to each other, creating rhythms with shakers, clapping and smiling and drawing apart the imaginary clouds in the sky.

The detox unit has a quiet room, with a lamp of moving colours, calming music and giant beanbags. Four or five come, not to dance or move, but to breathe, to come to self, to quietness, allowing the beanbag to take one's whole weight, sinking down. Breathing is itself language, laying something down and receiving it back. We can hold our consciousness on this going and coming of breath. We cannot control the mind or the heart, our 'addictions' of all kinds (i.e. what dictates to us) but we can bring attention to this other controllable pace of breath within our being.

Detox clients risk this silence and breath, they risk what may come in the protected quietness of the room. Zen wisdom teaches first to expire, to let go, to allow surrender, vacuum and possibility. 'Pause,' it counsels, 'in that deepest place of letting go, pause to leave something there' ... only then breathe in to take in what has changed and become something else.

We *take* what we need for life, often when we want and how much we want. There is no 'receiving' on supermarket shelves or on the internet: we choose, take, reject, consume or dispose of. Breath is different: it lays down and receives back.

Breath may simply be discovered during these sessions: 'I never knew I could breathe.' New muscles may be discovered moving our ribs and pushing out in our backs. 'I did not know I had these muscles.' Detox may be a journey into facing vulnerability and loss, breath may become a friend, a tool to recognise where we are and where we may be, for once a thing we can control. One asthmatic began to breathe in the quietness: 'I never thought I would breathe again.' Literally, breath was given back in breathing.

The light in the lamp with all its colours moves up and down, like the breath, at times we listen to the recorded sound of waves on the shore, allowing tides to come and to go. Breath itself allows being and becoming. Often the quietness simply welcomes us in, in seconds there is sleep, a hand on the belly, a body and mind cradled into another rhythm. Insomnia is a huge fear and power in detox. Quiet breathing in this sheltered place suddenly brings sleep and relieves pain. I have heard the unbelieving voice say with such relief 'no pain, no pain, no pain.' The breathing, the session, does not accomplish this for ever, not for any of us, but breath can be learned, in some small way, as a tool for the journey ahead.

The expiring is to release, let go, forgive. In the quietness I speak words that can be received within their own breathing, words linked to the breathing, to the long sound of an outbreath:

> *I release myself, and everyone else in my*
> *life, I forgive myself and everyone else,*
> *I give myself another chance,*
> *I give everyone else another chance.*

Each life is unique. Addiction may bring all of us in different ways to patterns of life we have not wanted. The sound of breath, of tide, the sense of our bodies moving with each breath is a powerful possibility of letting something go, and letting something come, allowing new creative concepts to emerge. In the quietness we can truly 'imagine'. We can see not what we have been, but what we have become. The whole past is not to be closed and consigned to nothing, but kept as roots in a dark pond when the lotus flower opens to light. Whatever has been is still part of our life university, the learning place which has its value now as precisely that.

Within the breath going and coming, we can all speak of what we want to relinquish, name energy verbs to come into the vacuums, imagine what we can be, and move into a place of discovery. 'The past does not dictate the future,' the flow is not towards a 'recovery' of something which has been, but a discovery of what we may be.

The breath and the quietness,
the willingness to drop into the breath, is itself
the great undertaking,
moving us to the possibility of a tomorrow,
different from what has always been.

The clients do this for themselves, coming into this willingness. They create these sacred enclosed moments.

In the dance we move around,
stilling of body into breath leaving and
returning, requires another courage.

Darkness, death, loss, friends gone in early years, shame, guilt, tears, comfort, all may come up from within, and the breath allows feelings to flow, not here as destructive powers, but within the tides that breath allows. The breath is a *beginning* of a becoming.

When the session finishes we breathe deeply, stretch up our arms and hands and fingers to receive whatever has been given, rubbing our hands together, bringing their warmth to our eyes and faces.

We sense that in our own breath is everything, then we can grasp our own shoulders with love, and emerging say 'I have come this far, I have come this far.'

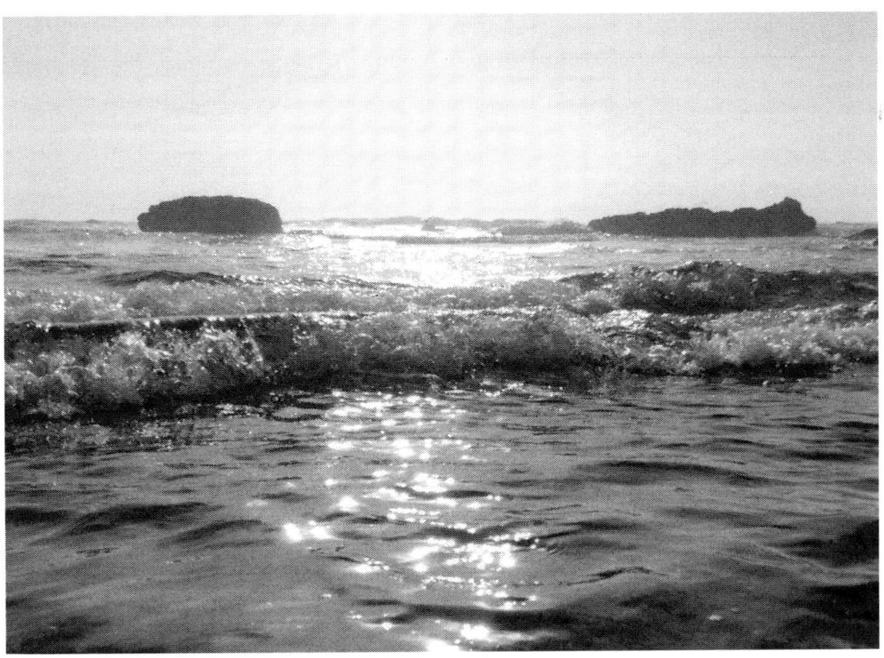

A dance for Buddug: 'listening beyond the listening'

from Cai Tomos

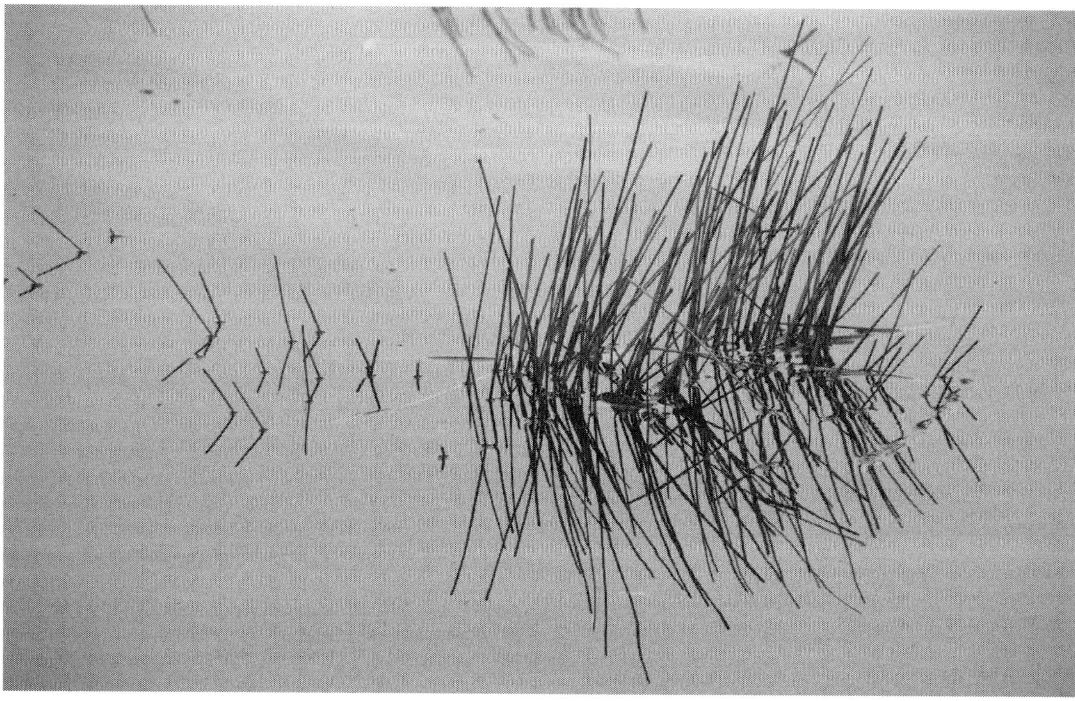

In 2010 I began running a regular movement group for elders in Caernarfon, North Wales. Five years later and the group is still going strong. At the beginning, the sessions were simply about getting people together to move and enjoy each other's company. But over the years I noticed that, the more we addressed people's own creativity and imagination and let them follow their own instincts and movement, the more people seemed to gain from the sessions.

One member of that group was Buddug. I was curious about Buddug's dancing; she had such a unique way of using her body, listening so deeply to her own movements. Buddug began losing her sight ten years ago. A few years later she also lost her husband Geraint to cancer. Over the years of working with the movement group, Buddug found that dancing was giving her a freedom that she relished. So over a year we began making a piece together, and the result of this was a solo, called 'Listening beyond the listening'.

When I asked Buddug why she danced, she stated, 'for freedom'. She said: 'This dance is about shadows and light. When I began losing my sight, I began to notice the shadow, not only in my vision, but in my life. Dancing is where I am free.' This feeling of freedom drew us deep and close together in our work, regardless of the 35 years age difference between us, our love of freedom in movement became the ground of our meeting.

We take time – moving and listening – to find a common language. We build this language slowly, together. For me there is something less about trying to dance but to find and convey something of what we feel, to illuminate our humanness. Often this involves an undoing of our usual body patterns, so that we drop inward to sense of essence. This reveals itself in the small details, a quiver, a reach of a hand, a rise and fall of a breath, the softening of the face to the air. This sense of essence always seems to appear when we slow down. Something is communicated that transcends but also includes the personal.

As we worked together, Buddug taught me about how without sight she listens, how she feels her way into the world. She would often hear the sound of the sea from the studio, it was as if her whole being was inviting the sea towards her. Her dance seemed about making this listening visible. Its title came from Buddug saying one day that as she goes about in the world now, she is 'listens beyond the listening'.

Buddug thought about significant moments in her life as she began to lose her sight. I asked her if there were any phrases or words that came with these memories as she moved?

Where do I go ... I need to listen ... I must keep going ... I must see

Buddug worked with these phrases and allowed further images and memories to come in response to these words. Each memory was of a different time in her life, like rooms in the house of her memory. She would enter each one and inhabit that place and time. She would move from these memories and slowly began to develop gestures that somehow held all that she felt then and now, both the memory and the feeling and sensations of her body now in this day.

Gradually each gesture became infused with deeper meaning and intention. There was a sense that Buddug was becoming moving self-portrait, slowly revealing herself. Reaching a hand up to the air, her eyes seeking upwards, she would breathe into each emerging gesture.

Buddug's own words

I was very, very nervous and very unsure what I was letting myself in for. It was very difficult to learn to listen to my body ... and to keep on breathing and listen to my breath, but as the work got on, the more I listened. I realised I felt better, less stressed, and I was able to relax in the dance, and the dance got better, using the breath work. I have to continue thinking about it and doing it.

I use my ears a lot, because I've lost my sight. Listening is the thing I do every day. But the type of listening you encourage is to listen using my whole body. Not only listening to the noise within the room, but further out. I realised that by standing still and breathing I could hear my own breathing, but I could also hear the sea. This way of listening is very powerful, when you start, you realise that you are listening with the whole of your body, working with it, it gives you power. Internal power.

I realised I was less tired at the end of sessions; I was relaxing into the dance. I felt I could do two then three hours then more ... and at the end of the day still feel exhilarated by it all. Because most probably, my fitness was improving, but also because I wasn't tensing up as much within my body.

I was looking forward to coming into the studio more and more – and feeling happy dancing – and looking forward to the sessions. I felt relaxed after the sessions although it was very, very emotional at times. Having let go of that emotion that needed to come out, it felt really good, to let it go, and to be able to face it, which I'm doing now.

The dance gives you the freedom that you can't have when you're walking along the streets, tied to my guide dog, or using my white cane. When I'm dancing ... I'm really free...a sense of openness really, like suddenly I blossom, like a flower, it feels very beautiful... a nice feeling...of beauty and openness and honesty..

I feel better in myself through the last few months, I feel better not only in the dance but in other parts of my life, I feel more confident and more at ease in myself, and really I know where I'm going, I want to carry on leading my life this way... Dancing through it... Yes, dancing through it.

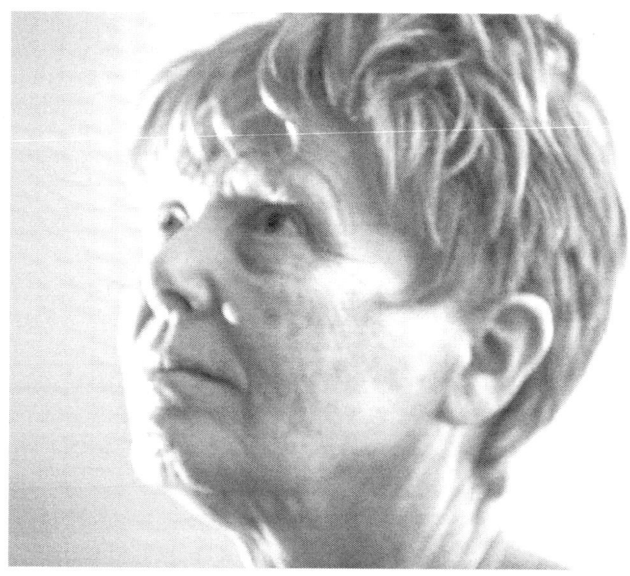

What is health ...

Tackling physical inactivity is recognised as a high priority for public health. It contributes to 1 in 6 deaths in the UK, equal to smoking, and costs the NHS an estimated £8.9 billion a year.

The overwhelming number of complaints to GPs are headaches, somatic pains, heart conditions, apathy, depression, obesities, emotional and physical stresses – these could be called 'dis-eases' of lifestyle. Currently life expectancy for the poor is nine years less than for the rich.

Antidepressant prescribing has nearly doubled since 2006 from 30–54 million monthly prescriptions, with four million patients on such medication despite the government

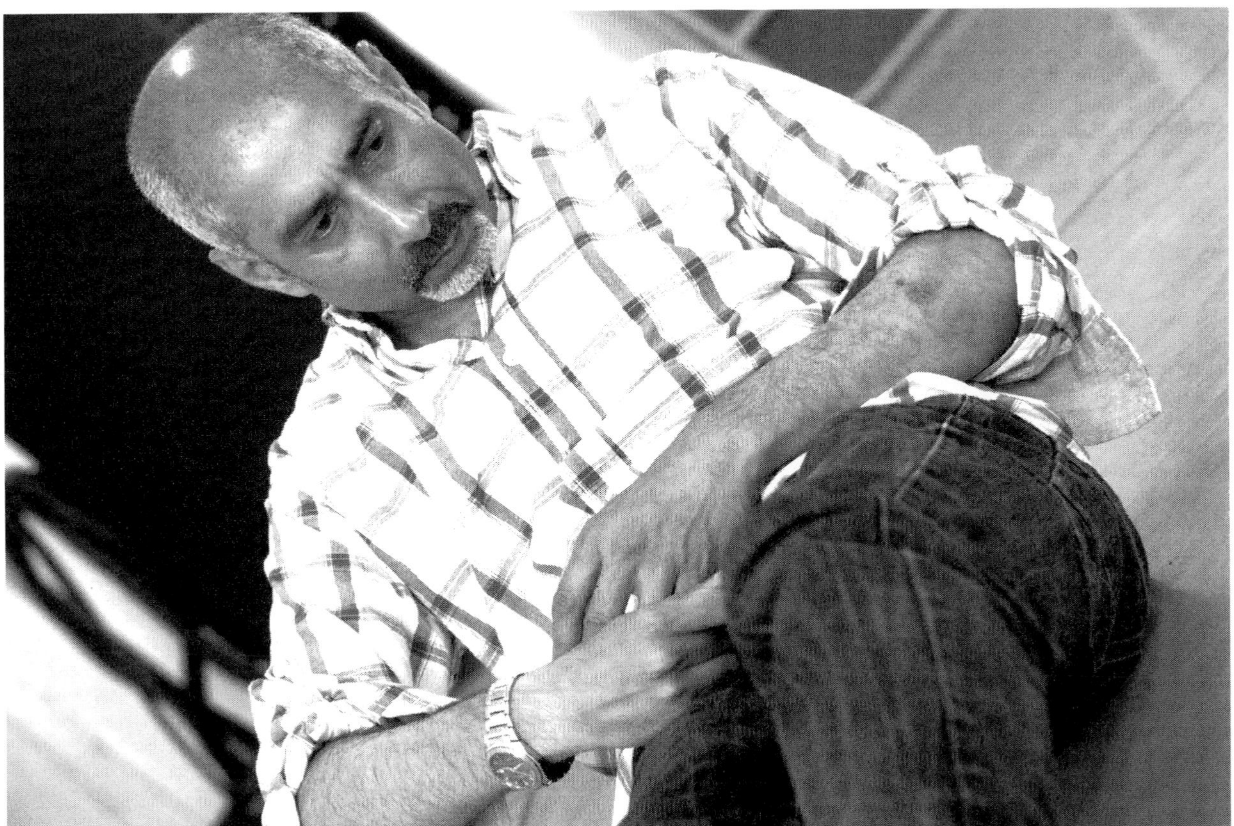

recognising the need to 'end the Prozac nation' and improve access to talking therapies as an alternative to antidepressants.

A poll of 2,000 GPs (*Pulse*, June 2013) showed that 97% 'did not think they were positively influencing people's lives or accomplishing much in their role', and 43% were 'at very high risk of burnout'. They are overwhelmed by 40 patient contacts per day, and 'six out of ten are considering early retirement'. Over 100 practitioners are reported to be quitting (*Pulse*, Aug 2014).

'Not only is life expectancy linked to social standing, but so is the time spent in good health; the average difference in "disability-free life expectancy" is now seventeen years between those at the top and those at the bottom of the economic ladder.' Randeep Ramesh, *The Guardian* (11 Feb 2010)

'The World Health Organisation predicts that in ten years' time mental ill health will be the second greatest cause of morbidity in populations within advanced economies, second only to heart disease
Depression affects one in three of the population at some time in their lives and yet only two per cent of the national health budget is spent on interventions for depression.' Mike White, *The Guardian* (11 Feb 2010)

A study in 1973 by Harvey Brenner showed that a 1% rise in unemployment was followed by a 6% increase in admissions to psychiatric hospitals, a 4% rise in suicides, an increase in admissions to prisons and a 6% increase in murders.

The NHS spends approximately £400 billion a year on our illnesses. Mental health costs the UK economy £75 billion in loss of earnings and in healthcare. The World Health Organisation predicts that by 2020 depression will be the biggest cause of ill health worldwide.

Wellbeing assessment from Breath of Fresh Air project

At the end of the project we asked people to fill out questionnaires with a score out of five for their feelings about health, wellbeing, etc. In all domains people's sense of their own wellbeing had improved. We have presented the raw scores to show the differences they felt in each domain.

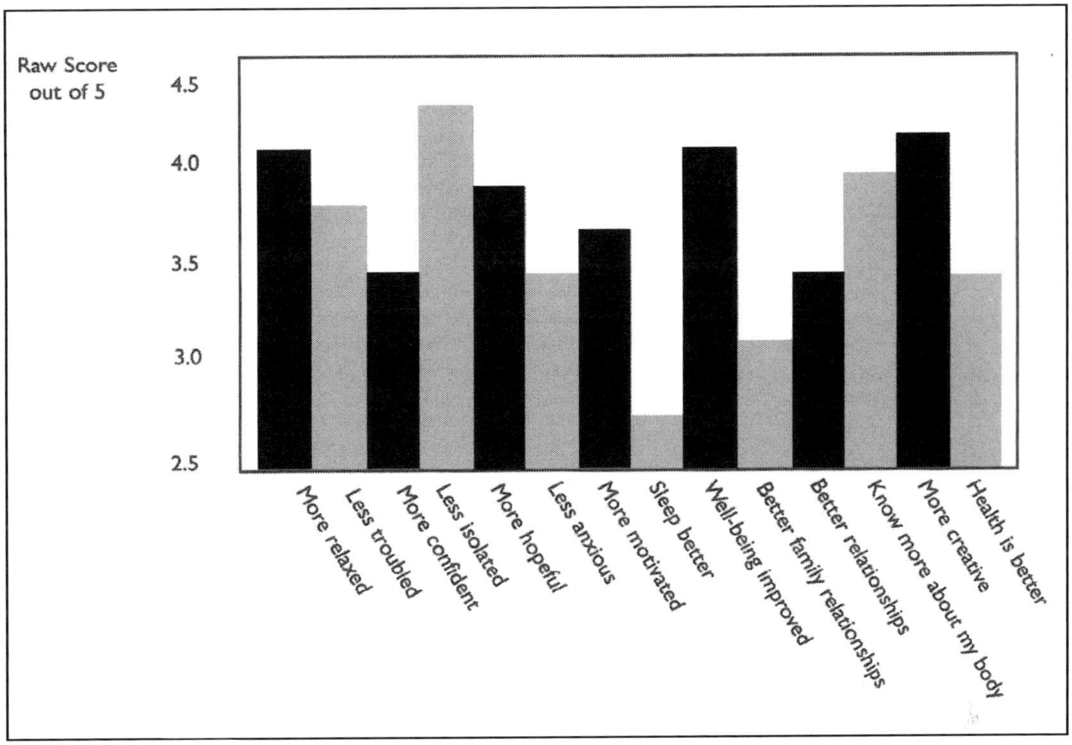

Collation of raw scores by Dr Wendy Macdonald, University of Manchester.

Permissions

Extract from: 'Introduction' from the book *Wild Geese - Selected Poems* by Mary Oliver. Bloodaxe Books. © Mary Oliver. Used by permission of the author via Charlotte Sheedy Literary Agency.

'reading the Japanese poem Issa' from *New and Collected Poems: 1931-2001* by Czeslaw Milosz (Penguin Classics 2005), © Czeslaw Milosz Inc., 1988, 1991, 1995, 2001.

Extract from: *The Assumptions of the Rogues and the Rascals'* by Elizabeth Smart, © Elizabeth Smart, 1980. HarperCollins. Reprinted by permission of HarperCollins Publishers Ltd.

Quote from: '*Winter Pollen*' by Ted Hughes, © Ted Hughes, 1995. Faber and Faber. Used by permission.

Extract from: *'And our Faces, My Heart, Brief as Photos'* by John Berger, © John Berger. Pantheon Books. Used by permission of Penguin Random House.

Excerpt from: *A Poetry Handbook* by Mary Oliver, © 1994 Mary Oliver. Reprinted by permission of Houghton Mifflin Harcourt Publishing Company. All rights reserved.

Poem: '*For a New Beginning*' from: *Benedictus*, written by John O'Donohue, © John O'Donohue. Random House. Used by permission of Penguin Random House.

Extract from: '*The Betrayal of the Body*' by Alexander Lowen © Alexander Lowen, is used by kind permission of the Lowen Foundation. www.lowenfoundation.org

Excerpts from: *The Spell of the Sensuous: Perception and Language in a More-Than-Human-Word* by David Abram, © 1996, David Abram. Used by permission of Pantheon Books. All rights reserved.

Excerpt from: *Becoming Animal: An Earthly Cosmology'* by David Abram, © 2010, David Abram. Used by kind permission of David Abram via The Spieler Agency, New York City and Pantheon Books. All rights reserved.

'Being', was taken from: *Orpheus: A version of Rilke's Die Sonette an Orpheus* by Don Paterson, © Don Paterson. Faber and Faber and used by permission of Faber and Faber.

Lines from: *Mental Fight* by Ben Okri © 2000. Reprinted by kind permission of Ben Okri.

Extract from: *'The Human Effect in Medicine'* by Michael Dixon and Kieran Sweeney. Taylor and Francis. Reprinted with permission of Taylor and Francis.

Extract from: *'Nature as Creativity'* by David Bohm, Nobel prize-winning physicist and R. Webber, from *ReVision* journal vol. 5, no. 2, Fall 1982. Used with permission from ReVision publishing.

Extract from: '*The Figure a Poem Makes'* is reprinted from *Selected Prose of Robert Frost*, ed. Hyde Cox and Edward Connery Lathem, © 1939, 1966, 1967. Henry Holt and Co. Used by permission of Henry Holt.

Extract from: *Arctic Dreams* by Barry Lopez. Vintage Classics. © 2014. Used by permission of Penguin Random House.

Poem: 'somewhere i have never travelled, gladly beyond', © 1931, 1959, 1991 by the Trustees for the E.E. Cummings Trust. © 1979 by George James Firmage, from *Complete Poems: 1904-1962* by E.E. Cummings, edited by George J. Firmage. Used by permission of Liveright Publishing Corporation.

Reprinted by arrangement with The Permissions Company, Inc., on behalf of Shambhala Publications Inc., Boulder, Colorado, www.shambhala.com.

Extract from: *Art Heals: How Creativity Cures the Soul* by Shaun McNiff, © 2004 by Shaun McNiff.

Extract from *New Self New World* by Phil Shepherd © 2010. North Atlantic Books. Used by permission.

Extract from *Send* by Kay Syrad, © Kay Syrad 2015, is used by kind permission of Kay Syrad and Cinnamon Press.

'A Short Story of Falling' is taken from *Falling Awake* by Alice Oswald, © 2016. Jonathan Cape. Used by permission of Penguin Random House.

Artwork

Illustration: 'Anatomy Image cambrai 1678' from: Ame Bourdon: *Nouvelles Tables anatomiques* was found at: https://www.nlm.nih.gov/exhibition/historicalanatomies/bourdon_home.html.

Illustration of a 'Diaphragm' is from: *Anatomy for* Movement by Blandine Calais-Germain. La Liebre de Marzo.

Illustrations

Cover image: Antonia Bruce, Harvest, maize rootball. Cyanotype on treated paper, 2015.

xi **Preface** Study for *Wing* photo: Caroline Lee

p. 1 **Introduction** artist and photographer: David Ward
*The Reverend Robert Walker, Skating on Duddingston Loch (Glider)*1993 Light projection. Collection: the artist. Photographed in the exhibition *David Ward: Keepers of Light* at the Arthur M. Sackler Museum, Harvard University, 1993.Based on the original painting by Sir Henry Raeburn (1756 -1823). Courtesy of the National Galleries of Scotland, Edinburgh.

Breath of Fresh Air
p. 6 poster by The Moose Factory, Alston Cumbria
pp. 14, 18, 21, 25, 31, 33 photos: Sharon Higginson.

Breath
pp. 42/43 Antonia Bruce part of series Maize – First Food Residency, see biographies
pp. 51, 66 photos: Christian Kipp *Pneuma* dancers, Eeva Maria Mutka and Cai Tomos performance collaboration, Miranda Tufnell, David Ward, Sylvia Hallett-Natural History Museum Oxford, Nov 2015
pp. 53, 62 photos: Tomo Brody from Filipa Periera Stubbes working in Addenbrookes Hospital
pp. 54, 55 photo: Chris Drury *Way of White Clouds* looped video of white clay water entering into a still black lake
pp. 56, 61 Pari Naderi *Redefining Beauty* Lucinda Jarrettt and Rosetta Life. Performance with elders at British Museum and Victoria and Albert Museum
p59 diaphragm Anatomy for Movement, Blandine Calais-Germain

Touch
pp. 69, 84, 85, 89 photos: Michael Reinhart
p. 71 photo: Filipa Periera Stubbs
p. 73 photo: Miranda Tufnell
pp. 72, 75, 77, 80, 82, 83 photos: Tomo Brody, Filipa Pereira-Stubbs, Dancing for dementia, Moving with Memory and Mood (2013) a project bringing together a group of adults living with or affected by dementia.
p.86 photo: Chris Lewis work with Daphne Cushnie/ Susie Tate *Dancing Recall*
p.87 Pari Naderi *Redefining Beauty*

The Practice of saying Yes
pp. 90, 93, photos: Christian Kipp, Eva Karczag in Promenade 3 with Chris Crickmay, Coventry, 2010.

Between You and Me
pp. 94, 106, 113 photos: Michael Reinhart
pp. 96, 97, 99 photos: Leila Romaya Small Things project Alder Hey hospital
pp. 102, 115 photos: Antonia Bruce Maize
pp. 105, 111 photos: Tomo Brody, Filipa Pereira-Stubbs, Dancing for dementia, Moving with Memory and Mood (2013) a project bringing together a group of adults living with or affected by dementia.

Getting Your Bearings
pp. 120, 127 149 Chris Drury artist p120 ***Medicine Wheel*** *'one natural object for each day of the year the wheel follows the seasons… but it also marks my inner year, reflecting its joys and tragedies …and the very basis of my work – the movement between inside and outside'* p127 ***Shelter for Dreaming,*** *'A shelter is a basic human need and a manifestation of human presence it is a dwelling place within the movement of a walk'.* p149 ***Life in the Field of Death*** *text drawn with permission from* ***Silent Spaces*** *and Chris Drury website www.chrisdrury.co.uk*

pp. 124, 128, 143, photos: Michael Reinhart

p.130 photo: David Ward artist installation *Light on the Feet (Footfalls for Samuel Beckett)* 2015 One image from a folio of nine. Archival prints on acid-free cotton rag paper. Collection: King's College, Cambridge. (Originally commissioned as a light projection by King's College, Cambridge for *Somewhere there where: Samuel Beckett in dialogue with King's College Chapel* in 2015.)

p.134 photo: Tomo Brody *Carpe Diem* a performance project with Lucinda Jarrett, Rosetta Life, in partnership with The Place and British Museum

p.135 Angel on Bike photo: Popperfoto

p.137 photo: Pari Naderi *Redefining Beauty*

p.139 Anatomy Image Cambrai 1678 Ame Bourdon Nouvelles Tables Anatomiques

p.144 photo and artist Antonia Bruce

Self Care in times of chaos and violence

p.116 photo: Youval Hai. Artist Arvital Cnaani scraped acquatint (2012) Jerusalem print workshop

Towards Meaning

pp. 150, 158 photos: Michael Reinhart

p.154 photo: Tomo Brody *Carpe Diem* a performance project with Lucinda Jarrett, Rosetta Life, in partnership with The Place and British Museum

p.156 photo: Christian Kipp *Pneuma* dancer Eeva Maria Mutka performance collaboration Miranda Tufnell, David Ward, Sylvia Hallett 2016

Chance of Fair

p. 160 photo: Michael Reinhart

Laying the Foundations

p.164 photo: Edmund Blok '*Roxy Dancing*'

p.167 photo: Miranda Tufnell *Minnou*

p. 169 photo: Anni Mctavish

What is this pill called dance

pp. 184, 186, 188, 191 photos: Tomo Brody for Filipa Pereira-Stubbs Dancing for dementia, Moving with Memory and Mood (2013) a project bringing together a group of adults living with or affected by dementia.

Harry: the story of a child in hospital

p. 193 photo: Miranda Tufnell

Dancing Recall

p.198 photo: Chris Lewis

Moving Forward with Parkinsons

p. 202 photo: Michael Reinhart

Breath and becoming in mental health and addiction

pp. 206, 209 photos: Michael Reinhart

A dance for Buddug

p. 210 photo: Michael Reinhart

p. 212 photo: Cai Tomos

What is health

p. 213 photo: Tomo Brody *Carpe Diem* a performance project with Lucinda Jarrett, Rosetta Life, in partnership with The Place and British Museum

p. 217 Cover image: Antonia Bruce, Harvest, maize rootball. Cyanotype on treated paper, 2015

Biographies of contributors

Diane Amans is a dance artist, choreographer, author, training consultant.
She has over thirty-five years experience of leading dance activities with diverse community groups both in the UK and Europe. For 15 years up till 2006 she was artistic director of Freedom in Dance – a company she founded in order to offer accessible opportunities for people of all ages to participate in dance activities. She currently works as a freelance dance artist, lecturer and consultant offering professional development, arts and health projects, evaluation and mentoring. She writes regularly for a range of professional journals and presents papers at national and international conferences. Her textbooks *An Introduction to Community Dance Practice* and *Age and Dancing: Older People and Community Dance* are set books on undergraduate community dance programmes in the UK, Europe and United States.

Karen Adcock Doyle: Karen's background is as a learning disability nurse, she studied Waldorf Steiner education and worked for ten years as a therapeutic worker in Barnardo's. She currently works in a York primary academy, supporting children of 2-11 years old and their families in the school, Children's Centre and Enhanced Resource Provision. Karen supports children with social, emotional and mental health needs and works with movement to children to develop sensate language and have greater agency over their body, and has seen how this can help children to self regulate and be an active and positive member of their school community. She studied Dance and Somatic Well Being at UCLan, and with Dan Leven in Massachusetts.

Penny Collinson(MA, Dip IBMT, RSME)is Course Leader of *MA Dance & Somatic Wellbeing: Connections to the Living Body*, an ISMETA Approved Training Programme at the University of Central Lancashire, Preston, UK, and is Senior Lecturer on the New York City sister programme. Penny has worked as a contemporary dance performer (*Ludus, Motionhouse, Penny Collinson & Co*) and lecturer since 1992. She has trained for many years with Linda Hartley and holds a Diploma from the Institute for Integrative Bodywork and Movement Therapy (IBMT). Penny is a registered Somatic Movement Educator with ISMETA and runs a private practice from her home in Lancashire.

Kathy Crick teaches Improvisation, Contact Improvisation, Choreography and Performance at Trinity Laban Conservatoire, London. Over the last twenty years she contributed to many dance and performing arts programmes in Higher Education in the UK. She has facilitated creative projects in diverse educational and community settings, for example working with artists with learning disabilities with Mind the Gap performing arts, Heart'n'Soul and more recently with Lucinda Jarrett (Rosetta Life) at Trinity Hospice as part of the Art of Touch Project.

Daphne Cushnie is a dance artist and neurological physiotherapist working part time for the NHS in Cumbria and has specialised in running classes and projects in dance for neurodegenerative conditions (NDC) since 2003. Since then she has taken part in and observed with great pleasure the growth of this field from tiny acorns to a wealth of interest, diverse practice and exciting research across the UK and beyond. She continues to work alongside others to ensure excellent access to dance for all living with NDC

Lisa Dowler (MA, SME) is a dance artist with experience of facilitating dance and creating performance in diverse settings. Her inclusive, somatic approach to dance has enabled her to explore and evolve her practice by engaging through the arts with young people in socially and economically deprived areas, asylum seekers, disabled children, pregnant women and older people. In 2003 she began a long term collaboration with Cath Hawkins initially as a performer with Small Things Dance Collective. In 2006 Lisa became the first dance artist in residence at Alder Hey Children's NHS Foundation Trust, Liverpool and with Small Things and Alder Hey Arts has evolved ongoing pioneering research into the effects of improvisation for children and young people in hospital across acute wards including Neuromedical, Cardiac and Orthopaedic.

Amanda Fogg trained in classical ballet followed by working in Community Dance field with elderly people. She specialised in dance for people with Parkinson's and is a founder member of Dance for Parkinson's Network U K.

Sister Bridget Folkard, S.R.N., M.A, is a Sister of St. Mary of Namur. She joined the order 50 years ago, and has spent most of her life nursing in Congo and Rwanda. She returned to UK in 2008 following an accident, and has since worked in acute mental health and addiction services in Liverpool whilst co-ordinating prayer, life-discerning and Bible groups. Creative writing, movement and dance are intrinsic to her ongoing journey.

Lucinda Jarrett is a performance maker and writer. She works at Marie Curie Hospice, Solihull, The National Hospital for Neurology and Neurosurgery and across London. She has delivered performance engagement for the British Museum She is also co director of Rosetta Life and is producing Stroke Odysseys a performance practice as research project for stroke rehabilitation. She has extensive experience in leading participatory performance and dance in healthcare and has initiated and led complex science engagement programmes for The Welcome Trust, The Science Museum and BBC. She has also led patient engagement campaigns for End of Life Care in Scotland and England and for the NHS in West Midlands and the South London Hospitals.

Eva Karczag is an independent dance artist. For the past four decades she has practiced, taught and advocated for explorative methods of dance making. Performs solo and collaborative work internationally, many of her collaborations involving links across the arts. Danced with Strider (UK, 1972-75), Dance Exchange (Australia, 1976-79) and the Trisha Brown Dance Company (NY, 1979-85), all leading groups in the field of experimental dance. Was on the faculty of the European Dance Development Center (EDDC), Arnhem, NL (1990-2002), and is a certified teacher of the Alexander Technique. Received her MFA (Dance Research Fellow) from Bennington College, VT. Her performance work and her teaching are informed by dance improvisation and mindful body practices that engender trust in the body's innate capacity for ease, efficiency and integrated openness.

Brenda Mallon is a psychotherapist/counsellor, a creative writing tutor, workshop leader and an author.Based in Manchester, Brenda offers one to one work with both adults and children and specialises in working with bereavement, loss and separation. She was on the Board of Directors of the International Association for the Study of Dreams (IASD) and was formerly the vice chair of Manchester Area Bereavement Forum, (The Grief Centre). She is the author of eighteen books including '*Creative Visualization with Colour*', '*Dreams, Counselling and Healing*' and '*The Dream*

Bible'. Her latest book '*Working with Bereaved Children and Young People*', as with all her works, deals with the importance of creativity at the heart of relationships and personal well being.

Jasmine Pasch is a freelance movement practitioner, a professional dancer, teacher and counselor. She has worked across the arts, health and education sectors for over thirty years, and has written several pieces for publication. She works in the London Boroughs of Tower Hamlets and Brent with babies, toddlers, young children and their families, and supports early years educators to develop their understanding of the particular developmental, learning and play needs of this age group in both indoor and outdoor environments. Jasmine runs 'Wiggly Jigglers' at Rich Mix Cultural Foundation where infants just a few weeks old through to boisterous toddlers approaching their second birthday come together to move and play freely.

Filipa Pereira-Stubbs is a movement artist, dance teacher, and creative practitioner with over twenty years experience in dance and the arts. She is the Director of DanceMoves, delivering dance programmes at Addenbrooke's Hospital with the Department of Medicine for the Elderly, the Lewin Stroke unit and with the neuro-rehabilitation ward. DanceMoves runs integrated dance groups in the community for people living with dementia and their carers. Filipa worked as a dance/movement therapist with the NHS in psychiatry of old age. She has worked in the field of palliative care with Rosetta Life, co-founding Rosetta Life with Lucinda Jarrett, and then working as artist-in-residence at the Arthur Rank House in Cambridge. Filipa runs Barefoot Dance – teaching dance to all ages, from babies to octogenarians, privately, in school and in early years centres, including an annual integrated dance project for children with special and complex needs. Filipa is a core artist with Cambridge Curiosity and Imagination, and works as an independent artist with Kettles Yard and the Fitzwilliam Museum.

Susanna Recchia is an Italian dance artist, performer and teacher based in London since 2001. She trained at Laban,(Award of Best Performer in 2004) and did a Foundation Course in Dance Movement Therapy at Goldsmiths University, and MA in Dance and Somatic Well-being at Lancashire University. Her practice shifts between performing, teaching and researching in academic, artistic and health contexts. She worked with Candoco, an integrated dance company with able and disabled dancers, performing, teaching and touring internationally. As a performer, she has collaborated with internationally known choreographers, and has devised her own work joining practitioners from different disciplines, such as music, photography and film.

Tim Rubidge trained with Sigurd Leeder in Switzerland. Since 1975 he has explored and devised many dance works, presenting solo and small ensemble works nationally and internationally in the UK, Europe, USA and South Africa. He has developed ground-breaking participatory and community-based projects and since 2005 conceived and directed site-specific performances. He was Visiting Fellow in Performing Arts at Northumbria University 2008-2011, and a frequent participant in the cultural exchange programme between North East England and the Eastern Cape of South Africa 2005-2009. He is currently researching relationships between choreographic practice and refugees' experience of displacement. www.timrubidge.net

Michal Shahak is a dance artist and Somatic Movement therapist working in Tel Aviv and Jersualem. She has over twenty five years experience of teaching creative movement and awareness through the body self in adult and youth education settings. She has a private practice based on

Body Mind Centering, Somatic Experiencing and other healing trauma approaches.

Kay Syrad is a poet and novelist. She is the Poetry Editor of ENVOI and in a creative partnership with the artist Chris Drury. www.kaysyrad.co.uk

Susie Tate is a dance artist and education practitioner working in the field of health and wellbeing in Northumberland and Cumbria.Following ten years working in the education departments for number of leading dance companies, including English National Ballet, The Place and The Royal Ballet, Susie began to focus her work within the dance and disability sector. She held the post of Director for the Foundation Course in Dance for Disabled people at Candoco from 2005 – 2007. Now based in Northumberland, Susie is working freelance for Dance Art Foundation under their dance and health programme, Breathing Space, and for a Cumbrian county-wide project for people living with dementia, Dancing Recall led along side dance practitioner and neuro-physiotherapist, Daphne Cushnie.

Cai Tomos is movement artist and choreographer who began dancing in North Wales. He has worked both nationally and internationally as dancer, choreographer and maker. He has toured as a performer and presented his work in festivals in South and North America, Spain and mainland Europe. Currently he works with 'older' people both in London hospitals and in theatre settings. He runs an Elders Performance Company in Wales and offers workshops in the UK and abroad. Improvisational practices are at the heart of his work supporting people to develop and discover their own movement language and vocabulary.www.caitomos.com/www.sensingself.org

Katherine Zeserson is a cultural activist, singer, trainer and thinker. She was Director of Learning and Participation at Sage Gateshead and has an international reputation as a trainer, music animateur and educator, having led programmes in a wide range of community, educational and social contexts; from pre-school settings to post-graduate and professional development training programmes. Her current work focuses on strategy, practice and professional development in the fields of music / cultural learning /voice and arts for social justice. She believes in the power of reflective artistic practice to inspire human development and build compassionate communities.

Visual Artists and Photographers – Accompanying Images

Tomo Brody is a documentary film maker and photographer who has worked in hospitals in Gaza, pioneering prisons in west coast Canada and with many artists, musicians and institutes around England. He has also previously worked with Miranda Tufnell on her dance performance '*Pneuma*'.

Antonia Bruce is an artist who engages with many processes in her work. Emerging from a commitment to drawing, she has taken her work into print processes, movement and dialogues. In 2011, she curated '*Infinitas Gracias*' with Wellcome Collection, an exhibition looking at the role of faith in healing. Currently she is leading a project in Mexico, 'First Food Residency,' which invites artists to engage with food cultures in each other's countries. Her images in this book stem from an exploration of Maize, the staple food in Mexico, its stature, cultural history and contemporary identity. Corn is the food staff of life, the 'first food' for many. Mexico holds a key to the security of crop diversity with its the rich variety of seeds currently threatened by the growing pressure of mono-crop systems. *'I worked with plants picked fresh from the field and laid them swiftly on prepared paper where they left an imprint of a fleeting moment before the sun destroyed them.'* Surrounding the growing of corn are the many rituals, offerings, music and dance that have evolved since man first cultivated crops. Antonia's cyanotypes capture the corn cobs that tower above the farmers, moving like dancers, in the spirit of freedom. Laid against heavy duty watercolour paper which she paints with a solution of iron compounds, the silhouettes of her subjects are developed in daylight, creating exquisite shadows on blue. www.firstfoodresidency.com

Chris Drury is an environmental artist, making site specific nature based sculpture, often referred to as Land Art or Art in Nature. He also works in art and Science making installations inside, with maps, digital and video art, and with mushrooms. His work makes connections between different phenomena in the world, specifically between Nature and Culture, Inner and Outer and Microcosm and Macrocosm. *'I wanted to see the world with openness, not from a fixed point of view. So I began using the very stuff of the world.'* He collaborates with scientists and technicians from a broad spectrum of disciplines and uses whatever visual means, technologies and materials best suit the situation. www.chrisdrury.co.uk

Christian Kipp is a photographer based in Essex. He balances his photography between landscape work, mostly locally and in Scotland, and establishing long-term collaborations with a variety of artists. The two areas frequently merge and feed each other. www.christiankipp.com

Pari Naderi is a Dance Artist, Photographer and Teacher.www.parinaderi.co.uk

Michael Reinhart is a singer-songwriter, and photographer. He studied at The Ontario College of Art (1976), in Toronto, Canada and the studio school Art's Sake Inc., where he explored painting, drawing and printmaking. His creative experience includes painting & drawing exhibitions; internationally published illustrations and photographs; lighting, video and set design; and musical soundtracks and improvisation for contemporary dancers in Canada, USA and the UK. He lives in both Montréal and Edmonton in Canada.
'Photography, for me, is primarily the end product of near-incessant walking, something of an obsession, having temporarily lost the ability to do so for a period of time in the past. Walking is the crucible for creation and ideation for many artists and thinkers. Walking, for me, is looking. It is observing with the trained eye of a draughtsman in motion. In the last dozen years or so, I have tended toward making a photographic record of what I see with a focus, more often than not, on anomalies. The weird and the unordinary. Art that is waiting to be found.'

David Ward works in a wide range of media and has made numerous collaborations with choreographers, composers, architects and other artists. Ward has been Artist in Residence at King's College, Cambridge (1991), Harvard University (1994), Durham Cathedral (1997–98) and was a Research Fellow at the Henry Moore Institute in Leeds (1995). Current projects include a solo exhibition at Wolverhampton Art Gallery (until 9 July 2016), and co-curating the major summer exhibition, *Seeing Round Corners: The Art of the Circle*, at Turner Contemporary, Margate (2016). www.davidward-artist.co.uk

Bibliography and suggested reading

Abram, David, *The Spell of the Sensuous* (Vintage Books, 1997); *Becoming Animal: An earthly cosmology* (Pantheon 2010)

Achterberg, Jeanne, *Imagery and Healing: Shamanism and modern medicine* (Shambhala, 1985)

Adams, Patch, *Gesundheit* (Rochester: Healing Arts Press, 1998)

Berger, John: *And Our Faces, My Heart, Brief as Photos* (Random House, 1992)

Berger, John and Jean Mohr, *A Fortunate Man: The story of a country doctor* (Allen Lane, 1967)

Brenner, Harvey, *Mental illness and the Economy* (Harvard University Press, 1973)

Carel, Havi *Illness: The Cry of the Flesh (*Acumen, 2008)

Dixon, Dr M & Dr Kieran Sweeney, *The Human Effect in Medicine: Theory, research and practice* (Radcliffe Medical Press, 2000)

Drury, Chris, introduction by Kay Syrad, *Silent Spaces* (Thames and Hudson, 1998)

Frost, Robert, *The Figure a Poem Makes* (essay) (Modern Library ed., 1946)

Gersie, Alida and Nancy King, *Storymaking in Education and Therapy* (London: Kingsley, 1992)

Gintis, Bonnie D.O, *Engaging the Movement of Life* (North Atlantic Books, 2007)

Greenland, Penny, *What dancers do that other health workers don't* (Jabadao, 2000)

Halprin, Anna, *Dance as a Healing Art: Returning to health with movement and imagery* (Life Rhythm, 2000)

Hartley, Linda *Somatic Psychology: Body mind and meaning* (Whurr Publishers, 2004)

Heath, Dr. Iona, *Matters of Life and Death: Key Writings* (Radcliffe Publishing , 2007)

Hillman, James, *The Soul's Code; in search of character and calling,* (Grand Central Publishing,1996)

Ho, Mae-Wan, *The Rainbow and the Worm: The Physics of Organisms* (Singapore: World Scientific, 1998)

Hughes, Ted, 'Myth and Education' in *Winter Pollen: Occasional Prose*, (Faber and Faber, 1994)

Johnson, Mark, *The Meaning of the Body: Aesthetics of human understanding* (University of Chicago Press, 2007)

Juhan, Deane, *Job's Body: A Handbook for Bodywork* (New York: Barrytown Ltd, 1987) *Touched by the Goddess: The physical, psychological and spiritual powers of bodywork* (Barrytown /Station Hill Press, 1994)

Katie, Byron, *Loving What Is* (Rider, 2002)

Keown, Dr Daniel *The Spark in the Machine: How the science of acupuncture explains the mysteries of western medicine* (Singing Dragon, 2014)

Kern, Michael, *Wisdom in the Body* (North Atlantic Books, 2001)

Levine, Peter A and Maggie Kline, *Trauma-Proofing Your Kids: A Parents' Guide for Instilling Confidence, Joy and Resilience* (North Atlantic Books, 2008)

Lewis, John, *A.T. Still: From the Dry Bone to the Living Man* (Dry Bone Press, 2012)

Lopez, Barry, *Arctic Dreams: Imagination and Desire in a Northern Landscape* (Charles Scribner's Sons, 1986)

McNiff, Shaun, *Art Heals: How Creativity Cures the Soul* (Shambhala, 2004), *Art as Medicine, creating a therapy of the Imagination (*Shambhala, 1992)

Mehl-Madrona, Dr Lewis, *Narrative Medicine: The Use of History and Story in the Healing Process* (Bear & Co, 2007) *Coyote Medicine: Lessons from Native American Healing* (1998)

Milner, Marion, *On Not Being Able to Paint* (1950), *A Life of One's Own* (1934) Routledge, 2011 reprint)

Montagu, Ashley, *Touching: The human significance of skin.* (Harper and Row 1971)

O'Donohue, John, *Benedictus: A Book of Blessings* (Bantam Press, 2007)

Okri, Ben, *Mental Fight* (London: Phoenix House, 1999)

Oliver, Mary, *Wild Geese: Selected Poems,* (Bloodaxe Books, 2004) *A Poetry Handbook: A Prose Guide to Understanding and Writing Poetry* (Mariner Books, 1994)

Oswald, Alice, *Falling Awake* (Cape, 2016)

Sacks, Oliver, *A Leg to Stand On* (Picador, 1991) *Awakenings,* (Pelican Books, 1976)

Schwenk, Theodor, *Sensitive Chaos: The creation of flowing forms in water and air* (Rudolf Steiner Press, 1965)

Servan-Schreiber, Dr David, *Healing Without Freud or Prozac* (Rodale International, 2004)

Shepherd, Phil, *New Self, New World: Recovering Our Senses in the Twenty-First Century* (North Atlantic Books, 2010)

Smart, Elizabeth, *The Assumption of the Rogues and Rascals* (HarperCollins, 1978)

Syrad, Kay, *Send* (Cinnamon Press, 2015)

Todd, Mabel Elsworth, *The Thinking Body* (Dance Horizons, 1959)

Tufnell, Miranda & Chris Crickmay, *A Widening Field: Journeys in Body and Imagination* (Triarchy Press 2023) and *Body Space Image: Notes Towards Improvisation and Performance* (Triarchy Press, 2023)

Sutherland, Janet, *Hangman's Acre,* (Shearsman Books, 2009)

Van Der Kolk, *The Body Keeps the Score: Mind, Brain and Body in the Transformation of Trauma* (Penguin, Random House, 2014)

White, Mike, *Arts Development in Community Health: A Social Tonic* (Radcliffe, 2009)

Wilson, Michael, *Health is for People* (Darton, Longman & Todd, 1975)

There are many organisations that are engaged in this territory – here are a few useful ones:

MA in *Dance and Somatic Well Being: Connections to the Living Body,* University of Central Lancashire
www.theknowingbodynetwork.co.uk
www.communitydance.org
Dance for Parkinson
www.ae-sop.org
www.independentdance.co.uk

Also available from Triarchy Press

A Widening Field: journeys in body and imagination ~ Miranda Tufnell & Chris Crickmay

Body Space Image: Notes towards improvisation and performance~ Miranda Tufnell & Chris Crickmay

Skinner Releasing Technique: A Movement and Dance Practice ~ Manny Emslie

Rock Songs: story about walk about story about walkabout story ~ Nick Sales

Suomenlinna | Gropius: Two Contemplations on Body, Movement and Intermateriality ~ Paula Kramer

The Roots of Amerta Movement: An introduction to the movement improvisation of Suprapto Suryodarmo ~ Lise Lavelle

Before the Curtain Opens: Alexander Technique in the Actor's Life ~ Kate Kelly

Embodied Lives: Reflections on the Influence of Suprapto Suryodarmo and Amerta Movement ~ edited by Katya Bloom, Margit Galanter & Sandra Reeve

Attending to Movement: Somatic Perspectives on Living in this World ~ edited by Sarah Whatley, Natalie Garrett Brown & Kirsty Alexander

Nature Connection: A handbook of practices for therapy & self-exploration ~ Margaret Kerr and Jana Lemke

Ways of Being a Body - a three-volume series

Body and Awareness ~ edited by Sandra Reeve

Nine Ways of Seeing a Body ~ Sandra Reeve

Body and Performance ~ edited by Sandra Reeve

www.triarchypress.net/movement